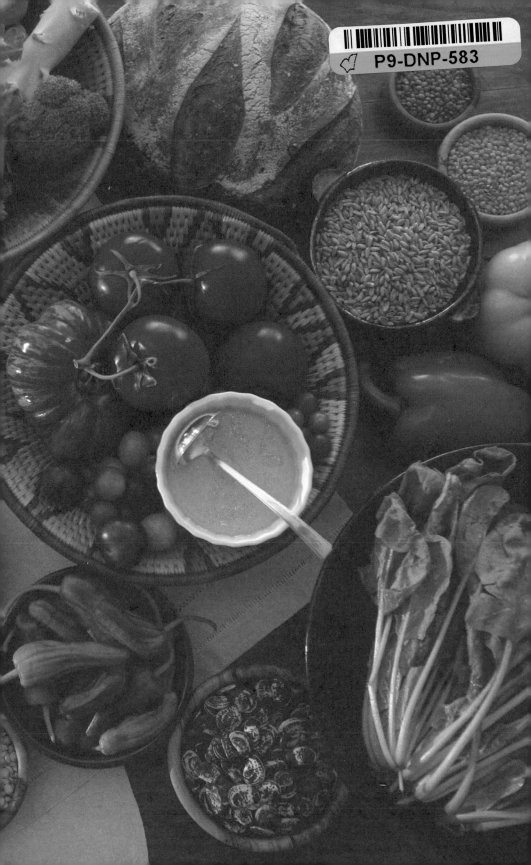

Praise for
THE NEW SONOMA DIET™

"What a sensible and workable diet ... The payoff is pleasure, both on the palate and looking in the mirror at the thinner and healthier person you have become."
—JOYCE GOLDSTEIN, chef, author, and culinary consultant

"If you're looking for a healthy lifestyle change, start here!"
—DAVID KIRSCH, CEO of MadisonSquare Club and
New York Times best-selling author of *The Ultimate New York Body Plan*

"Connie has done an amazing job of translating science into actionable advice for people interested in making lasting changes to their eating and activity habits."
—AMY MYRDAL MILLER, MS, RD, program director for
Strategic Initiatives, The Culinary Institute of America at Greystone

"Connie's common-sense approach to diet and, more importantly, lifestyle is a breath of fresh air ... I've personally adopted a number of her suggestions in my own cooking." —JOHN ASH, James Beard Award-winning chef and author

"Connie's 'Sonoma' approach of treating each meal as a celebration of life ... is indeed the recipe for achieving optimal health, weight, and a fulfilling life!"
—GEORGIA KOSTAS, MPH, RD, LD, nutrition consultant
and author of *The Cooper Clinic Solution to the Diet Revolution*

Praise for
THE SONOMA DIET®

"No calorie counting, no points, no weighing, no measuring, no obsessing about low-carb or low-fat foods. Just small portions of sun-drenched California-style cuisine, accompanied by red or white wine. Think gourmet, not gourmand."
—*Time* magazine

"The Sonoma Diet is a dynamite, healthy plan ... A tighter, portion-controlled interpretation of the Mediterranean diet, which has been touted for its ability to limit heart disease, cancer, obesity, and diabetes and prolong life."
—JOY BAUER, NBC nutritionist

"Just about everything the author advises—like eating whole grains instead of refined and watching your portion sizes—has been scientifically proven to improve your health and aid weight loss." —*O, The Oprah Magazine*

"On the Sonoma Diet, you can pretty much eat anything, including steak, bittersweet chocolate, and a glass of wine every night." —*New York* magazine

"Get skinny on Sonoma. Eat well and be happy. Unlike other weight loss programs, the Sonoma Diet doesn't require you to give up your favorite foods." —*Parents* magazine

"This is not another low-carb diet that frowns on whole grains and some fruit. Instead, Guttersen believes dieters need to break their refined sugar and starch addictions before slowly bringing complex carbohydrates back into the picture... Dieters will be relieved to know that Guttersen allows for a daily glass of wine later in the program." —*The Los Angeles Times*

"We love it! The Sonoma Diet proves that dieting can be delicious... Add flavor, experiment with vinegars and nut oils, seek out new varieties." —*Fitness* magazine

"Why we like it: As a dietician and consultant to the Culinary Institute at Greystone, the author pumps up the pleasure factor, saying flavorful food is a missing element to the long-term success of most plans. You'll find tons of tasty-looking recipes and detailed meal plans." —*The Chicago Tribune*

"If you want to lose weight without sending your kids the wrong message about food, here's a taste from the Sonoma Diet: a weight loss plan for people who love to eat." —*Child* magazine

"Finally a weight loss plan where bread, cereal, and even wine are allowed. After just 10 days, you'll watch pounds disappear." —*Family Circle* magazine

"The Sonoma Diet is a unique weight loss plan that brings together the art and science of food." —*More* magazine

"It offers some realistic strategies including how to handle cravings and how to dine out...The food plan is balanced and the recipes seem doable."—*USA Today*

"If Dr. Atkins were still around, he'd have one eye on Connie Guttersen... The key to this diet is fixing your plate with more grains and veggies and less protein." —*The New York Daily News*

"It's a way of eating that's realistic, not rigid... Radical concept: food is your friend, not your enemy." —*The Dallas Morning News*

THE NEW SONOMA DIET™

A Simple, Healthy, More Delicious Way to Live

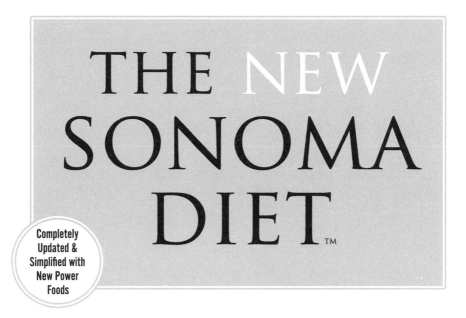

THE NEW SONOMA DIET™

Completely Updated & Simplified with New Power Foods

Trimmer Waist, More Energy in Just 10 Days

Connie Guttersen, RD, PhD

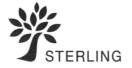

STERLING

New York / London
www.sterlingpublishing.com

2 4 6 8 10 9 7 5 3 1

Published by Sterling Publishing Co., Inc.
387 Park Avenue South, New York, NY 10016

© 2010 by Connie Guttersen, RD, PhD

Distributed in Canada by Sterling Publishing
c/o Canadian Manda Group, 165 Dufferin Street
Toronto, Ontario, Canada M6K 3H6
Distributed in the United Kingdom by GMC Distribution Services
Castle Place, 166 High Street, Lewes, East Sussex, England BN7 1XU
Distributed in Australia by Capricorn Link (Australia) Pty. Ltd.
P.O. Box 704, Windsor, NSW 2756, Australia

Sterling ISBN 978-1-4027-8118-6

For information about custom editions, special sales, premium and corporate purchases, please contact Sterling Special Sales Department at 800-805-5489 or specialsales@sterlingpublishing.com.

ACKNOWLEDGMENTS

Many thanks and much gratitude are due to the individuals who made this book a reality. Their vision, energy, and remarkable talents are a big part of the Sonoma Diet® philosophy and the value in enjoying healthy living. You have all inspired me with your tremendous talents and friendship throughout this project.

A sincere appreciation to the entire *Sonoma Diet* team at Sterling Publishing; your partnership has been essential in this amazing journey. Thank you, Marcus Leaver, Jason Prince, Michael Fragnito, Karen Patterson, and Jennifer Williams for supporting and believing in my endeavors and in *The New Sonoma Diet*. A special thanks to Elizabeth Mihalste, Jeff Batzli, Leigh Ann Ambrosi, and Anwesha Basu for your long hours and dedication to the project.

To Edward Ash-Milby at Barnes and Noble, you were the spark behind the return of Sonoma; thank you for your insight and enthusiasm.

To the Culinary Institute of America at Greystone, for the ongoing experience of keeping the state of science and nutrition in perspective with the enjoyment of wholesome, flavorful foods: Thank you for many wonderful years of learning and inspiration. A special thanks to my dear friend, mentor, and colleague of almost twenty years, Chef Toni Sakaguchi, whose passion and creativity for delicious meals are to be praised.

Thank you to Lary Rosenblatt, Laurie Lieb, Michael Burgan, and Fabia Wargin for sharing your excitement and vision. Your engaging language and organization of information is a result of many hours of proofing and guidance. So much effort went into finding a favorite image for this beautiful wine country—thank you, Faith Echtermeyer, for capturing the essence of the amazing Sonoma region.

I am indebted to Mindy Feinsheld and Vicki Saunders, whose tedious dietary calculations translate the exciting science into practical guidelines.

To the dynamic and energetic Sonoma KRUPP team led by Heidi and Darren Lisiten, Chanel Graham, and Li Wang—everything is possible with your vision and talents. A special thanks for my friend and agent, Heidi Krupp Lisiten, whose ideas set the course for an amazing and fulfilling future.

Finally, to Shawn, my husband, and our children, Gigi and William: without your patience, support, and inspiration, this project would not have been possible. The love and respect that stem from family are the foundation of health, success, and happiness. ◼

CONTENTS

· A Letter ·
FROM THE
AUTHOR

Five years ago, *The Sonoma Diet*, a *New York Times* best seller, changed the way Americans think about food, flavor, and weight loss. People experienced amazing results, and their success went beyond shedding pounds.

Besides getting down to their healthiest weight, Sonoma dieters reduced their risk for heart disease, arthritis, and diabetes while renewing their day-to-day energy and rediscovering their motivation to lead a more fulfilling life. Those vital improvements put them back on course toward personal satisfaction, career success, and better relationships. Not to mention they gained a new appreciation for flavorful food—and yes, good wine—as part of a great *life*, not simply a great *meal*.

All of which raises an obvious question: Why a new Sonoma Diet?

It's an excellent question, with some equally excellent answers that you're going to love. Let me start by telling you what I've been doing in the half-decade or so since The Sonoma Diet first swept across America.

I've worked in the nutrition field for more than twenty years, the last fifteen with the renowned Culinary Institute of America at Greystone in California's Napa Valley (a stone's throw from Sonoma County). I've had the good fortune of immersing myself in a world of flavor, working side by side with some of the most talented and creative chefs in the world. The experience transformed my nutrition philosophy into one that celebrates wholesome, nourishing foods coming together in a feast of bold flavors as part of a healthy eating style in which meals are enjoyed. That's the philosophy I used to create The Sonoma Diet.

Since then I've redoubled my research efforts and toured the country several times over. The more I investigated, the more I became aware of the broader sense of healthy eating and living, of the connection between enjoying meals and losing weight, of the futility of technical "miracle diets," and of the world of infinite possibilities that awaits all of us when advances in nutrition science are wedded to the deep and lasting pleasures of truly savoring delicious, wholesome meals.

In other words, I became more convinced than ever that the Sonoma way of losing weight while regaining health has little to do with a traditional "diet" that you "go on" and then move away from. Wholesome, joyful eating the Sonoma way is a lifestyle, fueled by ongoing quests for new and better nutrition secrets (my job) and new and better ways to enhance the pleasure of healthy eating (your job, with my help).

So it became clear to me that a one-and-done diet book was not the way to go. This revised Sonoma Diet is the next step in my personal commitment to help everybody, whether Sonoma veterans or newcomers, embrace a way of eating that encourages healthy habits, mindful choices, and an appreciation for the best nourishment available.

· · · · ·

WHICH BRINGS US BACK TO THE ORIGINAL QUESTION: WHY A NEW Sonoma Diet? One reason is that this new edition incorporates new discoveries in nutrition science that make the Sonoma eating plan even more effective for weight loss and overall health.

I explain these breakthroughs briefly and simply in the pages ahead, because I believe everybody benefits from knowing a little bit about the "why" of what they eat, as well as the "what" and "how." More important, I've adjusted some of the food and meal guidelines accordingly, adding effectiveness and variety without adding complexity.

The discoveries included in this new edition are truly exciting. For example, I've adjusted the plan to reflect new knowledge about the way some foods influence how we store or burn fat, with obvious weight-loss implications. Also, it turns out that certain nutrients have previously unknown health benefits for our minds, our appetite, and our energy levels. Other nutrients play a key role in controlling inflammation, a much more important risk factor for heart disease and other serious health issues than previously thought.

New research has also upgraded the health-enhancing roles of substances we already knew were beneficial. Three examples are omega-3 fatty acids, probiotics, and dark chocolate. I've tweaked the diet accordingly. In fact, one of the changes you'll notice immediately is the addition of two new Sonoma Power Foods—beans and citrus fruit—bringing the total of these weight loss heroes to twelve.

Speaking of fruit, its prohibition in the first ten days of the Sonoma plan has been repealed. While forgoing fruits' natural sugars during the initial transition phase speeds up the loss of those first few pounds, eliminating natural, nutrient-rich fruits for even a day contradicts the spirit of Sonoma. Of course, you can eliminate them for ten days if you wish, but I'm convinced that it's more beneficial in the long run to adhere to the Sonoma approach of enjoying wholesome, healthy foods instead of avoiding them.

I've also ratcheted up the emphasis on what I call whole-body health— that is, going beyond mere weight loss from "dieting" to a focus on living for overall health, increasing the potential of your mind and body to reenergize and revitalize. To that end I've expanded the section on exercise as a way not only to facilitate weight loss, but also to keep your mind, body, and spirit in balance.

·　·　·　·　·

THERE'S ANOTHER REASON WHY THE TIME IS RIGHT FOR A NEW edition of The Sonoma Diet. As I traveled around the country, I was inspired by the success stories of everyday Americans who for the first time in their lives had begun to experience the profound pleasure of enjoying meals while they were losing weight. But I also talked to those who didn't do so well.

The reasons for their problems were usually variations on a common theme: It was difficult for them to change the way they eat. This had nothing to do with the old-fashioned diet complaints of feeling dissatisfied and deprived. Nobody feels dissatisfied or deprived on The Sonoma Diet. Rather, it has to do with the practical difficulties of adjusting to a new way of thinking about meals, not to mention shopping for them, making time for them, and preparing them.

In this new edition, by popular request, I've addressed this issue with a major emphasis on time-saving and budget-saving strategies that collectively I call Sonoma Made Simple. You'll find Sonoma Express recipes that offer faster preparation and a new concept, Cook Once/Eat Twice recipes, that will make your life even easier. Based on the pantry items, you'll be able to prepare meals that don't require any shopping or cooking. The Sonoma approach asks you to spend more time enjoying your meals, but that doesn't mean you have to spend more time making them.

There's also an expanded collection of selections for people with special dietary preferences, including vegetarians and gluten-free eaters. I've also added information on the glycemic load for the recipes, an easy and convenient way to keep your blood sugar levels in check for easier weight loss and better health.

And then, of course, there's the most welcome addition of all—dozens of brand-new, super-flavorful, and wholesome Sonoma Diet recipes that turn any meal into a festive celebration.

All these additions complement the basic concepts of The Sonoma Diet that appear intact in this edition. Calorie and portion control are still built-in, so you can eat instead of count. The meal plans, food lists, and combination strategies are still the same, guiding you toward weight loss and improved health without burdening you with complicated instructions. And the emphasis is still on enjoying delicious, satisfying meals every day.

· · · · ·

I'D LIKE TO LEAVE YOU WITH A BIT OF PERSONAL HISTORY THAT I think will explain the spirit of The Sonoma Diet. My parents, being Italian, always stressed the importance of family meals. My mother would prepare a variety of fresh, seasonal dishes with vegetables, fruits, grains, and lean meats. At the table, we never talked about whether the food was healthy or not, or whether our meals contained certain antioxidants. We simply enjoyed the food and the pleasant conversation, sharing laughter and an appreciation for my mother's passion for wholesome meals.

Did these daily meals reflect a "perfect" diet? It really didn't matter. We knew we were nourished by genuine food prepared with love and by our warm family life.

Later, I saw my family lose its common-sense approach to eating, along with the pleasures of the table—all in the name of dieting. My father, an experienced medical doctor, wanted to lose the extra pounds wrapped around his waist. From different types of diets with strange food combinations to liquid diets that contained no food, our satisfying family meals faded away—and so did the special times we shared at the table. Our daily celebrations of food and each other were replaced by confusing discussions about what my father or the rest of the family should be eating.

I have sad memories of watching him not enjoying one of his favorite activities—having friends and family at the table sharing a glass of wine and a great meal. In his desperate urge to be "healthier" and trimmer, he counted how many days he would follow one diet before trying another and then another. All the while, the numbers on the scale kept getting higher.

I wouldn't wish that way of living, or eating, on anyone. The Sonoma Diet and my entire career reflect the lessons I learned from my family experience. No one should suffer those feelings of discouragement and deprivation based on a misguided notion of what it means to "eat healthy." I offer you this new and improved version of The Sonoma Diet so that you can achieve your weight loss goals and be happy and healthy as you enjoy delicious, satisfying food at festive meals that are full of the warmth and joy of life itself.

— CONNIE GUTTERSEN, RD, PhD

To Health
WITH GREAT TASTE

|————————————————————|

RETURN TO
SONOMA

The Sonoma Diet is a lifestyle.

It's a way of living that infuses you with health and energy, so you can feel great, look your best and do everything you've always wanted to do. It's a way of eating that treats meals as celebrations, that encourages you to indulge in the healthy pleasures of delicious, super-flavorful foods. It's a way to lose weight quickly and permanently while, perhaps for the first time in your life, you will truly cherish your meals.

And make no mistake about it—you lose every ounce of excess weight that you need to. But you'll do it the Sonoma way—not by avoiding food, but by enjoying satisfying amounts of the best foods on the planet.

There's no "diet food" on The Sonoma Diet. No specialty foods. Nothing out of the ordinary. Just wholesome, fresh, and delicious everyday foods that are affordable, easy to find, and even easier to prepare.

In fact, because Sonoma is as much a lifestyle as it is a diet, you can forget about having to eat different foods than the other people at your table. The health benefits and exquisite dining experiences offered by the recipes in this book are for everybody, overweight or not.

But if you do need to lose weight, the results are phenomenal. You'll shed pounds quickly at first, then steadily until your weight is right where you always wanted it to be—and maybe never dared to hope it could be. And the weight loss will last a lifetime.

Every step of your journey from overweight to perfect weight will be comfortable, pleasant, and simple. You won't have to track calories, keep score of any "points," or constantly weigh and measure your food. You don't have to count, plan, analyze, or worry.

That's because all the science has been done for you, down to the last nutritional detail. All you have to do is select from a huge variety of food choices, using the recipes in this book or improvising your own dishes following simple Sonoma guidelines. The main thing is to enjoy your meals.

The Sonoma lifestyle focuses on more than losing weight. It's all about a healthier and more energetic you. Sure, if you're overweight, weight loss itself will dramatically improve your health. But with the Sonoma plan, improved health isn't just a side effect of weight loss. It is the very route to weight loss, because Sonoma meals are designed to provide maximum health benefits, delicious flavors, and weight loss simultaneously. So you'll feel your new vibrancy well before you lose that last pound.

The Sonoma Diet is based on the very latest discoveries about nutrition, health, and weight loss. Behind every meal plan and food recommendation is cutting-edge research that goes beyond the now-dated notions of low-carb or low-fat. You will fill up on "Power Foods" that deliver maximum disease-fighting nutrients with a minimum of calories. You'll be eating meals in carefully planned combinations that not only bring out flavors but also maximize your body's absorption of essential nutrients. This is a big reason you'll be discovering a new vibrant health as well as a slimmer shape.

FRESH FROM THE COAST

The Sonoma Diet emerged just after the turn of the twenty-first century, leading a food and flavor renaissance that's still sweeping across America. It started on the West Coast, where a coastal California way of eating rediscovered the culinary delights of fresh, health-inducing ingredients, intensely pleasurable flavors, innovative but simple meal preparation, and the lost joy of a leisurely meal that emphasizes savoring your food and appreciating the people you are sharing it with.

The Golden State has a rich epicurean tradition, which today has evolved into a cuisine that stresses locally grown ingredients from its coastal counties and international inspirations from southern Europe,

Asia, and Latin America. The result of this fusion is a healthy and sensual way of eating that was once associated only with southern Europe—a feast for the senses and a boon for health and longevity. That's exactly how you're going to eat, Sonoma-style.

And that's exactly why you will succeed this time in reaching your ideal weight. You'll feel pleased and satisfied all day long, because The Sonoma Diet does not invite frustration by artificially limiting any category of food. That makes it the perfect eating lifestyle for everyone who's tried and failed to stick to a low-carb or low-fat diet. Sonoma is not "low" anything. It is a balanced meal plan that provides your body with everything it needs.

It is not a deprivation diet. Grains, meat, fish, beans, eggs—they're all there for you. Snacks? Of course. Wine? Sure, if you like. In moderation, it's good for you, and it's part of the California meal-celebration tradition that Sonoma exemplifies.

Instead of banning whole categories of foods, Sonoma helps you eat reasonable amounts of the leanest, healthiest foods in each category. You'll learn to satisfy your hunger without overeating. You'll learn to eat slowly and savor every bite. And you'll learn how to finish a meal feeling content, never deprived.

Sonoma is not a low-carb diet. On the contrary, it stresses a huge variety of plant-based, carbohydrate-rich energy food. Do you like rice or other grains with your main course? Enjoy them, as long as they're the best-tasting, whole-grain, fiber-rich version. Bread? You bet, and from Day 1 of your diet. Cereals? Every day if you like. Fruits and vegetables? In abundance.

Sonoma is not a low-fat diet, either. Heart-healthy and flavor-enhancing olive oil can be an everyday feature of your meals, bringing out nutrients and flavors in many of the foods you eat.

You'll be encouraged to take advantage of other healthy dietary fats as well. A variety of nuts and avocados, for example, and the heart-protective natural oils in fish will help you lose weight and keep you satisfied as you do it.

The Sonoma secret to weight loss is rediscovering the joy of eating. It's about the sensual pleasure of savoring a variety of fresh, wholesome, and delicious foods. In other words, you'll be adopting a new eating lifestyle. You'll find it far more pleasurable and satisfying than the one you'll be leaving behind. The Sonoma lifestyle will be a part of you long after you've reached your target weight. It will keep you slim, healthy, and enjoying every meal for the rest of your life.

THE SONOMA REGION

The name "Sonoma" is synonymous with the spirit of the healthy meal plan you'll be following. To understand it, you need to do a little elementary geography work.

Pull out a world map and find the Mediterranean Sea. Trace your finger along the sea's perimeter and notice what the countries you cross— among other places, you'll pass through coastal Spain, southern France, Italy, Greece, Lebanon, Algeria, Tunisia, and Morocco.

What are these lands known for? Ideal climates, fresh fruits and vegetables, fine wines, lean meats, abundant fish, and heart-friendly olive oil. In fact, the eating habits and the active lifestyle in this part of the world are so beneficial to human health that science has a name for them—the Mediterranean diet.

Now follow the line straight westward from the Mediterranean across the Atlantic and the United States until you come to the California coast. You're in Sonoma County, north of San Francisco Bay.

Here the waves break on rocky coasts that give way to majestic redwood forests covering coastal mountains. Further inland, rolling hills are dotted with olive trees and apple groves.

On countless slopes lie some of the most lauded vineyards in the world, the grapes gleaming green and purple in the California sun. Along Sonoma's rustic trails and rural back roads, hikers and cyclists exercise as they take in the beauty of the surroundings.

This breathtakingly scenic region shares more in common with the Mediterranean than latitude and climate. Its fruits and vegetables are just as fresh and delicious, its wine as fine, its meat as lean, its fish and other seafood as abundant, its homegrown olive oil just as heart-friendly. The lifestyle? Even healthier.

The people of Sonoma are no different from any other Americans from Juneau to Miami. But they've set in motion an eating renaissance by tapping the health and weight-loss potential of the agricultural abundance they've been blessed with. Here there's a coast teeming with seafood, and fertile hills and valleys yielding olive oil, all kinds of berries, avocados, dates, figs, persimmons, a huge variety of greens, almonds, walnuts, citrus fruit, peaches, strawberries, beans of all types, and much, much more.

Here an artisan community has grown, turning this cornucopia into something more than a commodity to be traded. Bread bakers, cheese makers, small farmers, organic produce growers, and winemakers have cultivated a new way of appreciating food, and they are changing the culinary culture of the entire nation.

Out of the farms and restaurants and home kitchens of this idyllic land of healthy, sensuous eating comes The Sonoma Diet.

WEIGHT LOSS PLUS DELICIOUS FOODS

To repeat, the Sonoma way of losing weight is not to avoid good food but to eat the best foods on the planet. Here are some of them:

Lots of the best fresh fruits and vegetables instead of processed foods and sugary sweets. Generous allotments of whole grain bread and cereals instead of refined white flour products. Poultry, lean red meats, lamb, pork, veal, eggs, nonfat dairy, soybeans, and plenty of fish for your protein. Olive oil and nuts as your main dietary fat sources. Unlimited herbs and spices. A little wine. It doesn't matter if you live in Los Angeles, Dallas, New York, Atlanta, Seattle, Denver, or anyplace in between. Sonoma can be your way of eating anywhere.

Sound appealing? Then you're already in the Sonoma spirit.

The sections that follow will take you through the eating and weight loss plan step-by-step. The first thing you'll notice is how simple everything is. There's no rule that says good eating has to be complicated.

After a summary of the major points of the diet, you'll be introduced to the huge variety of foods you'll be eating. The emphasis will be on the Power Foods that deliver the most health-imparting nutrients with the fewest calories.

Then you'll be guided through the eating plan itself, with guidelines for choosing foods, preparing them, and eating them in the right proportions and amounts. You'll find recipes, specific meals to prepare, and tips for making things easy and for getting the most from your diet.

There are also sections dedicated to helping you through the inevitable rough spots—the cravings, the hurdles, the frustrations that pop up from time to time whenever you change your way of eating. You'll see exactly how to deal with any problem, so you can leave it behind and move on to your weight loss goal.

Within days of starting, you'll already notice a change for the better in the way you feel and the way your clothes fit. You will begin losing weight immediately.

You'll also notice a difference in the way you think about food. As you leave the old bad ways behind and adopt the new good ways, you'll discover an amazing thing. The new way tastes better! You're feeling better, you're losing weight—and you're enjoying your meals more than you ever thought possible.

That's what The New Sonoma Diet is all about. Let's get started. ▪

WHAT IS

THE NEW SONOMA DIET™

?

The Sonoma Diet is a unique weight-loss plan that brings together the latest in food science and a celebratory, pleasure-packed approach to healthy eating inspired by the flavorful cuisine and active lifestyle of one of the most beautiful places on earth.

There are two essential components to The Sonoma Diet that have made it such a popular and surefire way to lose weight since its inception. One is the generous selection of delicious foods that you'll be eating in satisfying amounts and healthy combinations, all meticulously designed for you to shed pounds safely and easily until you reach your best body weight.

The other is a festive, joyous approach to eating that turns every meal into a celebration of life. At the core of The Sonoma Diet is a true heart-felt love of delicious food. Consciously savoring every bite of the wide selection of flavor-rich recipes is essential to your success. You're going to find that an appreciation and enjoyment of flavorful meals makes for a healthy, slimming eating style that soon becomes second nature.

The guidelines that you'll be reading about in the pages ahead—and then following as you ease yourself into the Sonoma eating plan—make it easy for you to discover that heady sense of the good life every time you sit down for a meal. The foods and recipes have been carefully selected to make you healthier and happier as you lose the weight. The latest knowledge from the fast-evolving world of nutritional research is reflected in that food selection as well as in the meal preparations. Simple guidelines for amounts and combinations of foods make the plate your guide for eating satisfying amounts as you shed pounds.

THE PLEASURES OF SONOMA

The vitality-radiating residents of California's Sonoma County may not have invented the notion that an intense enjoyment of an abundance of delicious food is the best path to a happy, fulfilling life and a trim, healthy body. But the area's culinary creativity, its love of fresh, wholesome ingredients, and its abundance of great-tasting, sun-drenched foods exemplify the spirit of this idea perhaps more than anywhere else west of the Mediterranean. It's an idea that has helped make Sonoma a paradise of healthy eating and a center for active lifestyles.

It's also an idea that inspired The Sonoma Diet.

And it's an idea that will introduce you to a style of eating based on enjoying the bounty of nutritious, unprocessed foods that Sonoma is famous for—fresh vegetables, whole grains, nuts, olive oil, lean meats, poultry, fish, fruits, herbs, spices, and wine. They all come together in the Sonoma style of cuisine that is unique, varied, and intensely flavorful, yet amazingly quick and simple to prepare.

Keep in mind as you read through the basics of The Sonoma Diet presented here that the word "diet" has two meanings. In its most basic use, the term refers to your daily eating habits, what you eat on a regular basis. In that sense, it doesn't necessarily have anything to do with losing weight, though of course a healthy daily food regimen in proper amounts will usually keep you at your ideal weight.

The more common use of the term today is simply a shortened version of "weight-loss diet," a specially adjusted daily food regimen designed to induce weight loss. Anybody who says, "I'm on a diet" almost always means "I'm eating in a special way so I'll lose weight."

Both senses of the word apply to The Sonoma Diet. It's a weight-loss plan, but it's also a healthy and immensely pleasurable way to eat on a daily basis. That's why, since its inception, Sonoma has been popular even with those who don't need to lose weight, as well as with those who do. If you're happy with your current weight, simply skip the guidelines in Waves 1 and 2 and start enjoying the Sonoma recipes, and the health and vigor they bring.

PARADOX LOST

Decades ago, researchers started pondering a seeming paradox. Why is it that Mediterranean populations live healthier, longer lives with lower rates of heart disease, cancer, obesity, and diabetes compared to people in many other parts of the world? When Americans or northern Europeans eat what they consider pleasurable meals, they're told they're raising their risk of heart attack. When southern Europeans eat their versions of the same thing, they get healthier. What's going on?

The answer lies in the flavorful, nutrient-rich foods of the Mediterranean diet, as well as the way those foods are eaten. The cuisines of southern Italy, Spain, Greece, southern France, and other Mediterranean lands are diverse, but they have a lot in common.

The dishes are largely plant-based, which means that seasonal vegetables, whole grains, fruits, beans, and nuts play leading roles. Dairy is played down, but meat—especially poultry and fish—is prominent. Olive oil is a mainstay, not just for cooking but to provide flavor for all those vegetables, legumes, and salads that are so much a part of Mediterranean meals. Red and white wine are key components of many meals. Herbs and spices are used freely.

These foods, simple and unpretentious as they are, form the cornerstone of healthy eating. Especially when they're selected according to seasons, processed minimally, and prepared in beneficial combinations and reasonable amounts, these nutrient-packed foods boost your vitality, protect your heart, and improve your overall health.

Perhaps you've already guessed that everything I've just written about the Mediterranean diet could be written about Sonoma as well. Not that Sonoma cuisine is some kind of knock-off of the southern

European diet. On the contrary, it's distinctly American, a unique result of coastal California's privileged geography, agricultural abundance, and health-conscious population. But the two share so much in common that the advances in nutrition and weight-loss science that have resulted from studying the Mediterranean diet apply virtually 100% to Sonoma.

And make no mistake about it—an ongoing flood of research has consistently confirmed the health advantages of following a Mediterranean-style diet. Just recently, for example, researchers who followed some 23,000 Greek men and women for more than eight years found a compelling connection between the Mediterranean diet and a longer, healthier life. So not only does Mediterranean-style eating boost energy, facilitate weight loss, fight killer diseases such as diabetes and heart disease, and increase overall health, but it also appears to increase longevity as well. There's also emerging evidence that a Mediterranean-style diet improves your cognitive capacity, including memory.

Those are your benefits with The Sonoma Diet as well. Though Sonoma is uniquely its own, much of the underlying nutritional science I have tapped to put the Sonoma eating plan together is based on discoveries stemming from research into the Mediterranean diet. In general, the emphasis in both the New World and Old is on enjoying a generous variety of satisfying, nutrient-rich, health-inducing foods rather than lamenting what you must avoid.

One way you'll do that is by focusing on the Top Twelve Sonoma Diet Power Foods that will be introduced. Many foods stack up as power foods, but these twelve are exceptionally beneficial, delivering maximum nutrition with minimum calories. Eating these miracles of nature is as important for weight loss as not eating those processed or sugar-loaded "foods" that have so damaged the health and waistlines of modern mankind. As miraculous as these Power Foods are, there's nothing out-of-the-ordinary about them. You're already familiar with every one.

THE SONOMA SPIRIT

A typical diet book will inevitably instruct you at some point to change your relationship with eating. And you know what? That's exactly what I'm going to do here.

But instead of the usual advice along the lines of "downplay the importance of food in your life," I'm going to urge you to do just the opposite. I want you to *increase* the importance of food in your life, to celebrate your meals, and to savor each and every flavorful bite of the Sonoma foods and recipes you'll be eating.

That's the Sonoma way, and it's absolutely essential to losing weight on The Sonoma Diet. How you eat is as important as what you eat. It's no secret that the obesity epidemic in the Western world has coincided with the widespread tendency to eat on the run, to eat mindlessly while doing something else, and to eat impulsively to satisfy bad habits. Sonoma provides you with a way to leave all that behind and rediscover "the pleasures of the table."

Adding Sonoma foods to your meal repertoire, then, is only half the story. You need to use them to rediscover the pleasures of truly

To Lose Weight ...

Eat slowly ... so you'll feel more satisfied on less food, so you won't out-eat the signaling mechanism that takes twenty minutes for your brain to get the message that you're full, and so you can enjoy your meal more.

Eat with others ... because research shows that when you share meals with family or friends, you are more likely to eat healthier, feel more nourished and connected, and lose weight.

Eat in a relaxed setting ... as opposed to eating under stress or on the run, which is when you tend to overeat or eat poorly.

Eat with pleasure ... instead of micromanaging your meal or worrying about its effect on your weight. Sonoma Diet meals are designed for healthy weight loss, so just enjoy them.

Eat mindfully ... by paying attention to what and how much you're eating. You'll eat better, eat less, and enjoy it more.

Eat without distractions ... because multitasking, texting, television, and the like interrupt mindfulness, causing you to eat longer and more, even when you're not hungry.

appreciating delicious and healthy food, as well as the profound experience of celebrating a meal as an affirmation of life itself.

As Michael Pollan, the brilliant food journalist, put it:

> "Food is more than the sum of its nutrients and a diet is more than the sum of its foods…Food is about pleasure, about community, about family and spirituality, about our relationship to the natural world, and about expressing our identity."

Your ideal Sonoma meal will be eaten in the company of family or friends or both. It will be enjoyed slowly, with every bite savored and appreciated, and with everybody's attention on the food or on each other. We don't always have the time or the access to company to reach this ideal, of course, but I'm convinced that most people could reach it much more often than they do now. Even when you're eating alone on a short lunch break, you can slow down, relax, and be mindful of the meal you are eating.

Though most people assume the opposite, treating your meals as a celebratory feast shared with others helps you eat less, not more. Slowing down to savor your food as you commune with others at the table means you are less likely to overeat. This has been proven in the lab, where researchers have found that slower eating results in a higher release of hormones signaling fullness to the brain. It's also been proven every day at the restaurants and home tables of Sonoma and the Mediterranean.

Eat wholesomely…by choosing natural, unprocessed foods. The more a food is processed, the more nutrients and natural flavors are lost.

Eat seasonally…Because the growing seasons can inspire your menus and give you flavorful rewards.

Eat locally and sustainably… as much as possible. Just knowing where your food comes from and how it's produced makes you a more mindful eater.

Eat with wine…because, unless you don't drink alcohol at all, a glass of wine enhances your enjoyment of a healthy meal, is heart-friendly in and of itself, and embodies the Sonoma spirit.

THE NEW SONOMA DIET IS ALL ABOUT ...

BALANCE. It has nothing to do with low-carb or low-fat.

WHOLE GRAINS. You'll be eating bread and cereal from Day 1.

POWER FOODS. Generous amounts of delicious, nutrient-dense foods help you lose weight.

HEALTH. Like the Mediterranean diet, The Sonoma Diet stresses the kinds of ingredients and food combinations that protect against heart disease, diabetes, and other killers.

PLEASURE. You'll slow down to savor and enjoy your meals, Sonoma-style.

OLIVE OIL. This heart-healthy, nutrition-boosting, flavor-enhancing plant oil shatters the myth that dietary fat is evil.

SIMPLICITY. You don't count calories or anything else. You don't measure or analyze. Just select, prepare, and enjoy.

VARIETY. You can pick and choose the foods you want each day from generous lists of meats, seafood, fruits, vegetables, grains, and other food types.

EASY, MOUTHWATERING RECIPES. The recipes—simple, elegant, and delicious, including Cook Once/Eat Twice meals and meals that require no shopping or cooking—come straight from the culinary masters of California's Sonoma County.

AFFORDABILITY. These simple foods are readily available from supermarkets and farmers' markets.

SIMPLE PORTION CONTROL. Just fill your plate or bowl according to the proportions given on page 93 for Wave 1 and 107 for Waves 2 and 3.

FRESH WHOLE FOODS. The emphasis is on sun-drenched, flavor-packed, nutrient-rich treats like the ones from Sonoma's farms and ranches, and from your own community supported, local food producers.

WINE. It enhances your heart's health and your weight-loss effort as well as your meal. After the first ten days, you can enjoy a glass of wine with your main meal.

SATISFACTION. The meals are complete, satisfying, and won't leave you feeling hungry.

WE EAT FOODS, NOT CATEGORIES

One subject inevitably comes up when The Sonoma Diet is introduced: Is it low-carbohydrate or low-fat?

The short answer is "neither." But the most accurate answer may be this: "The question is irrelevant."

The very fact that it arises is a sign of the times. These days popular wisdom holds that weight loss depends on drastically upsetting the balance between carbohydrates, fats, and proteins. So diets swing like a pendulum from low-fat to low-carb.

That leaves a lot of diet dropouts feeling unsatisfied and confused. The low-fat diets tell us that food should taste dull and leave us hungry. The low-carb diets deny us our daily bread and turn vegetables and fruits into the enemy. Either way, losing weight becomes an exercise in self-denial.

Sound familiar?

The Sonoma Diet has nothing to do with low-carb or high-carb. It has nothing to do with low-fat or high-fat. Artificially low levels of dietary fat are neither pleasing nor healthy. There's even recent evidence that low-fat diets contribute to depression. You need fat, especially in the form of plant oils.

The food choices and portion control built into The Sonoma Diet are calculated for the best balance of proteins, carbohydrates, and fats. That balance will keep you satisfied at every step of your weight loss journey.

ESSENTIAL FATS

Plant oils are absolutely essential to a healthy diet, especially when you're trying to lose weight. Even if they did no more, plant oils add flavor to increase the pleasure of good foods. I'm convinced that one reason so many people don't eat enough vegetables and legumes is that they don't prepare them in flavorful ways. That's even more the case with those on a low-fat eating plan who must forgo the healthy pleasure of olive oil as a flavoring agent. That won't be a problem on the Sonoma Diet.

Of course, healthy fats offer a lot more than flavor. They help your body absorb nutrients, so you can get more nutritional benefit without eating more. They create a feeling of satiety at meals, so you don't leave the table feeling hungry. And many, like olive oil and certain fish oils, offer heart-healthy nutrients on their own.

SONOMA CARBS

Across-the-board limits on carbohydrates doom even the most dedicated dieters to failure. Low-carb is a strategy that cannot be maintained because it's unhealthy and unsatisfying.

As most people know these days, carbohydrates are the foods most directly converted to energy in the body. They're found in whole grains, vegetables, and fruits—all great foods.

Carbs also contain fiber. Fiber is not only essential for digestive and cardiovascular health, but it's also a key player in the physiology of weight loss.

Clearly, you need energy, nutrients, and fiber. That's why you need proper amounts of carbohydrates.

It's illogical for a diet to severely limit a category of food that includes healthy whole grains, vegetables, and fruits. It sends a message that there's a contradiction between losing weight and reaping the health benefits of high-fiber, nutrient-rich foods. It's a false message. Dieters sense that intuitively, which is another reason there are so many low-carb dropouts.

On The Sonoma Diet, you'll eat bread and cereals from the very first day. You'll have your fill of meat and fish, of course, but you'll also be encouraged to enjoy a variety of fruits and tastily prepared vegetables from Day 1.

LEAN AND MEAN PROTEIN

The Sonoma Diet is generous with protein from a lot of sources—beef, poultry, seafood, soy, nuts, seeds, some dairy, and even some of the high-protein whole grains such as quinoa. The common denominator is that the protein is lean regardless of the source, including the protein from red meat.

Protein is no more artificially restricted on The Sonoma Diet than fat or carbohydrates. In fact, studies have been showing lately that moderately higher-protein diets aid weight loss. Protein improves your body composition, sustaining muscle mass as you lose weight. It also improves your physical fitness, enhances your body's ability to control blood sugar levels, and helps keep your hunger in check as you adjust to eating less.

BACK TO BALANCE

Now that I've run down the Sonoma approach to the protein/carb/fat issue, you might want to just forget about it. Worrying about how much carbohydrate or dietary fat you're consuming is a distraction. Keeping track of nutritional categories such as "carbohydrate," "protein," and "dietary fat" just isn't the way normal folks go about planning their meals. And that's true whether you need to lose weight or not.

True, eating too many carbohydrates, especially refined ones—along with eating too much of anything—definitely contributes to being overweight. Carbohydrates are the most likely to be overconsumed because of their effect on blood sugar metabolism (which we'll get into later).

But the solution is not to compensate for too much carbohydrate (or fat) with too little. After some initial success, your body will rebel at the carb deprivation. So will your mind. You run the risk of becoming another low-carb (or low-fat) diet dropout. You're even a candidate for the infamous rebound effect, which leads you to weighing more than when you started the restrictive diet.

Rebounding is much less likely with The Sonoma Diet. As mentioned, the food guidelines and meal plans already have the ideally balanced carb/protein/fat ratio built into them. The calculations are calibrated to the three stages, or "waves," of your weight loss program. The amounts are set at the levels most conducive to losing weight without creating an artificial shortage of carbs or anything else that leaves you feeling deprived.

You'll never have to think about whether you're eating too many or too few carbohydrates. In fact, you'll see the word *carb* only occasionally in the rest of this book. Instead, you can turn your attention to the soul of The Sonoma Diet—enjoying the best-tasting and healthiest foods in amounts and combinations that will get you to your target body weight quickly, safely, and permanently.

In other words, the choices you'll be making are not between scientific categories such as carbohydrate, protein, and dietary fat; instead, you'll be choosing the healthiest, nutrient-rich foods within those categories.

You'll be eating controlled amounts of healthy fats. This is especially true for olive oil, an amazingly heart-healthy and flavorful oil that's a cornerstone of The Sonoma Diet. Olive oil is not a fat that you are reluctantly "allowed" to eat. Instead, you are actively encouraged to include it with your meals as a key component in your weight loss strategy.

It's the same with carbohydrates. The Sonoma Diet includes bread and cereal from the start, while other diets spurn them. But white bread and other foods made from refined white flour (many crackers, pasta, and cereals) will indeed be virtually eliminated, for reasons that will be explained beginning on page 48. At the same time, though, you will be urged to enjoy healthy amounts of breads, crackers, pastas, and cereals made from whole, unrefined versions of grains, such as wheat, oats, rye, and barley.

White bread and whole-wheat bread are both mostly carbohydrates. But they're not the same. The first will sabotage your weight loss program faster than any other food except sugar. The second, on the other hand, is a fiber-rich, nutrient-loaded pleasure food that is so beneficial for your weight loss goals that you'll find it listed with olive oil among the Power Foods in this book.

Add the starring role of fruits and vegetables and you get a pretty good idea that The Sonoma Diet isn't about

WHAT'S A "DIETARY FAT"?

It could be animal fat such as the marbling in prime rib, a dairy fat such as butter, or the trans fats typically found in margarine and in many processed foods. It could also be the oils in fish, avocados, olives, seeds, and nuts. You will not be given the unrealistic and unhealthy instruction to "severely limit" your consumption of all of those fats. Instead you'll be encouraged to choose the last five while moderating animals fats and eliminating trans fats, mostly because of their proven harm to your overall health.

low-carb or low-fat. It's about eating controlled but satisfying amounts of healthy, great-tasting foods, regardless of their category.

What people are saying about Sonoma...

"Speaking from a food lover's point of view [as a chef]—this is a lifestyle! It is a different approach to eating healthy which does not feel restrictive or where you don't feel hungry. The easy-to-follow Sonoma plate guidelines were great to keep me in tune with the best combinations of wholesome ingredients. One of my favorite tips to share, toasting whole grains and cooking them in flavorful liquids, was essential to enjoying the many different whole grains. My personal challenge—learning how to cut out the extra sweets; it was not easy, but I did it! The most remarkable change I noticed in myself was how quickly my waist size dropped. I really feel more youthful and have so much more energy. I am still working on losing the next 20 pounds—stay tuned Sonoma!"

—Andy, lost 30 pounds

LET'S GET REAL

Before these words reached your eyes, The Sonoma Diet was conceived, designed, tested, adjusted, and retested by experts to ensure maximum efficacy for its twin goals of weight loss and improved health and vitality. The result is a proven plan that will help you lose weight—quickly at first and then steadily until you reach your goal.

But no diet will work if you can't stay with it. And you won't stay with any diet that's too complicated, too challenging, or too boring. That's why volunteers struggling with the same weight issues you do have tested The Sonoma Diet. It's not enough for a diet to be scientifically sound. It has to work in the real world.

Let's face it: Most of us already have enough to worry about. We have jobs to do, spouses to keep happy, children to raise, a home to maintain, and a life to live. The last thing we need is a demanding food regimen that turns mealtime into a stress-filled ordeal of complicated rules and "diet dishes" that nobody likes.

The Sonoma Diet is none of those things. Everything about this diet is enjoyable, simple, and satisfying. Most of all, it's realistic. You don't need to be an amateur nutritionist to follow this diet. All the thinking has been done for you. You won't count carbs and you won't count calories. They've already been counted. All you have to do is choose foods from long lists of options and put them on your plate in the proportions given in the book.

Preparing the meals will be easy too. The recipes provided are not only quick and simple to follow, but they're also based on the Sonoma cuisine that's among the most praised (and healthiest) in the world. You'll be amazed at how great a cook you've become.

In fact, preparing Sonoma meals is even simpler than before. I've added some "Sonoma Made Simple" approaches that give you the option of streamlining your meal prep. In the pages ahead you'll find ways to prepare express meals and Cook Once/Eat Twice recipes—two days' worth of meals you can make in one session, cutting your cooking time in half.

No matter how you choose to prepare your meals, the ingredients are affordable and easy to find. You'll do best on the diet if you try foods and dishes from the lists that are new to you. Variety is your ally. But there's nothing on the lists that isn't readily available at your local farmers' market or supermarket.

You Make the Call

The list of protein choices includes a wonderful variety of fish, shellfish, lean meat, poultry, soy, and eggs. You fill a certain percentage of your plate with something from the protein list at most meals. Though I make suggestions and encourage variety, I don't insist on any particular protein to fulfill that requirement, as long as it is lean.

Conversely, you may choose never to eat meat, instead fulfilling your protein requirement by eating fish or eggs or even going with soy or bean dishes. This "you make the call" method is the only realistic approach to a weight loss plan. Dedicated carnivores can no more be expected to do without meat than vegetarians can be expected to eat it.

Snacks? They're fine on the Sonoma Diet. If a snack keeps you from feeling hungry, by all means have one. You can't eat just anything between meals, of course. Like everything else on the diet, you need to snack on the right amounts of the right things. Look for some suggestions on pages 100 and 117. More options are listed with the meal plans beginning on page 207 and 266.

There's another reality-based touch that you'll appreciate. The Sonoma Diet asks you to abandon your bad eating habits, but not your personal eating preferences. The variety on the food lists and the flexibility in choices make sure you can eat the way you always have. You'll eat less, you'll eat healthier, and you'll eat slower. But you'll still choose the foods you like best.

SIMPLE FOR BUSY LIVES

You'll find The Sonoma Diet amazingly easy to follow.

The three basic factors that determine your weight loss are food selection (what you eat), food combination (what your meals consist of), and portion control (how much you eat). The unique "plate-and-bowl" concept you'll be using makes each of those a very simple proposition. At the same time, so much variety is offered that you may never repeat the same meal twice.

What people are saying about Sonoma . . .

"The ease of the program . . . no counting, just watching the plate size, is huge for me. I love how healthy the food is, I'm allowed wine, and I haven't struggled to lose weight. I don't feel like I'm on a diet . . . the food is just so good I feel like I'm cheating! I knew this was the plan I could stay with the rest of my life and I love it!"

—Ed, lost 61 pounds

Food selection couldn't be simpler. It's merely a matter of lists. For example, every grain that is okay to eat is listed under "Sonoma Grains." Every acceptable fat appears on the list "Sonoma Fats." There are also lists of approved choices in the following categories: proteins (meats, fish, beans, etc.), dairy, fruits, vegetables, flavor boosters, and beverages.

Your fruit and vegetable options are divided into levels, or "tiers." Tiering simply recognizes that some foods in a category are more conducive to weight loss than others. Tier 1 vegetables, for example, may be enjoyed often in all stages of the diet. These include asparagus, eggplant, spinach, and tomatoes, among others. Vegetables from Tier 2 (such as artichokes and carrots) and Tier 3 (including corn and sugar snap peas) will be eaten more sparingly—and not at all during the initial wave of the diet. A similar tiering system applies to fruit.

When the diet instructions call for a certain amount of proteins or grains or anything else in a meal, all you have to do is consult the appropriate list and choose what you're in the mood for that day.

On the other side of the coin, there are two lists of foods that you'll be limiting. These are the foods that will sabotage your weight loss progress and raise your risk of heart disease and other illnesses. You'll see that they're mostly trans fats from partially hydrogenated oils, saturated fats, sugar, and refined flour products such as white bread, cakes, and cookies.

REDEFINING THE AMERICAN PLATE (AND BOWL)

How much do you eat at each meal? That's where the plate-and-bowl concept comes in. This concept brings the most recent nutrition science to your plate. It redefines the common American plate, heavily criticized for its super-sized portions, calories, and fat. The emphasis is a shift in focus, so that more vegetables and grains take center stage in the company of lean meats. You'll be using a seven-inch plate or a two-cup bowl for your breakfast and a nine-inch plate for your lunch and dinner. The diet instructions (which are explained and illustrated beginning on page 83 for Wave 1 and page 105 for Wave 2) will tell you how to fill those plates and bowl.

For example, a typical Wave 1 dinner will call for filling your nine-inch plate with 30% protein, 20% grains, and 50% Tier 1 vegetables. So you might want to fill half your plate with a raw spinach and vegetable salad. A salmon fillet can fill the 30% protein segment and wild rice the rest.

You'll welcome this concept as a lot easier than counting grams or ounces. Because the plates are set in size, the portion control is automatic. You don't measure; you just fill. And because the amount of each food type that goes on the plate is specified, you're assured of getting the best combination for healthy weight loss. This is a style of eating that will make you more mindful of what's on your plate, long after you reach your target body weight.

In addition to the fat found naturally in your food (in meats, salad dressings, and so on), you'll choose additional fats to add flavor to your food and keep you satisfied. Your daily fat allotment is measured in teaspoons of plant oil or individual nuts, so they won't appear as percentages on your plate diagram. Your flavor boosters don't need to be measured at all—they're limitless.

WHEN TO STOP

The Sonoma plate-and-bowl concept takes the guesswork out of portion control, but it's still up to you to stop eating when it's time. Remember to:

• Stay mindful and pay attention to your internal cues, not just the plate.

• Aim for 80% satiety, not "feeling full." The other 20% will take care of itself.

• Keep in mind that people tend to underestimate how much they're really eating.

LOSING WEIGHT IN WAVES

The way you'll feel when you start the Sonoma plan is not how you'll feel as the weeks pass by. This is good news, because you'll feel better. Healthy eating gets easier as time passes, not harder. There are lots of reasons for this. Two stand out.

One is that you'll be enjoying your meals more than you did before. Remember, the recipes you'll use are inspired by Sonoma cuisine—a style of cooking that's as noted for its full, robust flavors as for its healthy goodness.

OUT OF SIGHT, OUT OF MIND, OUT OF MOUTH

Stock your kitchen and pantry with healthy foods so you're not tempted by undesirable choices. Then, organize your cabinets so that less-desirable foods—especially snack foods—are also not easily visible or accessible.

The other is that somewhere around ten days into your Sonoma plan, perhaps earlier, you'll realize that the portions determined by The Sonoma Diet plate-and-bowl concept are big enough to satisfy you at every meal. You'll wonder how you managed to eat those huge servings you helped yourself to before.

For these reasons, the Sonoma plan is divided into three distinct "waves." Wave 1 lasts for the first ten days. It's during this period that you'll be overcoming your habit of consuming large amounts of sugars, refined flour products, and other fast-absorbing foods that most likely led to your weight concerns in the first place.

The list of restricted foods may appear fairly long in Wave 1. But you'll still have full, rich meals—with whole-grain bread or cereal, meat or fish, fruit, and plenty of vegetables.

In Wave 1, you're naturally recalibrating your body and turning around bad eating habits a lifetime in the making. This challenge comes right at the beginning, when your enthusiasm and confidence are in high gear. You'll be thrilled with the results, since this is the period of fastest weight loss. And right when you're fully adjusted to your new healthy eating habits, your portions and choices increase.

Now you're in Wave 2. This is the main leg of the plan, where you'll stay until you reach your target weight. Weight loss is not as quick as it was in the first wave, but it comes steadily. During this wave you'll continue cultivating the Sonoma approach to eating, savoring each meal slowly with an emphasis on health and pleasure.

MISSING NUTRIENTS

Government figures show that the content of a number of vitamins and minerals in various crops has declined by as much as 20% in the last half century. During the same period, there's been a sharp increase in the consumption of processed foods with their empty calories. The bottom line is that most Americans are getting less nutrition per calorie than they used to. The result is more obesity and more vitamin and mineral deficiency. That's why The Sonoma Diet's emphasis on nutrient-rich Power Foods and food combinations that emphasize maximum nutrition per calorie is so important for weight loss.

For Waves 1 and 2, you're provided with a daily meal guide that gives precise dishes (with recipes) that match the instructions for filling your plate or bowl with the right balance, variety, and combinations of food. This meal guide will tell you exactly what to eat for breakfast, lunch, and dinner for each of the ten days in Wave 1 and for fourteen-day cycles in Wave 2.

These meal guides make your meal planning easy, since all you have to do is prepare what the guide suggests. But as long as you follow the plate-filling instructions and food lists, you also have the option of choosing whatever you want. Specific instructions or freedom of choice? It's up to you.

Wave 3 starts the day you reach your target weight. Since congratulations will be in order, your wine choice for the day just might be a bit of the bubbly. Now it's time to convert your new appreciation of healthy eating from a weight loss diet into a lifestyle.

By Wave 3, you'll know what works best for you. Your portion control and food choices will come naturally, and you won't need percentage instructions. Unlimited fruits and vegetables are yours to enjoy. You'll also want to give yourself a special treat now and then. If at any point you find your weight starting to creep up, just pull out those plates and bowls and start back on Wave 2. ∎

· *The Top Twelve* ·
SONOMA DIET
POWER FOODS

The success of The Sonoma Diet is based on eating good foods, not avoiding them. Deprivation can't be the focus for the simple reason that it won't work. Moderation, balance, and a mindful approach to making smart food choices are the keys to losing weight and gaining health. So is recognizing the broad strokes of what it really means to be healthy.

The Top Twelve Sonoma Diet Power Foods help you create a core of earthly delights that not only promotes health, but also is the key to your success in losing those extra pounds. These delicious foods aren't the only power foods, but they're the ones that offer the most exceptional nutritional value with the fewest calories. Their nutrient richness gives you the most nutritional bang for their calorie buck. They're an object lesson in why health and weight loss go hand in hand with The Sonoma Diet.

They are also part of this book's "stealth health" approach to weight loss, where the science is behind the scenes so that you can focus on eating the delicious and wholesome recipes inspired by the most flavorful cuisine under the sun. In other words, you don't need to master any nutrition science to reap their benefits; you just need to eat them. But I believe that you deserve at least to be aware of the reasons these foods are so helpful to your weight loss plans, so I've included some basic nutritional information in the descriptions that follow.

THE POWER AND THE GLORY

All twelve Sonoma Diet Power Foods are plant foods, because they're rich in health-promoting chemical compounds known as phytonutrients ("phyto" means "plant" in Greek). Besides giving fruits and vegetables their unique personality of vibrant colors, pleasing flavors, and interesting textures, many of these plant compounds act as antioxidants in the body, quelling free radicals and preventing cell damage that could lead to heart disease, inflammation, diabetes, cancer, Alzheimer's disease, and even premature aging. There are hundreds of phytonutrients (or phytochemicals), creating an overwhelming vocabulary of hard-to-pronounce terms. But you don't have to say the names correctly to reap their amazing health and weight loss benefits.

Eating The Sonoma Diet Power Foods has been found to be one of the best ways to reverse metabolic syndrome—the dangerous accumulation of symptoms that includes extra pounds around your waist. For that reason, these same foods have been shown to reduce your risk for heart disease and diabetes.

Your twelve Sonoma Diet Power Foods also act as anti-inflammatories. An emerging theory in medicine today identifies inflammation as both a warning sign and a trigger of a number of health problems, such as coronary disease, cancer, obesity, autoimmune diseases, and Alzheimer's disease. In fact, inflammation is so widely linked to heart disease that many physicians routinely order tests for a key marker of inflammation, known as c-reactive protein (crp), as readily as they do cholesterol tests.

Inflammation is your body's way of defending itself against harm or infection, such as that which occurs as a cut or scrape heals. But when inflammation becomes long-term, beyond what your body needs, problems set in. Extra pounds around the waist create a vicious inflammatory cycle—they promote inflammation in the body, which in turn provides the perfect environment for gaining more weight.

The food you eat can induce inflammation or reduce it, depending on your choices. Saturated fats (from full-fat animal products), trans fats in partially hydrogenated oils (from commercial cakes, cookies, crackers, and other processed foods), and refined starches and sweets make inflammation worse.

Inflammation-quenching foods include cold-water fish, flaxseeds, canola oil, and walnuts (for their omega-3 fatty acids); nuts, olives, canola oil, and avocados (for their monounsaturated fats); and a wide variety of vibrantly colored fruits, vegetables, nuts, and seeds.

The best foods to protect against inflammation? Not by coincidence, they're the Top Twelve Sonoma Diet Power Foods, including the two newest members, citrus and beans.

POWER PAIRINGS

Eating the recommended seven to nine servings of produce daily would certainly improve the health of most people in the Western world, not to mention their waistlines. As you follow the Sonoma guidelines, however, you'll do much better than that. For one thing, your fruit and vegetable intake will include the Power Foods that you're about to be introduced to. But it will by no means be limited to them.

On the contrary, mixing and matching your fruits and vegetables to create a dazzling variety of tastes, colors, and textures not only makes your plate more appealing, but also magnifies its health and weight loss benefits significantly. When you include all colors of the rainbow when choosing your fruits, vegetables, grains, and nuts, you're multiplying the phytonutrients—not only their number but their health benefits, since they work together synergistically.

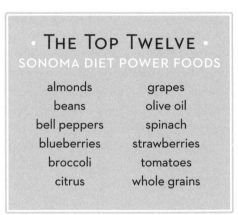

· THE TOP TWELVE ·
SONOMA DIET POWER FOODS

almonds	grapes
beans	olive oil
bell peppers	spinach
blueberries	strawberries
broccoli	tomatoes
citrus	whole grains

Variety is also key with the Top Twelve Sonoma Diet Power Foods, because it allows their nutrients to work together to enhance their protective qualities, not to mention their flavor. For example, extra-virgin olive oil drizzled over ripe tomatoes or included as part of a rich tomato sauce not only brings out the flavor but also helps your body absorb more of the disease-preventing lycopenes in tomatoes. The antioxidant flavonoids in spinach and other bitter greens are more available to your body when they're consumed with healthy plant oils from nuts or olives (cooking these greens with plant oils is also a natural way to mellow that hint of bitterness).

Another example: The many inspirations in your Sonoma Diet grain medleys offer appetizing combinations of protein-rich ingredients like beans, nuts, and whole grains, where the quality of protein is just as rich and complete as in your favorite lean meats.

What people are saying about Sonoma . . .

> *"I've been on the maintenance wave for about a month and have kept the weight off. More important for me is that my cholesterol lowered from 249 to 217 in one month! My energy level is up. I feel fantastic!"*
>
> —Karen, lost 7 pounds

ALMONDS: A MIGHTY NUT

All nuts are good for you and have a place in any variation of coastal California cuisine. But you will find almonds in a surprising number of dishes throughout Sonoma restaurants and homes. In the United States, they're grown exclusively in California. Their sweet taste is one reason they're so popular. But sweetness alone doesn't make almonds a Power Food; the marriage of great taste and nutritional benefits does.

It may surprise you that almonds, a food relatively high in calories, make the list of top Power Foods. The fact is all calories, especially fat calories, are not created equal. The fat in almonds is primarily heart-healthy

ALMONDS AND DARK CHOCOLATE

A dream team combo, almonds and dark chocolate go perfectly together to provide an antioxidant boost as well as a hunger-suppressing sweet treat. Almonds and dark chocolate both contain antioxidant flavonoids.

monounsaturated fat, the same type found in olives, olive oil, avocados, and other nuts.

Increasingly, science shows that almonds decrease the risk for heart disease. Recent medical studies found that eating one ounce of almonds daily (about a handful), as part of a healthy lifestyle, reduces LDL cholesterol (the bad stuff) and thereby reduces your overall heart disease risk. Other studies have shown that almonds are protective against cancer and diabetes as well. And eating almonds regularly may decrease other risk factors in the blood that are related to artery-damaging inflammation. An exciting discovery in these studies was that the addition of the extra daily calories from almonds didn't lead to weight gain.

Could there be some nutrients in almonds that actually help you lose weight? Research says yes! Populations who regularly eat moderate amounts of these nuts, averaging a handful a day, tend to have healthier body weights and live longer than people who don't. That may be because almonds provide just the right combination of protein, fat, fiber, vitamins, and minerals to curb hunger, but it also seems that our bodies may not absorb all their calories.

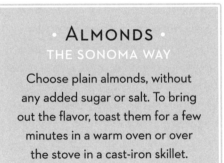

· ALMONDS ·
THE SONOMA WAY

Choose plain almonds, without any added sugar or salt. To bring out the flavor, toast them for a few minutes in a warm oven or over the stove in a cast-iron skillet.

ALMONDS' JOYS

Almonds stand out as especially rich in calcium—in fact, they're one of the best nondairy calcium sources. They also deliver plenty of protein, copper, zinc, potassium, magnesium, and B vitamins. And like all the other Power Foods, almonds supply antioxidant nutrients, most notably vitamin E.

The more we learn about almonds, the more they amaze. Ongoing research finds that almonds may have a prebiotic effect. Prebiotics (not the same as probiotics) are nutrients that your body can't digest, but that provide nourishment to the good bacteria in your gastrointestinal tract. Well-fed helpful bacteria in your gut mean better immunity and overall well-being for you.

Almonds provide a wonderful example of how focusing on eating good foods is a more direct route to your target weight than concentrating only on avoiding "bad" foods. A typical "low-fat" diet might discourage eating almonds. That's counterproductive. Almonds, in proper amounts, can help you avoid eating problem fats. A revealing 2004 study published in a British medical journal illustrated this. About eighty men and women were told to eat a quarter of a cup of almonds every day but were given no other diet instructions. After six months, on their own, the almond eaters had noticeably cut down on the amount of harmful saturated fats and trans fats they were eating. In other words, eating a smart fat—almonds—helps you avoid problem fats. That's exactly what you'll be doing on The Sonoma Diet.

MORE CHEWS, MORE HEALTH

Eating slowly doesn't just let you savor your food and make you mindful of how much you eat. With almonds, the slow approach boosts their health benefits. A recent study out of Purdue University suggests that the more we chew almonds—up to forty times—the greater the release of heart-healthy nutrients such as vitamin E and plant oils, and the more your hunger is curbed.

BEANS:
BIG BENEFITS, GREAT TASTE

Beans are a new addition to the Sonoma Diet Power Foods list, but they're one of the oldest—and healthiest—of cultivated crops. Part of a more general grouping called legumes, beans come in an assortment of shapes, sizes, and colors. Some of the most common legumes are soybeans, lentils, peas, peanuts, and chickpeas (garbanzo beans).

Mediterranean cuisines feature beans and other legumes in the company of olive oil, grains, nuts, and seeds. This culinary adventure, along with Latin and Asian cuisines, has inspired me to include beans in many of the Sonoma recipes you'll be eating. You'll find a variety of colorful salads, rich soups and stews, creamy spreads, salsas, and dressings—all given a boost of flavor and nutrition with legumes. Since there are literally hundreds of bean varieties, each with its own color, texture, and flavor, you can make the same dish with different beans, each variation offering an entirely new culinary experience.

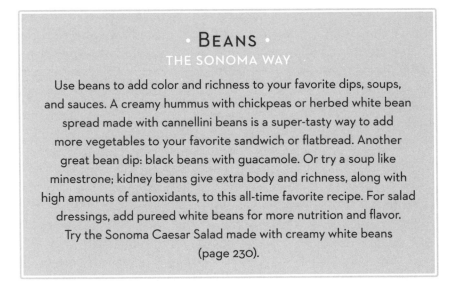

· BEANS ·
THE SONOMA WAY

Use beans to add color and richness to your favorite dips, soups, and sauces. A creamy hummus with chickpeas or herbed white bean spread made with cannellini beans is a super-tasty way to add more vegetables to your favorite sandwich or flatbread. Another great bean dip: black beans with guacamole. Or try a soup like minestrone; kidney beans give extra body and richness, along with high amounts of antioxidants, to this all-time favorite recipe. For salad dressings, add pureed white beans for more nutrition and flavor. Try the Sonoma Caesar Salad made with creamy white beans (page 230).

LOSING WEIGHT, FEELING GREAT

Beans and other legumes are nutritional superstars, providing many of the nutrients often lacking in the American diet. They're an excellent source of fiber, manganese, and folate, as well as a good source of protein, potassium, magnesium, and iron. As for weight loss, it's known that people who eat beans regularly tend to have lower body weight and smaller waist sizes than those who don't. Part of the reason may be that the types of fibers and carbohydrates found in beans help keep blood sugar levels in balance, keeping your hunger down and energy up. Fiber in general decreases hunger and possibly even increases satiety signals to the brain. And white beans have the added weight loss benefit of stimulating an appetite-satisfying hormone known as cholecystokinin, or CCK.

LEGUMES FOR LONG LIFE

Will eating beans help you live a longer, healthier life?

CANNED BEANS

Canned beans contain all the major nutrients of fresh beans. You can keep a variety of them on hand and use them interchangeably in most of the Sonoma recipes. Rinsing canned beans will reduce the sodium content by as much as 40%, or you can select varieties offered in a low-salt version. Canned beans are an easy addition to your favorite salads.

Recent research says yes. Scientists studied the eating habits of elderly people in Greece, Sweden, Australia, and Japan. Of all the dietary factors analyzed, eating beans was most consistently linked to reduced mortality risk. No other food or food group showed the same kind of life-prolonging effect.

Here in the United States, the National Health and Nutrition Examination Survey (NHANES) finds that people who eat legumes at least four times a week have a 22% lower risk of heart disease compared to those who eat beans less than once a week. For more than twenty years, the research has shown that beans can have a beneficial effect on several important risk factors for cardiovascular disease, including total blood cholesterol, LDL (the bad cholesterol), lipoproteins, and triglycerides. And research from the Department of Nutrition at the Harvard School of Public Health found that the consumption of just one serving of beans per day is associated with a 38% lower risk of heart attacks.

One more thing: Beans have more protein than any other vegetable (yes, beans are vegetables). In that sense, half a cup of beans is equal to two ounces of lean meat. People who eat more protein may tend to eat less overall. So beans, as a premier protein source, have the advantage over many other foods. You get not only the potential weight-curbing properties of protein, but also the protective qualities of phytochemicals and antioxidants. Try eating at least three cups of cooked beans each week.

BEANS FOR KIDS

Children who eat beans tend to have healthier diets, especially when it comes to how much fiber they eat. They also tend to have smaller waist measurements when compared to kids who don't eat beans. Sonoma recipes with beans that are sure to be favorites with the entire family include Black Bean Guacamole, Smoky White Bean and Tomato Soup, and White Bean Chile Verde with Sonoma Pesto.

BELL PEPPERS:
RINGING IN THE NUTRIENTS

How can such a seemingly lightweight vegetable be bursting with so much nutrition? Well, that's what makes bell peppers such a solid Sonoma Diet Power Food—lots of health-imparting nutrients and a minuscule amount of calories (about 35 each). And they're healthy and tasty raw or cooked.

They're also a classic Mediterranean vegetable—think stuffed bell peppers, or raw bell pepper strips in a brightly colored spring salad. Brought to southern Europe from the New World by the Spanish in the sixteenth century, bell peppers grow anywhere that's not too cold. That includes Sonoma, where locally grown versions are sold fresh at farmers' markets.

The power of bell peppers is right there in the colors. Green, purple, red, yellow, and orange are all phytonutrient-rich bell peppers (or sweet peppers, as they're also called). But the nature of some of the nutrients changes with the color, and so does the taste, subtly. Heart-healthy, cancer-preventive, sight-saving benefits abound with any hue. What all those colored peppers have in common are generous natural doses of the antioxidant vitamins A and C. These two vitamins protect against heart disease and inflammation. Two other vitamins abundant in bell peppers—B6 and folic acid—help out by lowering levels of a heart disease–related protein called homocysteine. One of the most important findings about heart health in recent years is the connection between high homocysteine levels and your risk for a heart attack or stroke.

FIGHTING CANCER

While peppers of all colors are rich in antioxidant carotenoids, the red ones pack a bonus in the form of lycopene. This is a powerful antioxidant that gives tomatoes and red bell peppers their color. Its specialty is fighting cancer. The evidence is clear that a daily dose of the lycopene found in bell peppers, along with their vitamins and beta-carotene (another carotenoid), reduces your risk of colon, cervix, bladder, pancreas, and prostate cancers.

Bell peppers' potent combination of carotenoids and antioxidant vitamins also appears to offer protection against lung disease and lung cancer. Here, too, the red and orange bell peppers may provide an extra boost because of a special carotenoid called beta-cryptoxanthin, which is found in other orange foods as well—from pumpkin to papaya.

SOME LIKE THEM HOT

Chile peppers are relatives of bell peppers. Despite their fiery hotness, chiles are popular for both flavor and health. They contain a powerful compound, capsaicin, which gives chiles their spicy kick and your health a solid boost.

VISION PRESERVATION

There's also evidence that the antioxidants in bell peppers help stave off age-related vision problems, such as cataracts. Once again, the red bell peppers may be the best choice for your eyes, because only they have some special nutrients thought to protect against macular degeneration, a common cause of vision loss.

The beauty of bell peppers is their built-in variety. You'll find all kinds of ways to enjoy bell peppers as you progress through your diet. And you'll start right in on them with Wave 1.

Blueberries:
Potent and Delicious

Everybody loves blueberries, but how often do people eat them? Some never do. Others only think about blueberries that are baked in muffins. Their loss. Blueberries are an especially potent Power Food on their own. If you've always thought of blueberries as a rare special treat, think of them now as something to eat often. Whether you buy them fresh (at a supermarket or farmers' market) or frozen, they're a superb investment for your health, your weight loss, and your taste buds.

ANTIOXIDANT POWER

The magic of blueberries comes from the astonishing amounts of antioxidants they contain. Government surveys have ranked blueberries at the top of the fruit list in antioxidant content. In fact, based on what we currently know, only one food on the planet (red kidney beans) offers more antioxidants per serving than blueberries.

Many of those antioxidants are the same flavonoids responsible for the heart-strengthening benefits of grapes and wine. That includes resveratrol, one of the true Hall of Fame nutrients on The Sonoma Diet team, thanks to its well-documented heart-protecting abilities. But blueberries, it turns out, pack even more resveratrol than wine.

Not surprisingly, that wine-like antioxidant action puts blueberries among the elite of Sonoma-style heart-healthy foods. But recent research has uncovered another amazing benefit. Eating blueberries regularly may slow down, and perhaps even reverse, the memory decline that comes with aging. That same brain-

> ### • BLUEBERRIES •
> #### THE SONOMA WAY
>
> In Sonoma fresh, sweet blueberries dropped into whole-grain cereals, topped with nonfat yogurt, or just popped into your mouth one by one are part of the healthy lifestyle. It's not uncommon for folks there to pick ripe blueberries right off the bush to take home to eat.

saving ability is also found in strawberries and spinach—two other Power Foods included in the Sonoma Diet.

The protective power in blueberries is also related to the antioxidants known as anthocyanins, the pigments responsible for their deep blue color. Blueberries reduce your risk of a whole slew of illnesses, including certain types of cancer, vision loss, and digestive disorders. Recent studies suggest that blueberries play a role in reducing waist size and risk factors associated with those extra pounds known as metabolic syndrome.

You may have heard about cranberries' ability to fend off urinary tract infections. Blueberries contain the same bacteria-inhibiting phytonutrients as cranberries. Investigators still need to find direct evidence that blueberries work against urinary tract infections as effectively as cranberries. In the meantime, though, the probability that they do gives you one more reason to indulge often in these sweet treats.

BROCCOLI:
A GOURMET POWER FOOD

Broccoli is about as Mediterranean as a vegetable can be. It was first grown in Italy; then the Romans spread it across Europe, and immigrants brought it to America. Raw or cooked, it's a super-player in The Sonoma Diet, something for you to eat in virtually unlimited amounts for the rest of your life.

VITAMIN C AND CALCIUM

You probably don't need convincing when it comes to broccoli's benefits. Its reputation as one of the world's healthiest foods is well established. But did you know that broccoli is one of the best sources of calcium and vitamin C?

Consider this. There's as much vitamin C in a serving of broccoli (that's half a cup in The Sonoma Diet) as in an orange. But an orange will set you back 60 to 70 calories—not a huge amount, but considerably more than the 20 or so in a serving of broccoli. That's why broccoli is a Power Food.

Same goes for calcium. A half-cup serving of broccoli delivers about 40 milligrams of calcium—a decent amount. Sure, you'll get more than that in a cup of milk, but you'll also get 85 to 150 calories, depending on what kind of milk you're drinking. And milk—even skim milk—has saturated fat. Broccoli has zero fat of any kind. That's right. None.

> ## · BROCCOLI ·
> ### THE SONOMA WAY
>
> Don't overcook your broccoli into a soggy, nutrient-depleted mush. Take advantage of the huge selection of herbs, spices, and other flavor enhancers you can use at any phase of the diet. Or you can eat broccoli raw, just like you'd enjoy carrots. Chomp away. You're doing your health and your body weight a favor.

CANCER FIGHTER

Beyond its role as a rich source of vitamin C and calcium, broccoli is a deluxe detoxifier. It clears away potentially carcinogenic toxins and inhibits tumor growth, making it a strong cancer fighter.

The big anticancer gun in broccoli's phytonutrient arsenal is a detoxifier called sulforophane. As the name hints, this is the substance responsible for the sulfur-like smell of broccoli as it cooks. But there's no sulfuric taste at all to broccoli. Properly cooking broccoli, such as lightly steaming it, enhances its flavor even more. Broccoli's a true gourmet vegetable as well as a cancer fighter and heart protector.

BABY BROCCOLI

Broccolini, also known as baby broccoli, is a cross between broccoli and Chinese kale. With more slender stems and smaller florets, it's more tender than regular broccoli and has a sweet and slightly peppery taste. Cook this tasty green with your favorite extra-virgin olive oil, a bit of garlic, some red pepper flakes, and finish it with a squeeze of fresh lemon juice and a pinch of salt.

CITRUS: A BURST OF HEALTH

The beautiful colors of citrus and their burst of sweet or tart flavors make them popular around the world. They were enjoyed for centuries in the Mediterranean region before Spanish missionaries brought the first citrus trees to coastal California. Today, a variety of citrus fruits turn up in Sonoma's Mediterranean-style dishes, as well as in the local Asian and Latin cuisines that sometimes influence them. Although grown in warm climates, these fruits are available year-round and will be part of your Sonoma meal plans for gaining health and losing weight.

NUTRITIONAL POWERHOUSE

Ask most Americans to name a citrus fruit and they'll most likely say "orange." The sweetness of most varieties makes them popular for snacks, dessert, and in the morning juice glass. And

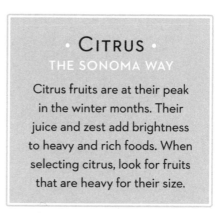

· CITRUS ·
THE SONOMA WAY

Citrus fruits are at their peak in the winter months. Their juice and zest add brightness to heavy and rich foods. When selecting citrus, look for fruits that are heavy for their size.

most people probably know that oranges are packed with vitamin C. Just one medium-sized orange provides more than 100% of the recommended daily amount for that essential nutrient. Recent studies have also shown that the vitamin C found in oranges and other citrus provides a boost to the immune system and decreases the risk associated with cardiovascular disease, cancer, and stroke. But oranges and vitamin C are just a part of the citrus Power Food story.

Along with vitamin C, citrus fruits have plenty of potassium, which helps regulate blood pressure and boost heart health. These fruits also have folate, which helps to prevent birth defects and may also protect against heart disease, depression, and some cancers. Different phytochemicals in citrus have antiviral, antioxidant, anticancer, and even anti-inflammatory benefits. Hesperidin is one of the key nutrients to offer anti-inflammatory protection and can reduce the symptoms of high blood pressure.

Exciting research also confirms that citrus fruits, grapefruit in particular, can help people who struggle with a health peril associated with extra pounds around the waist—insulin resistance. Fibers contained in the white fuzzy parts of the whole grapefruit, known as the albeto layer, help keep blood sugar levels stable and can curb hunger for up to four hours after eating.

> ### POWER COMBO
> ## LEMON & GREEN TEA
>
> Maximize the health benefits of citrus by pairing it with other nutrient-rich ingredients in Sonoma foods. For example, adding lemon juice to green tea increases the staying power of the tea's antioxidants and makes them even more available for the body to absorb.

> ### POWER COMBO
> ## SALSA & FLANK STEAK
>
> Adding a colorful Latin fruit salsa to a grilled flank steak makes it easier for the body to absorb and utilize the iron contained in the meat.

GRAPES: FRUIT OF THE GODS

The Greeks and Romans considered grapes a gift from the gods. And why not? There's something miraculous about a gnarly black vine creating generous clusters of bright pearls of fruit, each bursting with pure goodness. These ancient southern Europeans appreciated the health-imparting power of grapes themselves. But they positively worshipped the fruit's capacity to convert itself into that most sensuous of nectars—fine wine. The Greeks and Romans bequeathed their love of grapes and wine to their modern southern European successors, who turned both into cornerstones of the Mediterranean diet.

Grapes are equally revered in today's Sonoma. There the hillsides are covered with vineyards, their ripening fruit gleaming green and purple in the preharvest sun. The Sonoma Diet is indebted to this important part of the Sonoma economy.

GOOD NEWS FROM THE GRAPEVINE

What's wonderful about grapes as a Power Food is that they deliver virtually all the nutrients that wine does. That means you'll still reap most of the heart-protective and weight loss benefits of grapes' abundant phytonutrients even if you cannot (or choose not to) drink a daily glass of wine.

Grapes and wine are a big reason why modern researchers got curious about the Mediterranean diet in the first place. Why, they asked, did southern Europeans suffer so few heart attacks even as they ate so richly? A big reason, we know now, is the special potency of the heart-protective nutrients in the grapes and wine they consume so liberally.

The deep blue and purple hues of grapes hint at the powerful antioxidants found in their skins and seeds. Concord grapes and other varieties promote flexible arteries, thus improving blood pressure and circulation in the body. The polyphenol phytonutrients also team up with vitamin C to boost your immune system's capacity to fight off infection. One interesting new area of research suggests that many of the antioxidants found in grapes may also keep our minds healthy—especially as we age.

It would take an organic chemistry textbook to describe the myriad flavonoids that make grapes such a heart-healthy food. But you've already met an important one—resveratrol, the same wonder nutrient that powers blueberries. While there's actually more resveratrol in blueberries than in grapes, the supporting cast in grapes is unbeatable. Because the flavonoids and other antioxidant nutrients work

COLOR BLIND

Red and purple grapes are richer in flavonoids than the white and green varieties, but I'm not going to hold you to that. Grapes of any color are Power Foods.

GRAPE JUICE POWER

Concord grape juice yields more antioxidant power per serving than other common 100% fruit juices. And it provides many of the same heart-health benefits as red wine. For less sugar and more flavor, try a Sonoma spritzer, as described on pages 97–98.

together like a philharmonic orchestra, grapes have achieved elite status as a Power Food.

Surveys show that most people don't eat enough deep blue and purple fruits and vegetables, even though that color category happens to have one of the highest levels of natural antioxidant and anti-inflammatory powers. That's even more reason to include grapes and other dark blue and purple foods in your daily core of meals.

OLIVE OIL:
A WEIGHT LOSS BLESSING

In Sonoma County each year, there's a special festival called the Blessing of the Olives. That's how central olive trees and the foods they yield are to the economy and the eating habits of the region.

Olive oil, the most treasured gift of these blessed trees, is just as central to The Sonoma Diet. There's probably no food choice you'll make that does more for your health and weight loss efforts than olive oil. That's good news for your taste buds, because no other vegetable oil comes close to olive oil's rich, pleasing flavor. A dish prepared with olive oil announces to anyone who smells or tastes it, "I'm special."

HEALTHY FAT

The research is clear as can be that a major reason for southern Europeans' low rate of heart disease is their use of olive oil as their main source of dietary fat. By adopting olive oil in the same way, you'll get the same benefits. And because you'll learn to enjoy olive oil in healthy amounts in place of the harmful fats you may be used to, you will lose weight.

To appreciate olive oil as a Power Food, banish from your mind the

· OLIVE OIL ·
THE SONOMA WAY

Always buy extra-virgin olive oil. "Extra-virgin" simply means that the oil comes from the first pressing of the olives and therefore retains the most beneficial nutrients. It also has by far the most delicate and pleasing taste.

notion that it's the "least bad" fat. It is a heart-healthy food that is good for you. You need dietary fat to lose weight, but you need the right kind. Olive oil is one of the best. Choose extra-virgin olive oil and you'll also enhance the flavors of your meals.

Put simply, olive oil is mostly made of monounsaturated fat, the kind of fat that actually lowers your levels of the bad LDL cholesterol as well as blood fats called triglycerides. The fats you'll be limiting (saturated fat) and avoiding (partially hydrogenated trans fats) raise those levels. The healthy fat alone qualifies olive oil as a Power Food par excellence.

POWER COMBO

OLIVE OIL & SPINACH

A huge plus for olive oil is its special ability to interact with other foods. Try it as a dressing over a spinach salad. It not only improves the flavor by toning down the subtle bitterness of the leaves, but also boosts the action of all those beneficial phytonutrients in spinach.

A WEALTH OF ANTIOXIDANTS

But there's more. Unique among vegetable oils, olive oil—particularly extra-virgin olive oil—is rich in the same family of antioxidant phytonutrients that make all the other Power Foods on the Top Twelve list so effective in preventing heart disease. The same phenols that make olive oil taste so good also make up its main category of antioxidants. Olive oil also contains carotenoids (like beta-carotene) and vitamin E.

Emerging science is suggesting that some of these compounds help keep the mind healthy by reducing risk factors associated with the development of Alzheimer's disease. One of the most exciting studies pertaining to the antioxidants in extra-virgin olive oil suggests it has a preventive role in obesity, metabolic syndrome, and type 2 diabetes. Study after study confirms that eating an olive oil–rich Mediterranean-style diet (of which The Sonoma Diet is one) is better for heart health than a low-fat diet and specifically improves blood sugar control, blood pressure, cholesterol levels, and inflammation markers.

SPINACH: FULL OF SURPRISES

Spinach is the quintessential "green leafy vegetable" so often recommended for overall health. In fact, that's what spinach basically is—big green leaves (though the stems are great too). What's in those leaves borders on the miraculous.

Calorie for calorie, spinach is a valuable Power Food. The nutritional benefits are so abundant—and the calories so negligible—you can eat virtually all you want of this amazing plant. Like tomatoes, broccoli, and bell peppers, spinach is a Tier 1 vegetable that you can eat in unlimited amounts from the first day of your Wave 1 meals.

· SPINACH ·
THE SONOMA WAY

Raw and cooked spinach are almost like two distinct foods, their taste and presentation are so different. When cooking spinach, try lightly steaming it to preserve its phytonutrients. Raw is best, however, as in a tasty spinach salad. Drizzle on extra-virgin olive oil, add some toasted nuts, or check out the dressings in the recipe section. Raw or cooked, spinach is an all-star Power Food you'll be enjoying a lot.

NUTRIENT-RICH

Spinach is full of pleasant surprises. It's a natural, low-calorie source of iron, which makes it invaluable for pregnant, lactating, or menstruating women. And like broccoli and almonds, it's a rich nondairy source of calcium. The combination of calcium and vitamin K (which spinach also delivers in abundance) promotes bone health and prevents osteoporosis.

Keep in mind also that along with blueberries and strawberries, the flavonoids in spinach are thought to slow cognitive decline, meaning they may prevent the memory loss that often accompanies aging. Spinach is also rich in lutein, a carotenoid that a growing body of research has linked to eye health and a reduced risk of age-related vision problems.

Like most Sonoma Power Foods, spinach provides a generous and varied supply of antioxidant nutrients that fight heart disease by discouraging dangerous oxidation of existing blood cholesterol. But spinach also protects your heart in lots of other ways, making it stand out among heart-healthy foods. For example, spinach is especially rich in folate.

Another key recent discovery is the role of inflammation in heart disease. Spinach has well-known anti-inflammatory properties, so it's possible it protects your heart that way. (It certainly helps prevent inflammatory conditions such as arthritis and asthma.) There's also recent evidence that the protein in spinach contains components that help you avoid high blood pressure, a top risk factor for serious heart problems.

STRAWBERRIES: THE PLEASURE PRINCIPLE

Wash and slice enough fresh strawberries to fill a half-cup measure, and you're looking at maybe 25 calories, 30 max. You're also looking at a first-rate Power Food that delivers not only the fiber, vitamins, and minerals you expect from a fruit but also a generous dose of especially beneficial phytochemicals. That combination makes strawberries a surprisingly potent health booster for your heart, joints, and even your mind.

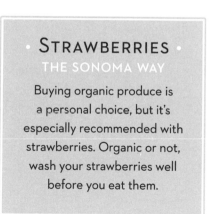

· STRAWBERRIES ·
THE SONOMA WAY

Buying organic produce is a personal choice, but it's especially recommended with strawberries. Organic or not, wash your strawberries well before you eat them.

DELICIOUS HEALTH

If you're like most people, you probably don't think of strawberries as "health food." They taste too good, for one thing. And they're usually associated with oversugared jams and jellies, ice cream packed with saturated fat, and cakes and pies made with refined flour.

But that's just the kind of thinking you'll leave behind as you shed pounds with The Sonoma Diet. Strawberries are a pleasure to eat and a boon for your health and weight loss efforts. Period. Once you realize there's more enjoyment in a half cup of fresh, ripe, nutrient-rich strawberries than in a strawberry pastry, you're well on your way to reaching your weight goal.

Eating strawberries provides your body with a unique assortment of phenols (a broad category of phytonutrients). These are antioxidants, acting like rust busters to keep cells healthy and minimize the harm of cholesterol accumulating in your arteries. Strawberries' special phenols have also been shown to reduce dangerous inflammation throughout the body, including the arteries. Their anti-inflammatory action appears to work much like aspirin. That provides even more heart protection, now that inflammation is considered such a major risk factor for heart disease.

Like blueberries and spinach, strawberries also contain special flavonoids that appear to have a brain-saving effect. Thus eating strawberries regularly may literally save your memory. There's also abundant evidence that eating strawberries regularly helps protect you from cancer, age-related vision impairment, and (because of their anti-inflammatory properties) rheumatoid arthritis.

FRESH OR FROZEN

Strawberries perish quickly but freeze (and thaw) well. So go ahead and buy a big sack of frozen strawberries to last you for a week or so. Also look for straight-from-the-farm berries that were picked ripe, visit a local farmers' market, or stop at a fresh fruit stand.

TOMATOES: PRIDE OF THE KITCHEN

Picture a kitchen with lots of ripe red tomatoes, sliced fresh on a cutting board or simmering in an aromatic sauce. The scene is common in Sonoma homes and restaurants, where vine-ripened and often homegrown tomatoes are key to the region's healthy and satisfying way of eating.

Your kitchen will look much the same from now on. Tomatoes are a top Power Food—nutrient-packed and great tasting, with barely 40 calories each. You're encouraged to eat plenty from Day 1 of The Sonoma Diet. And you'll find that it's easy to do. The beauty of tomatoes is their versatility.

PHYTOCHEMICAL POWER

What makes tomatoes such a strong ally in your healthy diet? Part of their power comes from their rich array of phytochemicals that work together to protect your cardiovascular system. That makes tomatoes a classic heart-healthy Sonoma food. Tomatoes' most powerful component is a phytonutrient called lycopene. This is the carotenoid that gives red tomatoes their bright color. It's also one of the most-studied nutrients in recent years. The evidence has repeatedly shown that lycopene in tomatoes reduces the risk of several cancers—including breast, cervix, prostate, pancreas, and lung cancers.

That puts tomatoes in a unique category. For most Power Foods, the scientific case for their heart-protective benefits is solid, while evidence for their cancer-fighting property is strong but incomplete. Not so for tomatoes. Their anticancer action is even more proven than their heart benefits. Eating tomatoes, then, will help you lose weight, keep your heart healthy, and stay cancer-free as you grow older. That's the mark of a true Power Food.

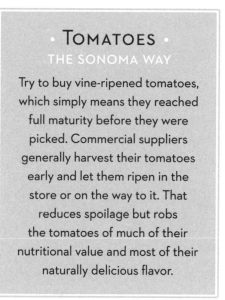

· TOMATOES ·
THE SONOMA WAY

Try to buy vine-ripened tomatoes, which simply means they reached full maturity before they were picked. Commercial suppliers generally harvest their tomatoes early and let them ripen in the store or on the way to it. That reduces spoilage but robs the tomatoes of much of their nutritional value and most of their naturally delicious flavor.

Eat tomatoes fresh, canned, as a sauce, or as a paste. All forms are high in lycopene. Fresh tomatoes are best in the summer, so stock up and enjoy them at their peak. In the colder months, make your own tomato sauces and soups with canned tomatoes. Some canned tomatoes come with added flavors, like Muir Glen's fire-roasted tomatoes, to make your cooking even easier.

WHOLE GRAINS: FOR WHOLE HEALTH

While some diets prohibit or severely limit any kind of grain or cereal, whole grains are the very heart and soul of The Sonoma Diet. Eating whole grains while eliminating refined white-flour foods boosts your health in countless ways and is a key element of steady and sustained weight loss.

Once you scan the list of The Sonoma Diet whole-grain products, you'll quickly see that your choices are almost unlimited. Anything made with refined grains can be made with whole grains—breads, cereals, pasta, crackers, you name it.

GREAT GRAINS

Here's a list of whole grains. Don't worry if you don't recognize them all for now. Just remember that any of them will provide great, healthful taste, and many are featured in the Sonoma recipes.

amaranth	corn	quinoa	teff
barley	farro	rice	triticale
buckwheat	kamut	rye	wheat
bulgur	millet	sorghum	wild rice
	oats	spelt	

A BOUNTY OF BENEFITS

A variety of recent studies highlight the many ways whole grains deliver better health. Harvard researchers followed thousands of women over ten years and found that those who ate whole grains regularly reduced their risk of hypertension by 11 percent. Eating whole grains has also been shown to reduce the risk of diabetes and inflammatory diseases in women. And everyone can benefit from the grains' proven ability to reduce weight, percentage of body fat, and the risk of cardiovascular disease. Eating whole grains can also reduce tooth loss and risk of gum disease, build healthier arteries, and boost your mood.

GO WITH THE GRAIN

What makes a grain "whole"? Whole grains contain all three parts of a grain: the bran, the germ, and the endosperm. The bran includes dietary fiber, B vitamins, and such important minerals as selenium, potassium, and magnesium. The germ, the embryo of the grain's seed, contains B vitamins, vitamin E, essential plant oils, and phytonutrients. Finally, the endosperm contains starch, B vitamins, and proteins.

In white, refined grains, however, the germ and the bran are stripped away, meaning most of the key nutrients are stripped away too. Worse, your bloodstream absorbs white flour so fast that your blood sugar levels first soar and then dive as the fat-producing hormone insulin rushes in as a response. Science also suggests that these spikes in blood sugar lead to more inflammation in the body, increasing your risk for heart disease and diabetes.

So a major difference between refined grains flour (or white flour) and whole grains (or flour made from them) is the speed of conversion to blood sugar. Today, researchers generally agree that the rate at which your body converts food into blood sugar (glucose) is a better indication of the food's healthiness than how much carbohydrate it contains. This rate is measured by the glycemic index (GI). The lower glycemic index of whole grains means a slower release of blood sugar and a healthier food choice. (More about that later on page 110.)

WHOLLY HEALTHY

Here's a quick look at just some of the health benefits of eating whole grains:

REDUCES THE RISK OF	BY %
stroke	30–36
type 2 diabetes	20–30
heart disease	25–36
digestive system cancers	21–43
hormone-related cancers	10–40

Another difference between whole grains and refined: Whole grains deliver lots of the best kinds of fiber; refined white flour delivers almost none. Fiber, as you'll see later, is one of your greatest health allies, as it slows cholesterol absorption and lowers blood fat levels.

WHEN WHEAT WON'T DO

You may have noticed the phrase "gluten-free" appearing on grocery items
and restaurant menus. The U.S. market for gluten-free breads, pastas,
cookies, crackers, cereals, and other foods is hovering around the $2 bil-
lion mark.

So what is gluten? It's a protein found in wheat and other grains, and
it's the source of celiac disease, an autoimmune disorder that damages the
small intestine and reduces the body's ability to absorb nutrients. About 3
million Americans suffer from celiac, many undiagnosed. Gluten intolerance also seems to play a role in a host of other ailments. People with
migraines, multiple sclerosis, or chronic fatigue see their symptoms
lessen when they avoid gluten. So do some children diagnosed with
autism or attention-deficit/hyper-activity disorder. Wheat or gluten
intolerance can also spark poor digestion, chronic congestion, and
skin rashes.

Though true celiac disease is relatively uncommon, gluten
sensitivity may affect as much as 20% of the population. Most of
those people have no idea they are gluten-sensitive, and they could

GRAINS WITH GLUTEN

barley	rye
bulgar	semolina
durum	spelt
farro	triticale
kamut	wheat

GLUTEN-FREE GRAINS

amaranth	quinoa
buckwheat	rice
corn	sorghum
Indian rice grass	teff
millet	wild rice

get relief from a number of bothersome symptoms if they simply reduced their consumption of gluten-containing grains from once a day to once every several days. That's why I've included gluten-free recipes in the Sonoma plan (for example, see pages 214, 226, and 355). And it's usually easy to substitute gluten-free grains in other recipes you like. ▪

What About Oats and Gluten?

Oats are naturally gluten-free, but they are often contaminated with wheat during processing or growing. So to be sure that you aren't getting gluten with your oats, look for oat products and other gluten-free varieties from these companies:

Bob's Red Mill
Cream Hill Estate
Gluten Free Oats
FarmPure Foods
Gifts of Nature

For more information about a gluten-free diet, go to Glutenfree.net.

A FOOD & TASTE TOUR
OF THE NEW SONOMA DIET

To lose weight, you have to love to eat.

If that sounds strange, consider the opposite side of the coin: Traditional diet thinking maintains that to lose weight you must downplay the role of meals in your life and avoid food as much as possible.

Now, that really is a strange statement. It runs counter to all the behavioral traits hardwired into our genes from millions of years of evolution. We know we need to eat to survive, and our happiest memories are of food, family, and friends. It's natural to resist any advice to the contrary.

If you've tried to lose weight before, you probably sensed intuitively that such an anti-food approach would be a problem. It's hard to defeat an "enemy" that you love.

The Sonoma lifestyle stresses enjoying food, not avoiding it. The secret, of course, is enjoying the right foods in the right amounts. That's the only healthy way to lose weight.

You will be choosing from a large variety of foods and recipes that have been shown to have the strongest of health benefits. By "health benefits" I mean that these foods make you feel better, increase your energy and vitality, and help protect you from killer diseases—mostly heart disease, but also diabetes, many cancers, and age-related conditions such as vision impairment, memory loss, and arthritis.

This connection between improved health and weight loss is at the core of the Sonoma way of eating. One reason for the link is obvious.

It makes absolutely no sense to adopt a weight loss diet that isn't healthy (although, sad to say, it's been done far too often).

The other reason is the key to your success. Sonoma-style eating stresses wholesome, great-tasting foods that satisfy your hunger while delivering an abundant supply of health-inducing nutrients in a minimum number of calories. By making every calorie count, the diet intertwines health and weight loss. One ensures the other.

THE SONOMA FLAVORS

Chefs and home cooks have long known the allure of a dash of exotic flavor in everyday meals. Spices and herbs enhance natural flavors, curbing that unhealthy tendency to reach for the salt shaker or to add butter for flavor. And their medicinal qualities are well documented. Many are packed with antioxidants, have anti-inflammatory properties, or provide antimicrobial effects. So whether it's cayenne, cinnamon, ginger, turmeric, garlic, or a host of other natural flavorings, herbs and spices play key roles in the Sonoma way of eating.

TRUE LOVE

You may have trouble thinking of healthy eating as something to enjoy. That's understandable. There's a long and sometimes deserved tradition of thinking of "health food" as flavorless, unappetizing, and a little odd. Let's disabuse you of that caricature. The Sonoma style of eating, like the Mediterranean diet before it, has shown that the healthiest of food choices make for the tastiest of dishes. Skip ahead if you like and thumb through the recipes you'll be eating (if you haven't already). You'll see what I mean.

Many people also wonder how much enjoyment is left in a diet that excludes three things they think they love the most. They're talking about sugar, saturated fat, and refined flour foods such as white bread, cereals, crackers, pasta, and cake.

That's a legitimate concern. And it's true that those ingredients, which are found exclusively in highly processed food products, are to be avoided. The simple fact is that if you want to shed pounds, you have to forget about those "foods" until you reach your target weight. And if you want to stay at your target weight and be healthy, those foods will be rare throughout Wave 3 of the diet—which is to say for the rest of your life.

You'll soon discover that you can easily do without white bread, fatty burgers, and sugary sweets. Because of the way processed foods such as white bread and refined sugar affect your metabolism, eating them is more a matter of habit than enjoyment.

You're going to break yourself of those habits beginning with Wave 1 of the Sonoma diet. That will liberate you to appreciate the true joy of fresh, healthy food. Trust me—the crunch of a cool fresh apple is a far richer delight than the crunch of the twentieth potato chip. The chewy taste experience of whole-grain bread or cereal goes way beyond the compulsive experience of gobbling down white crackers or sugar-laden cereal.

And once you've learned to truly savor the natural sweetness of fresh ripe berries, then cakes and cookies and candy bars will seem way too sugary.

Healthy pleasures last longer than guilty pleasures. You'll see.

What people are saying about Sonoma…

"I sing Sonoma Diet praises to family and friends who have commented on my success with it. This is a new food lifestyle for me—I will eat this way for the rest of my life. Even when I eat out, it truly astounds me how easy it is and the difference it makes. I have lost 33 pounds and have my last 5 to go!"

—Elizabeth, lost 33 pounds

WHOLE GRAINS

You've already been introduced to whole grains as one of the Top Twelve Sonoma Diet Power Foods. They qualify for the honor because of their rich fiber content and abundance of healthy nutrients, including antioxidants, vitamin E, selenium, magnesium, and B vitamins.

There's another major reason whole grains are so essential for weight loss. By eating whole grains instead of refined white flour, you are sharply reducing the top metabolic cause of weight gain. The process of milling grains into white flour (or white rice or white pasta) not only robs them of most of their nutrients, but also modifies an otherwise healthy food into a quick supplier of body fat.

Here's why: All carbohydrates—grains, fruits, vegetables, and other foods—supply energy by bringing sugars into the bloodstream. Your body releases the hormone insulin to process those sugars into usable energy. What can't be used in due time is stored as body fat.

That's all fine and natural. But refined foods such as table sugar and white bread are digested and absorbed much more quickly than whole grain, with damaging consequences. For starters, over time they increase the risk for inflammation, heart disease, and diabetes. Refined foods also make it easier for the body to convert extra calories to body fat. The other negative factor is that what was an excess of blood sugar minutes before is now a low blood sugar level. You're soon craving more of the same refined sugar and flour that caused the problem in the first place.

FINDING AND BUYING WHOLE GRAINS

We live in a refined-grain world, so it's not always easy to know if you're in fact getting real whole-grain bread or cereal. Here's what to know when you're shopping:

- Look for "100% whole grain" or "100% whole wheat" on the ingredient label.

- The first grain listed on the ingredients label should be identified as "whole," and there should be no grain listed not identified as "whole."

- Healthy-sounding words like "100% wheat," "multigrain," or "cracked wheat" have nothing to do with whether the bread or cereal is whole-grain or not.

- The best type of whole-wheat bread advertises the term "whole cracked wheat." But remember that wheat is not the only healthy whole grain for bread or cereal.

- Use the same guidelines when buying whole-grain flours. Reliable sources include King Arthur Flour, Arrowhead Mills, and Bob's Red Mill.

- Don't be fooled by dark brown coloring. That can come from molasses or food color.

Refined grains, then, are the opposite of a power food. They deliver very few nutrients at a high cost of calories that quickly become body fat. Substituting whole grains for refined grains subtracts a problem food from your diet and adds a healthy, satisfying food that's conducive to weight loss.

Symbols of Grain Goodness

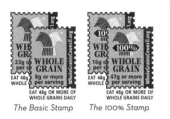

The Basic Stamp   The 100% Stamp

To help you find whole grains, the Whole Grains Council has come up with two handy seals of approval. When you see the basic Whole Grain stamp on a label, you know you're getting a product with at least 8 grams of whole grain per the labeled serving size—half of the recommended 16 grams per serving size.

For even better health benefits, look for the council's 100% Whole Grain stamp. It means all the grain ingredients in the food are whole grains, and you get a full 16 grams of whole grain per labeled serving size.

WHOLE GRAINS FOR YOUR HEALTH

If you're a typical American eater, white bread and crackers are old dietary friends. So switching from refined white flour products to natural whole grains may seem like a major change. But like any change for the better, the challenge comes only at the beginning. You'll soon see that whole grains are richer tasting, offer much more variety, have a chewy, substantial feel in your mouth, and help you feel full and satisfied sooner and for longer.

Whole grains offer health benefits as well. Because whole grains keep blood sugar and insulin under control, you not only avoid needless weight gain, you also reduce your risk of diabetes, cancer, stroke, and heart disease. The evidence for this is consistent and convincing.

For example, the Harvard School of Public Health conducted a six-year study of 65,000 women and found that those whose diets were high in white bread, white rice, and pasta had two and a half times the risk for type 2 (adult-onset) diabetes than those who ate a diet rich in high-fiber foods such as whole-wheat breads and other whole-grain items. Those who ate mostly whole grains (the daily equivalent of a bowl of oatmeal and two slices of whole-wheat bread) were 30 percent less likely to develop type 2 diabetes.

Whole grains also protect against heart disease, which happens to be the number one killer of American women today. Another team of Harvard researchers studied 75,000 women and concluded that those who ate more than two and a half servings per day were 30 percent less likely to develop heart disease than women who ate lesser amounts.

A third major study, the Harvard Nurses' Health Study, found that women who ate more whole grains weighed less than women who consumed fewer. Significantly, in this study weight gain was associated with eating more refined grains, the very grains that Sonoma shuns.

COOKING THE SONOMA WAY

Try a variety of cooking methods. For example, grains can be toasted in the oven for crispy treats, simmered or boiled (oatmeal-style), or stir-fried into "grain medleys" for salads, as a side dish, or even in a starring role as the main course.

FULL POWER

When selecting bread, read the label and make sure not only that the bread is 100% whole grain, but also that it contains at least 2 grams of fiber per slice.

Breakfast cereals offer a wide variety of healthful choices. Look on the nutrition label for choices that offer as high as 8 grams of fiber per serving and the lowest amounts of sugar, less than 5 grams per serving. Here is a start to finding some of these cereal brands: Uncle Sam, Ezequiel cereals, Post Shredded Wheat Bran, Kellogg's All Bran, the Kashi line of cereals, and Nature's Path.

GREAT GRAINS

Most of us hear the word "grains" and think of bread and cereal first, then maybe crackers and pasta. That's fine. The whole-grain versions of those foods can be regulars in your meals. Just make sure they are indeed whole grain and not refined and that you don't exceed the serving sizes recommended in the book.

But think about variety as well. Variety is not only the spice of life—it's the spirit of The Sonoma Diet. I'll be offering some alternative ways to prepare your grain allotment for each meal. You'll also want to try new and different whole grains, taking full advantage of the booming variety now available in markets. Even whole wheat, which is the most familiar whole grain, comes in different forms, such as wheat berries, bulgur, groats, and cracked wheat.

Those same variations are found in whole-wheat breads as well. In fact, with a little poking around, you can eat whole-wheat bread for months and never have the same kind twice.

FEELING YOUR OATS

Oatmeal provides soluble fiber, the kind that reduces your blood cholesterol levels. It's also rich in essential minerals like magnesium and it packs a considerable amount of antioxidants. Consider these different varieties when choosing your oatmeal.

Steel-cut oats: This is the best variety for keeping your blood sugar levels in check because it has been the least processed. That means the oats take longer to cook, but their nutty taste and hearty texture are worth the wait. A quick tip: Cook ahead and freeze in individual serving sizes.

Rolled oats (or old-fashioned oats): Also good for your blood sugar levels, these oats have been rolled and flattened into flakes so they'll cook faster than steel-cut oats.

Quick-cooking oats: These oats are rolled even thinner and finer so they cook even quicker.

Instant oats: These are the most processed oats, often with a very fine texture. This variety can contain more sugar and other added flavorings and ingredients, so beware.

For example, white whole-wheat flour, which is made from a special variety of white wheat, is light in color and flavor but has the same nutritional properties as regular whole-wheat flour. Whole-wheat pastry flour is milled from soft wheat. It contains less gluten than regular whole-wheat flour and helps ensure a tender crust in baked goods, while still providing all the goodness of whole grains.

And, of course, there are other whole-grain breads besides wheat, such as oat, rye, and pumpernickel. As long as it's whole grain and not refined, any one is fine.

Oat flour is an especially good whole grain. Made from finely milled whole oats, it is an excellent source of dietary fiber. It can replace a portion of all-purpose flour in many baking recipes and adds an oat flavor and texture. Also, any kind of "sprouted" whole grain offers all the goodness of whole grains while being more readily digested in the body.

Similarly, there are now many varieties of whole-grain rice available. These grains are minimally processed, just enough to sort and remove the inedible outer husk, leaving the nutrient-rich outer bran layer intact. All are superb vitamin B sources, and they also contain phytonutrients in the same

WAVES OF GRAIN

A Sonoma favorite, from the heart of California's Sacramento Valley, is the rice varietals from Lundberg Family Farms, a leader in producing high-quality organic and ecofarmed rice products in a sustainable manner. These products embrace wholesome goodness and tradition. Here are some delicious varieties to try:

Black japonica: With mild to sweet flavors, this blend of short-grain black and medium-grain mahogany rice has a moist texture, with flavors reminiscent of mushrooms and nuts.

Wehani: A red-grained rice developed in the United States, wehani is great for pilafs, casseroles, and rice salads.

Brown jasmine: First grown only in Thailand, this fluffy, long-grained rice has a sweet floral aroma and can be used as side dish, in pilafs, and in desserts.

Brown basmati: Basmati, a preferred long-grain rice in India, lends an exotic aroma to many dishes.

categories as some fruits and vegetables. Another option is wild rice, a wonderfully wholesome food you may have tried only in restaurants. Brown rice and wild rice take a little more effort to prepare than cover-it-and-forget-it white rice, but they're worth it—for your taste and for your waist.

A BETTER PASTA

Barilla Plus Pasta, made from multigrains and legumes, tastes and looks like traditional white pasta but with improved nutritional value, primarily due to a higher source of high-quality protein and omega-3 fatty acids. The real health advantage—better control of your blood sugar levels.

Pasta has a well-deserved bad reputation in weight loss circles, but that only applies to regular white pasta (and, of course, to any pasta in excessive amounts). Whole-wheat pasta and other variations made from multigrains are healthy and recommended. They're also enjoying something of a boom in popularity in recent years.

For a change of pace from typical pasta, try a Sonoma recipe featuring soba noodles. These are basically buckwheat noodles or pasta, an excellent whole-grain alternative to refined wheat flour noodles or pasta (buckwheat isn't actually wheat at all—it's a fruit seed from a plant related to rhubarb). It's a favorite in Japan and has caught on in North America as well in recent years.

You'll also notice on The Sonoma Diet grains list a perhaps unfamiliar entry called quinoa (pronounced keen-wa). It's a wheat alternative from South America with a nutty taste. Grains are primarily carbohydrate with some protein as a bonus, but quinoa offers something few grains can—the same high-quality protein you get with meat or eggs. It's usually prepared like a light, fluffy rice, but you can also toast quinoa on a sheet pan in the oven for a nuttier layer of flavor. If you haven't tasted quinoa yet, try the recipe for Toasted Quinoa Pilaf on page 244.

SPROUT IT OUT

There's another way to enjoy the goodness of whole grains: sprouted. Grains are seeds, and seeds are one of nature's marvels. Within each seed is the potential of a whole new plant, patiently waiting its turn in the sun.

Sprouted grains contain simple molecules of starch that are easy for the baby plant to digest. The same may be true for some people. Proponents of sprouted grains claim that grains that have just begun sprouting offer all the goodness of whole grains while being more readily digested.

What's more, the sprouting process apparently increases the amount and availability of some vitamins (notably vitamin C) and minerals, making sprouted grains a potential nutrition powerhouse.

FINDING SPROUTED GRAINS

Sprouted grains and products made from sprouted grain flours may be tougher to find than other whole-grain foods. These companies offer a wide range of sprouted-grain resources:

Alvarado Street Bakery (alvaradostreetbakery.com)

Essential Eating Sprouted Foods (essentialeating.com)

Food for Life (foodforlife.com)

Shiloh Farms (shilohfarms.com)

Silver Hills Bakery (silverhillsbakery.ca)

Sun Valley Rice (sunvalleyrice.com)

THIS FOR THAT

You can make substitutions when you bake or cook to add more whole grains to your diet. When making cookies, muffins, quick breads, and pancakes, for example, replace half the white flour with whole-wheat flour. Or you can substitute a third of the flour with quick-cooking or old-fashioned oats. Here are some other ideas:

- Add half a cup of cooked bulgur, wild rice, or barley to bread stuffing.
- Add half a cup of cooked wheat or rye berries, wild rice, brown rice, sorghum, or barley to your favorite canned or home-made soup.
- Use whole corn meal for corn cakes, corn breads, and corn muffins.
- Add three-quarters of a cup of uncooked oats for each pound of ground beef or turkey when you make meatballs, burgers, or meatloaf.

There are three main ways to enjoy sprouted grains: You can buy packaged sprouted grains, cook sprouted grains as side dishes, or bake with sprouted grain flours.

VEGETABLES

We can thank the chefs of Sonoma for showing us how to enjoy vegetables with contemporary flavors and preparations. Their vegetable dishes offer not only a treasure-trove of healthy nutrients but also culinary delights that are right at home on the menu of any gourmet restaurant.

KEEP IT LOCAL

A natural and easy way to move forward to better health and weight control is to eat locally raised food harvested at the pinnacle of ripeness. Calorie for calorie, locally grown food may offer more nourishment and flavor than foods that have traveled thousands of miles around the globe. When we speak of Sonoma Diet Power Foods, we really mean the power of fresh food.

Many Sonoma Diet recipes offer versatile tips to include seasonal variations as substitutions. A risotto can call for wild mushrooms and barley in the winter but offer summer variations with zucchini and tomatoes. Look for these helpful notes in many of the recipes in this book and see how easy it is to expand a few menus into a lifetime of healthy eating.

Despite the best efforts of southern Europeans and the chefs of Sonoma (not to mention medical researchers), Americans in general eat too few fruits and vegetables. What they do eat, they eat in insufficient variety. This has a lot to do with why so many people are overweight and undernourished.

Sadly, low-carb diets contribute to the problem by severely restricting fruits and vegetables, sometimes to the point of near elimination. The Sonoma Diet, on the other hand, puts vegetables at center stage. Like the Mediterranean diet, it is plant-based. That doesn't mean it's vegetarian—you'll have plenty of meat and fish—but it does mean that many of your calories will come from nutrient-rich foods such as vegetables, grains, fruits, nuts, and plant oils. Remember that all Top Twelve Sonoma Diet Power Foods listed in the book are from plant sources.

And nine of those twelve are fruits or vegetables. You'll lose weight because you'll be shown how to take advantage of these and other nutrient-rich power foods to supply your body with all the health-promoting nutrients it needs with a calorie count small enough to let you lose weight.

The secret to getting the full health and weight loss benefits of vegetables is to enjoy eating them. The days of considering vegetables a necessary evil on your plate are over. The recipes you'll be following stress the innate flavors of whole vegetables and the herbs and spices that go with them. You'll develop a new appreciation for the natural goodness of fresh vegetables.

Most dieters are vaguely aware that vegetables are "good for you." But eating more fruits and vegetables will also help you lose weight. To help you understand just how important they are in The Sonoma Diet, let's take a few pages to look at what they offer. I'll talk mostly about vegetables here. But most of the benefits apply to fruits as well.

WHAT EATING LOTS OF FRUITS AND VEGETABLES DOES FOR YOU

- Decreases your risk for stroke and heart attack
- Protects against several types of cancers
- Lowers blood pressure
- Improves digestion and discourages intestinal disorders
- Guards against cataracts and other age-related vision problems
- Saves your memory as you grow older
- Helps you lose weight by providing vital nutrients with a minimum of calories

COOKING VEGETABLES TO PERFECTION

Each vegetable has its own distinct personality when it's cooked. Stir-fried veggies may be fairly crisp, while braised or stewed vegetables seem to almost melt away. Pairing the right vegetable with the right type of cooking brings out the best flavor and texture. In many instances, cooking them properly preserves their maximum nutrient benefits. For example, stir-fried veggies should not be overcooked; delicate B and C vitamins can be depleted. In contrast, the slow and flavorful roasting of carrots, sweet potatoes, and eggplant develops their flavor and natural sweetness without compromising nutrient benefits. Here are some examples of the best ways to prepare various veggies to ensure the most flavor, texture, and nutrition.

Stir-frying: bell peppers, broccoli, carrots, green beans, mushrooms, Napa cabbage, peas, scallions, snow peas, spinach, sugar snap peas, zucchini

Sautéing, stewing, or braising: bell peppers, chard, collard greens, eggplant, fennel, green beans, kale, leeks, mushrooms, mustard greens, summer squash, tomatoes

Crisp and raw: baby field greens: arugula, endive, radicchio, spinach; bell peppers, broccoli, carrots, celery, fennel

Grilling and broiling: mushrooms, peppers, radicchio, sweet potatoes, tomatoes, zucchini

Roasting: beets, carrots, corn, eggplant, mushrooms, onions, potatoes, pumpkins, squash, tomatoes, turnips

WORKING TOGETHER

We've already seen how the health benefits of all power foods (whether they're in the top twelve or not) come from the abundance of plant nutrients—phytochemicals—they deliver to your cells. Research in recent years has been successful in identifying those phytonutrients, especially the ones that protect your cells by acting as antioxidants. So a question naturally arises: If we know what the beneficial chemicals in the foods are, why don't we just take them in capsule form?

As you probably know, such supplements exist. Quercetin, beta-carotene, and lycopene supplements are already popular. There are many others.

The whole idea of The Sonoma Diet is to satisfy your hunger by eating foods with a maximum of nutrients. Supplements certainly qualify as nutrient-rich—lots of nutrients, not many calories—but they hardly make for enjoyable eating. No hunger was ever satisfied by swallowing a pill.

The other problem with supplements in place of real food is that they isolate the most active nutrients or supply various nutrients in unnatural proportions. This sabotages much of the benefit of nutrient-rich vegetables. Why? Because nutritionists are convinced by the evidence that the vitamins, minerals, and phytonutrients in any one vegetable work in harmony to strengthen your cardiovascular system, slow age-related vision loss, prevent certain cancers, or deliver all their other health benefits. Separating out one phytonutrient, no matter how powerful it is, ruins this synergy. You have a solo player instead of the orchestra.

That's why whole, fresh vegetables are your best choice. This doesn't mean they can't be cooked or that some parts can never be removed for a more pleasing dish. But you want to leave the entire lineup of phytonutrients intact as much as possible.

MORE FLAVOR IN YOUR VEGGIES

When cooking your fresh wholesome vegetables, follow these tips for bringing out their delicious flavors:

Season veggies with moderate amounts of kosher salt and freshly ground black pepper during the cooking process, not at the end. Seasoning during cooking adds better flavor through the whole vegetable, not just on the surface. And you'll end up using less salt.

Use fresh herbs—thyme, basil, dill, mint, parsley, cilantro, oregano, tarragon, chervil—as part of a marinade, dressing, or sauce. Add a bit of lemon zest with the fresh herbs, then drizzle a bit of extra-virgin olive oil, and you have simplicity at its best.

Add healthy, flavorful oils: extra-virgin olive oil, sesame seed oil, and nut oils help to retain moisture and add flavor for salad preparations, grilling, or marinades.

Brighten flavors with a little acid. Wine-flavored vinegars, herb-infused vinegars, balsamic vinegar, fresh lemon juice, white wine, pomegranate molasses, and ginger can be used for marinades, dressings, and sauces.

Toward that end, frozen vegetables are usually okay. But most canned vegetables—not all—have been processed at the expense of their nutrients. They may also contain added ingredients, such as salt, preservatives, or even saturated fat. If you must choose canned vegetables, check the ingredients list carefully. Two canned options that will fit nicely into a Sonoma-style pantry are canned tomatoes (including tomato sauce and tomato paste) and the many different varieties of canned beans.

IN PRAISE OF VARIETY

Not only do phytochemicals work synergistically within the same vegetable, but their health benefits accumulate with each kind of vegetable you eat. That's the biggest argument for the variety I advocate so strongly in The Sonoma Diet. The wider variety of vegetables you eat, the bigger the roster of plant nutrients you benefit from. Another reason for eating lots of different vegetables: the variety of ingredients and subtly different cooking styles makes every meal a taste adventure.

If you look at the three lists of recommended vegetables in The Sonoma Diet, you'll be able to group them by colors roughly according to the following categories.

GREEN VEGETABLES

If you remember what spinach and broccoli offer as two of the Top Twelve Sonoma Diet Power Foods, you have a pretty good idea of the potency of the phytonutrients in green vegetables. Besides protecting against heart disease and cancer, eating green vegetables keeps your vision sharp and your bones and teeth strong as you get

COLORFUL VARIETY

The easiest way to get variety into your vegetable selection is to choose a variety of colors. Generally speaking, vegetables in one color group—red, yellow, green, etc.—contain distinct types of phytochemicals, though there is much overlap. Putting different-colored vegetables on your plate and changing colors again with the next meal ensures the widest variety of nutrients while keeping your palate entertained. For example, try the recipes for Veracruz-Style Fish or Broccoli Salad with Dry Figs, Walnuts, and Mint.

older. Leafy greens are also rich in folate, a B vitamin that is linked to better memory and hearing and is even protective against several cancers.

The strongest members of the green team are the cruciferous vegetables—broccoli, Brussels sprouts, cabbage, kale, and bok choy. (Cauliflower is also a cruciferous vegetable, but it plays for the white team.) These vegetables are especially rich in vitamins, minerals, and a huge variety of antioxidant phytonutrients.

BAG IT

A quick and easy way to get a variety of fresh greens is to pick up different versions of the bagged salad blends available at supermarkets.

Another subcategory consists of green, leafy vegetables that are usually used in salads but can also be sautéed, stir-fried, or steamed. Spinach is the top power food among these greens, but there are many others, such as collard and mustard greens and the tops of turnips and beets.

Many of the green vegetables and dark leafy greens, such as chard, kale, Brussels sprouts, arugula, and dandelion, have bitter tastes that will mellow into mouthwatering flavors with some basic culinary tips you'll find in the pages ahead. These bitter flavors are the trademark taste of their powerful antioxidants. When they are prepared in the right company of ingredients, the bitterness mellows to a delicious flavor and your body can absorb these antioxidants better. Try preparing these vegetables with ingredients such as olive oil, nuts, lemon juice, or small amounts of flavorful cheeses. Look through The Sonoma Diet recipes for more ideas.

RED VEGETABLES (AND SOME FRUITS, TOO)

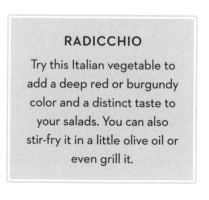

RADICCHIO

Try this Italian vegetable to add a deep red or burgundy color and a distinct taste to your salads. You can also stir-fry it in a little olive oil or even grill it.

Most red vegetables and fruits get their color from one of two phytonutrients—lycopene or antho cyanins. Lycopene, found in foods such as watermelon, pink grapefruit, and tomatoes (especially canned and cooked), has been linked to

Salads That Satisfy

A tossed salad of fresh vegetables mixed with greens is an ideal food for The Sonoma Diet. It works to fulfill the vegetable requirement in any meal instruction. Consider these tips when making your salads:

Be sure to power-pack your salads with nutrient-rich raw vegetables. Experiment with different ingredients to wake up that salad and turn it into a tasty treat.

The darker the green you use, the more nutrient-rich it usually is. Romaine and watercress, for example, have eight times more beta-carotene and twice the calcium and potassium than that old stand-by, iceberg. It's the least nutrient-rich lettuce there is. Essentially it's just an empty vehicle for salad dressing.

Other good dark green leaf choices are spinach, kale, beet greens, turnip greens, collard greens, and mustard greens.

Try the unfamiliar. A number of European or Asian greens are now available in American markets. Arugula, sorrel, chicory (also called curly endive), escarole, mizuna, and tatsoi are delicious, nutritious, and a worthwhile change of pace.

There's no rule saying that salad greens have to be green. Try radicchio (wine red) and Belgian endive (purple).

Include mâche (also known as lamb's lettuce) as another alternative to greens. Its soft texture and sweet flavors are a tasty addition to soups and salads.

Add those raw Sonoma Power Foods into your salads—bell peppers of all colors, beans, almonds, broccoli (or broccoli sprouts), tomatoes, spinach, even sliced grapes or toasted grains or seeds.

Olive oil and/or vinaigrette-based dressings are key to Sonoma cuisine. Remember that extra-virgin olive oil improves the flavors of all greens and helps your body absorb their nutrients. Or try using nut oils and flavor-infused vinegars to add some variety to your salad dressings.

a lower risk of cancer. A 2009 study found that men with the highest blood level of lycopene were 45% less likely to develop any type of cancer. There is also evidence to support a protective role for lycopene in cardio-vascular disease.

Anthocyanins are compounds that give strawberries, raspberries, and red grapes their color. Their antioxidant properties help defend cells against damage and may even protect vision.

Tomatoes, rich in vitamin C and lycopene, may be the most powerful red vegetable. Keep in mind that to get the most benefit from tomatoes' antioxidant lycopene, it's better to cook them (skin and all) and accompany the stew or sauce with olive oil. That helps your body's absorption of the lycopene and also boosts the flavor and sweetness of the tomatoes themselves.

TOMATO TIPS

- Fresh tomatoes picked in season, from June through October, may have twice as much vitamin C and more healthful nutrients than those picked from November to May.

- Heirloom tomatoes—grown from older seed varieties—are cultivated for their flavor and texture. Unlike mass-market varieties—bred for consistent look and durability—heirlooms come in all shapes, sizes, and colors.

- Buy tomatoes as close to home as possible in your local markets. Look for those that are plump, shiny, and aromatic.

- Store tomatoes at a cool room temperature, away from sunlight.

- Here are some delicious favorites to try: brandywine, Cherokee purple, golden jubilee, red currant, San Marzano, and yellow pear. They can be served with a drizzle of your favorite extra-virgin olive oil, a sprinkle of sea salt, and fresh basil.

WHITE VEGETABLES

White does not mean colorless. There are powerful antioxidants behind the pale color, called anthoxanthins.

Cauliflower, turnips, onions, and mushrooms jump to mind when you think of white vegetables. So do some flavor enhancers such as ginger and garlic. All are excellent Power Foods—lots of great taste and healthy nutrients for a tiny amount of calories.

Onions are especially good heart protectors. They share with garlic a powerful phytonutrient called allicin, which helps prevent atherosclerosis, or hardening of the arteries.

Jicama (HEE-ka-mah) is a fleshy white root (under a brown skin) that can be steamed, baked, or boiled like a potato. It's also a light and tasty treat eaten raw. Cut it into cubes and try it as a snack with fruit or mixed with green salads. Try cutting jicama into sticks and dipping it in hummus, a recipe from The Sonoma Diet seasonings section on page 189.

Parsnips are low on the glycemic index, making them beneficial for keeping blood sugar stable.

YELLOW AND ORANGE VEGETABLES

These are especially effective in protecting your vision and immune system. Carrots, corn, pumpkins, rutabagas, several squashes, and the yellow or orange versions of tomatoes and bell peppers are members of this color family.

Here you'll find some of the most beneficial phytonutrient categories, such as the antioxidant carotenoids and flavonoids. These are also examples of vegetables that contain antioxidants, which will perform better for you when combined with healthy types of fats. Interestingly, some of the

SWEET POTATOES

Sweet potatoes get their healthy color from beta-carotene, which is about three times richer in the skin than in the rest of the tuber. What most Americans call "yams" are actually orange-colored sweet potatoes. True yams are starchy vegetables that belong to a different family than sweet potatoes and are much lower in beta-carotene than sweet potatoes.

yellow and orange vegetables are relatively high in natural sugars, which is why they are Tier 2 or 3 vegetables.

PURPLE VEGETABLES

Yes, there are purple vegetables. Had you forgotten eggplant, Belgian endive, and purple cabbage? You'll also find purple bell peppers, purple asparagus, purple carrots, and even purple potatoes—which happen to have three times the anthocyanin content of white ones. The phytonutrients responsible for the color (usually in the phenol or anthocyanin category) seem to be helpful in slowing down the ravages of aging. Urinary tract health and memory function benefit from purple vegetables. If you're looking for a tasty way to fix eggplant, the Grilled Vegetable Rolls on page 239 are a good start.

FIGS

Although considered a fruit, a fig is actually a flower that is inverted into itself.

Tender and sweet, figs range in color from the golden skin of the calimyrna to the rich black mission fig, with many more in between. Figs provide more fiber, calcium, and potassium than most common fruits. They are also an important source of polyphenols, the same heart-protective antioxidant found in wine and tea.

FATS

Dietary fat is what you eat. Those extra pounds of body fat are what you want to eliminate. Dietary fat can lead to body fat, but not as directly or inevitably as you may have assumed.

The Sonoma Diet fat philosophy is simple. The right kind of dietary fat in the right amounts is not only good for your health but vital to your weight loss. Very low-fat diets will not work for most people. Researchers from Harvard found that people following a Mediterranean-style diet for weight loss were more successful than those following a low-fat diet. The types of fats eaten in a Mediterranean-style diet are primarily monounsaturated (for example peanut butter, nuts, and olive and canola oils). What is the message here? The tastier and more satisfying the food, the greater the overall success.

Another interesting find in this study was that the quality of the food eaten in the Mediterranean-style diet was far better and more nutrient-rich than the low-fat diet. You need to maintain the right balance between fats, proteins, and carbohydrates in order to shed pounds in a healthy way. The meal plans you'll be following on The Sonoma Diet are designed to do just that.

The reasons you need fats in your diet are many—mainly for health, flavor, and enjoyment. We've already seen how extra-virgin olive oil and nuts, the star fats from the Mediterranean diet, actually lower levels of the bad LDL cholesterol and deliver heart-healthy nutrients. Other fats, such as avocados, peanuts, and omega-3 oils (found in salmon, walnuts, and flaxseeds), also provide beneficial nutrients such as antioxidants and phytonutrients.

OMEGA-3 BENEFITS

Omega-3 oils protect the immune system and play a role in protecting the body from heart disease, depression, Alzheimer's disease, diabetes, inflammation, colitis, psoriasis, and arthritis.

FLAXSEEDS

These tiny seeds pack a powerful punch of omega-3 fatty acids, fiber, and phytonutrients. Grind your flaxseeds (a coffee grinder works great) to release the omega-3 fatty acids. Sprinkle onto yogurt, cereal, or salads. Add a half teaspoon to your pancake batter, oatmeal, and smoothies.

Just as important, fats help you feel just full enough as you finish a meal. Without that feeling of satiety, you'll eventually start overeating just to find some kind of satisfaction. Anyone who's been on a very low-fat diet knows that feeling well.

Fats also increase the benefits of other nutrient-rich foods. For example, lycopene, the super-nutrient in tomatoes, can't be properly absorbed in your digestive tract without some dietary fat in the vicinity. So whether it's for smart nutrient-boosting or culinary sense, don't underestimate the value of fat as flavor.

If you're not eating well and become deficient in nutrients, one of the first things to suffer is your mood, as well as your concentration and how you express your emotions. Half of the brain's weight comes from fat, so it's not surprising that the types of fat you eat can affect your mood and health. An interesting area of science relates to omega-3 fatty acids and how they help brain cells communicate. Studies suggest that omega-3 fatty acids keep the mind healthy and happy by having a positive influence on concentrations of brain chemicals called neurotransmitters—specifically dopamine and serotonin—which are important factors in emotional well-being.

RICH, DARK, AND CHOCOLATE

There's something enticing about dark chocolate, especially when it comes in precious tiny packages or lurks behind a well-lit glass case. It's the ultimate pleasure food, but the good news is that dark chocolate also provides health benefits. Studies suggest that the antioxidants in dark chocolate and cacao, called flavanols, may protect arteries and help them relax, thereby easing blood flow. Enjoying just a quarter-ounce of dark chocolate every day was found to lower blood pressure without increasing body weight, according to a fifteen-year Dutch study. The anti-inflammatory compounds of dark chocolate are just what the doctor ordered when the percentage of cacao is greater than 70%.

Dark chocolate products are composed primarily of cacao and sugar along with tiny amounts of vanilla and emulsifiers. To estimate the cacao content, also called the percent cacao, of semisweet, bittersweet, or dark chocolates (not milk chocolates), refer to the nutrition label. Find the total grams per serving and subtract the grams of sugar; most of the remaining grams are the cacao content. Most semisweet or bitter-sweet dark chocolates that do not claim a percentage are in the 45 to 50% cacao content range.

When it comes to baking cocoa, look for natural, rather than Dutch-processed varieties. Natural unsweetened cocoa is not treated with alkali; the Dutch is. Stay away from milk chocolate, since it typically has sugar as one of its primary ingredients.

THERE'S FAT AND THEN THERE'S FAT

As the heading suggests, not all fats are created alike. There are three naturally occurring types of fat—saturated, monounsaturated, and poly-unsaturated—as well as one manufactured fat, known as partially hydro-genated oil (commonly referred to as trans fat).

Most types of fat you should eat come from plant oils. The healthiest are monounsaturated fats, such as extra-virgin olive oil, nuts, canola oil, and avocados. Other healthy oils are found in the polyunsaturated cat-egory, such as rapeseed oil, sunflower oil, and the omega-3 oils found in some salmon, mackerel, tuna, flaxseeds, soy, and walnuts. Omega-3 oils are noted for being anti-inflammatory, thereby protecting your heart, brain, and immune system. There is also science to suggest that they play a role in healthy body weights.

The kind of fat you must limit eating is the saturated fats found mostly in animal foods, such as meats and dairy products, as well as those found in palm and coconut oils. This doesn't mean you can't eat meat or dairy. You can. But it does mean that you must seek the lean or nonfat versions of meat or dairy foods. You can recognize saturated fat because it's solid at room temperature or lower—the white rimming a steak, the marble in prime rib, the chicken fat that skims a soup in the fridge, a stick of butter. Its primary sin is raising the levels of bad LDL cholesterol in your arteries, inviting heart disease. In fact, saturated fat ups your blood cholesterol more than dietary cholesterol itself.

Partially hydrogenated oils should be avoided because they have far worse effects on your health and heart than saturated fats.

FAT BALANCE

The saying "you are what you eat" holds true for fats. A close look within your body reflects the types of fats you eat on a daily basis. These fats or fatty acids make up the outer covering of cells, known as cell membranes. The types, balance, and amount of fats you eat can influence your immune system, raising or lowering the risk for inflammation, heart disease, dia-betes, arthritis, cancer, and even depression.

What exactly does fat balance involve? You should eat primarily mono-unsaturated fats, consume lesser amounts of vegetable oils such as corn oil and soybean oil, eat saturated fats to an even smaller degree, and avoid hydrogenated oils.

In the last century, Americans have drastically increased their intake of processed foods and vegetable oils in relation to the intake of omega-3 oils. An increased consumption of vegetable-seed oils makes it difficult for the body to reap the benefits of the omega-3 oils. For many who already consume low amounts of these omega-3-rich foods, this poses an even greater disadvantage.

NUTS TO YOU

Eating nuts several times a week has been shown to reduce your risk of heart disease by 30 to 50%. How much should you eat? About a handful of nuts, or one ounce per serving, is a great source of protein (almost as much as you'll find in most meats), fiber, and antioxidants. Nuts are great as snacks and perfect taste boosters when sprinkled on salads or added to hot dishes. They're almost as calorie-rich as they are nutrient-rich, though, so you'll be eating them in measured amounts. You'll appreciate that. Small servings of nuts allow you to savor their special taste rather than gobbling them down thoughtlessly. Although

THE UGLY FAT

If extra-virgin olive oil is the good and saturated fat is the bad, then partially hydrogenated fat is the ugly. This altered fat is found in processed food, fried food, margarine, and many kinds of packaged baked foods, such as cakes, cookies, tarts, and pies.

Also called trans fats, partially hydrogenated fats are chemically altered oils that are solid and creamy. Originally conceived as an inexpensive alternative to saturated fats, partially hydrogenated fats are even more damaging to your heart and overall health. Medical studies now show that trans fats increase the risk of Alzheimer's disease, inflammation, type 2 diabetes, certain cancers, obesity, and even infertility.

Avoid them at all costs. Buy fresh foods and you'll never run across this type of fat. If you do buy packaged or processed foods, check the label. If the words "partially hydrogenated" fat or oil, "trans fat," or "trans fatty acid" appear on the ingredients list or label, put the package back on the shelf and buy something else.

nuts do contain a hefty number of calories, studies have found that regularly consuming nuts can be associated with healthy body weights and in some cases can provide an advantage in losing weight. Consider the portions in Wave 1 and 2 for the appropriate amounts in your meal plan.

You've already met nutrient-rich almonds, one of the top twelve Sonoma Power Foods. There are also other nuts on The Sonoma Diet fats list—walnuts, peanuts, and pecans (although other nuts can be substituted). Each contains all three kinds of fat, including the preferred monounsaturated fats.

Walnut trees abound in Sonoma, as they do along the Mediterranean. Walnuts are the richest plant source (as opposed to fish source) of omega-3 fatty acids. Besides cardiovascular protection, walnuts promote cognitive function (such as memory) and have an anti-inflammatory effect that fights respiratory problems, arthritis, and skin conditions.

Walnuts, almonds, peanuts, and extra-virgin olive oil are foods you'd be asked to eliminate on a low-fat diet. On The Sonoma Diet, you'll be encouraged to eat them often.

MORE OMEGA-3S

If you don't eat foods rich in omega 3s at least two or three times a week, you might consider a supplement. Go for the DHA (docosahexaenoic acid) plus EPA (eicosapentaenoic acid) combination. For adults, 1 to 2 grams is a good beginning range (a good children's dose would be 400 milligrams per day). Some of the strongest clinical evidence for fish oils shows that daily doses of 2 to 4 grams of EPA and DHA combined may help reduce elevated triglycerides by 20 to 40%. As little as 1 gram daily appears to reduce high blood pressure and improve cardiovascular risk factors.

As always, check with your physician to confirm if this step is right for you. Make your best selection among the many different brands by choosing supplements made from small fish, such as sardines, or algae, and brands that rated well in independent testing. Fishoilsafety.com can provide helpful information for selecting the best brands.

PROTEIN

Emerging research suggests that eating a little bit more protein than current dietary guidelines recommend will help your weight loss effort, as well as slow down age-related muscle loss. More protein as part of a balanced diet has also shown positive results in treating type 2 diabetes and reducing the risk of heart disease. The Sonoma eating plan delivers the protein you need in a variety of flavorful ways.

· LEAN MEAT ·
THE SONOMA WAY

One way to be smart about meat consumption is to limit yourself to the specific lean cuts of beef (or pork, lamb, or veal) designated on The Sonoma Diet Proteins and Dairy list (page 103 for Wave 1; page 121 for Wave 2). These have been carefully selected as lean cuts. A very lean cut of beef can have four times less saturated fat than a fatty cut and deliver more protein at half the calories. That's how you lose weight.

MEAT AND FISH

Meat is a perfectly acceptable protein choice on The Sonoma Diet. It has the advantage of being a "complete" protein, meaning it provides your body with the full package of the eight essential amino acids it needs. No individual plant protein source, with the exceptions of quinoa and soy, can quite do that. So if you're vegetarian, you need more variety to make sure all amino acids are covered.

Another health advantage of meat is that it provides dietary iron in a form easily absorbed by your body, along with other important nutrients such as zinc and B vitamins.

Your main consideration in choosing meats is leanness. Any cut of meat that's too high in saturated fat will do you and your diet more harm than good.

The "lean" requirement rules out a number of meat choices completely. Bacon, sausage, dark poultry, brisket, organ meats, and rib steak are just too fat-riddled, no matter how you cut them. You won't be eating them until you reach your target weight, and even then only rarely.

That still leaves a lot of meat choices—from lamb, veal, and venison to beef, pork, and white poultry meat (always without the skin). But none of those is going to automatically be lean enough to suit your weight loss needs. Make sure you choose the leanest cuts.

Fish, of course, is another protein choice. It's a lower-calorie alternative to meat, with all the protein, nutrients, and in some cases omega-3 oils. Don't forget shellfish for even more variety.

LEAN IS BEST

The best strategy to avoid overdoing the calories and saturated fat in meat is to choose cuts of lean meats and eat them in recommended amounts, three to four ounces cooked (about four to five ounces when raw). Keep in mind this is about 30% of your Sonoma Diet plate guideline.

A three-ounce serving of lean beef is an excellent source of protein, zinc, vitamin B12, and selenium, and a good source of niacin, vitamin B6, iron, and riboflavin. There's no question that lean beef, in the company of other wholesome, nutrient-rich foods, can be part of a heart-healthy diet. And it's not hard to find. There are no fewer than twenty-nine beef cuts that meet government guidelines for "lean." Here are some examples that make the "under 10" cutoff—that is, 10 grams of fat or less per three-ounce portion. For an easier way to identify these cuts, look for the cuts with the word "loin" or "round" in their names.

Extra lean: beef top round, beef eye round, beef top sirloin, pork tenderloin, ham (extra lean)

Lean: beef top round, beef flank steak, beef top loin (strip steak), beef tenderloin, ground beef (90% lean), pork loin, lamb loin chop, lamb leg

Vitamin Sunshine

Vitamin D is so critical to human health that nature designed a way for us to get it: the sun. Some foods—fatty fish, egg yolks, and fortified dairy products—do provide vitamin D. But the body itself can make vitamin D in response to sunlight. The problem is that we spend so much time indoors these days and (wisely) use sunblock when we go out that our bodies don't get a chance to make that vitamin D. That may be why research suggests that many Americans are not getting enough of it.

At the same time, other research suggests that we need even more vitamin D than current guidelines call for. That's because promising new roles for the vitamin are being uncovered. Besides protecting bones, vitamin D may help prevent certain cancers, multiple sclerosis, fatigue, diabetes, and heart disease. So supplements may be the answer. Your daily dose should be in the 1000 to 1500 international unit range, taken in the "D3" or "cholecalciferol" form.

EGGS

Another fine protein choice is eggs. They don't deliver quite as much protein per calorie as most meat cuts, but more of their fat is monounsaturated. What's more, the yolks turn out to be a good source of easily absorbable lutein, the eye-saving carotenoid found in spinach and other green vegetables.

By the way, eggs' undeserved reputation for increasing cholesterol levels in the bloodstream has been thoroughly debunked. One recent study found no difference in heart disease risk between those who ate one egg a week and those who ate one a day. Another study concluded that eating two eggs a day for six weeks had no impact at all on cholesterol levels. However, what is important is how you prepare your eggs. Large amounts of butter, cheese, and cream in the company of sausage and bacon don't lead to weight loss or healthy hearts.

OTHER PROTEIN CHOICES

Animal foods aren't your only protein choices. The Sonoma plan encourages you to put more plant proteins on your plate. When you get your protein from smart combinations of plants foods like beans, nuts, soy, and whole grains, you're simultaneously reducing your intake of harmful saturated fat and getting more fiber and more antioxidants. That's good weight loss strategy and another reason why plants are a major player in the Sonoma plan.

Soybeans are the top plant food for protein. They're also rich in genistein, a type of plant nutrient in the isoflavone phytonutrient category. It acts much like a plant-based estrogen and is thought to be protective against breast cancer in women and prostate cancer in men.

Soy also has the advantage of changing shapes and forms to suit any taste. Besides the beans themselves or tofu, there are any number of soy substitutes. Natural food manufacturers have been able to use soy to mimic the texture and taste of an amazing selection of meat products, including burgers and bacon. Edamame, which are fresh soybeans, are wonderful as a snack, in a salad, or with a grain medley.

You can also include legumes and beans (chickpeas, lentils, and lima, black, kidney, and pinto beans) as satisfying proteins. Beans and legumes are packed with nutrients beyond protein, including antioxidants, fiber, folate, magnesium, and iron.

Dairy foods such as cheese and milk pack plenty of protein. However, dairy is a minor player in The Sonoma Diet. Because many dairy products are full of saturated fat, your

THE FRIENDLY BACTERIA

Probiotics are a type of living bacteria that actually benefits your health. The most common are *L. acidophilus* and *Bifidobacteria bifidum*. These healthy bacteria enhance your immune function, discourage lactose intolerance, and prevent infections. There's also evidence that probiotics help with weight loss, especially around the waist. What's a good food source for these healthy bacteria? Yogurt. When you select a yogurt, choose nonfat, and look for words like "live and active cultures" on the label.

dairy portions are limited to the lower-fat varieties. You can put nonfat milk on your whole-grain cereal in the mornings or occasionally choose cheeses that are naturally lower in fat than other cheeses, such as parmesan, mozzarella, feta, goat cheese, and cottage cheese. You can also find low-fat versions of some common cheeses, such as cheddar. In addition, you can occasionally use small amounts of strongly flavored cheeses such as blue cheese to add richness and flavor to meals. These strong-flavored cheeses can go a long way in small amounts. ■

WAVE 1

I think you probably have a good idea by now of the special qualities that make this approach to eating work. You've learned the approach that distinguishes The Sonoma Diet from others. You've met the food. You know the emphasis on the vastly improved health that goes hand in hand with weight loss.

Now it's time to get started. Ready to shed some pounds?

You'll begin with Wave 1, the first of three diet segments. Each wave is designed slightly differently based on what works best for you and your body at each stage of your progress.

Wave 1 lasts only ten days. Its main goal is to introduce you to the pleasures of fine, but simple, meals. You will immediately start eating delicious breakfasts, lunches, and dinners prepared with healthy whole foods.

Your whole attitude about food will change. A meal will no longer be something to be consumed quickly without much thought. Your food will instead be appreciated as a treasured gift from nature to be savored slowly.

At the same time, Wave 1 will rid you of three destructive eating habits that cause weight gain. The first is an overdependence on highly refined foods that turn your metabolism into a body-fat production factory. Sugary desserts, white bread and crackers, sweetened cereals, and the like will be replaced by healthier but equally satisfying alternatives, mainly whole grains.

The second habit you'll lose is the haphazard eating of whatever happens to be available, easy, or familiar. This may be comfortable in the short run, but it's unsatisfying in the long run and keeps you overweight. Balanced meals with the right combination of food types are a prerequisite for healthy weight loss. Balanced meals are just as easy to make as the old grab-and-eat method because I've done the balancing for you. Your only job is to follow the simple meal plans or use the plate diagrams and food lists provided.

The third bad habit you'll be cutting out is eating too much. Overeating isn't something most people do intentionally. Most of us have no idea we are overdoing it with the portions. On the average, people tend to think they've eaten 20 to 40% less than they actually have. Your eyes, though, don't have to be bigger than your stomach. "Pre-plating" your meals according to the Sonoma guidelines is a smart and simple strategy to prevent the kind of mindless eating that so easily leads to overeating. Eating straight from a box, bag, or serving bowl is not going to help you reach your weight goals. The Sonoma way of enjoying meals will.

If you have pounds to lose, chances are pretty good your portions have crept up toward the generous side over the years. Wave 1 will set your meal sizes where they need to be to leave you satisfied but still on the road to weight loss. Portion control might be a bit of a challenge at first, but you can do it. In fact, one of the most common reactions from new dieters on The Sonoma Diet is genuine surprise at how filling and satisfying the adjusted portion sizes are after a few days. The perception of ease is important: Trying to lose weight with plans that are too restrictive increases stress levels in the body—and more stress leads to more weight gain.

To get you on the right track, I'll give you explicit and precise instructions about how much of each food type to eat with each meal. You'll even see exactly how much room each food type will take up on your plate. You can't go wrong.

The ten days of Wave 1 bring your most rapid weight loss. At first you'll be very aware of the adjusted portion sizes and the absence of long-familiar habit foods. But you'll also discover the pleasure of quality food and Sonoma-style recipes. And you'll be inspired by the quick weight loss—especially by the loss of inches around your waist. You'll feel your life changing for the better.

GETTING SONOMA-READY

The first day you start following the Wave 1 meal plans in this book will be considered Day 1 of your Sonoma diet. There will be ten such days in Wave 1. But even before Day 1 comes Day 0. This is the fun day.

Day 0 is the day you turn your life around—away from the unhealthy and disheartening old habits of weight gain and toward a new lifestyle of pleasurable, healthy eating for weight loss. You'll do this with a symbolic gesture that also serves as practical preparation for your new way of eating. You're going to convert your kitchen from a weight-gain factory to a creative space for the preparation of delicious, wholesome, and satisfying Sonoma-style meals.

I'm not talking about remodeling or anything difficult at all—just a little bit of rearrangement of the foods and ingredients you keep in your kitchen. One chart on the following pages indicates the foods you should be either tossing, donating, or hiding. Another highlights the foods that should replace them in your fridge, cabinets, and pantry.

Now, there's no need to be fanatical about this. There are some foods you won't be using on The Sonoma Diet—refined-flour breads, for example—that you might want to keep around for other family members. Understood. But let me suggest an out-of-sight, out-of-mind approach. Consider moving these "danger"

KITCHEN CLEANUP

The following items should be banned from your kitchen, or at least banished to dark corners:

- cake and cake mix
- candy and other packaged sweets
- chips (unless they're some of the healthy varieties now available—for example, black bean chips, stone-ground corn chips)
- cookies
- creamy salad dressings made with added sugars and/or partially hydrogenated oils
- margarine
- oils (except extra-virgin olive oil, nut oils, and canola oil)
- regular soda
- white rice

foods to one special area of the kitchen where you're less likely to see them.

The point here is that a smart pantry stocked with wholesome grains and pastas, spices, beans, flavorful oils, different vinegars, and a few more essentials will make it easier to prepare delicious meals and snacks on even the busiest days of the week. And trust me, you'll feel better just *being* in such a kitchen, stocked Sonoma-style, even before you eat your first Sonoma dish.

TIPS FOR A WELL-CARED-FOR PANTRY

Keep loose dry goods, like pasta, rice, cereals, and flour,
in airtight containers.

• • •

Consider how quickly you will use items when buying in bulk amounts.

• • •

Organize your shelves by putting the recently purchased items
in the back so the older ones get used up first.

WHEN TO TOSS

Despite what some people think, certain pantry items aren't meant to stay in a pantry forever. Over time, foods slowly spoil or lose flavor, so consider going through your cabinets and shelves to toss items that have passed their prime.

After six months:

baking soda and baking powder

nuts (stored in freezer)

nut butters

oil (stored in cool, dark area)

rice

After one year:

canned goods

dried beans

flour stored in airtight containers

grains (in airtight containers)

sugar

vinegar

YOUR SONOMA KITCHEN

Here are the kinds of foods and ingredients you'll want to
keep on hand for your Sonoma-style eating.

ON THE SHELF

artichoke hearts
    (canned or frozen)
broth, low-sodium
    (beef, chicken, vegetable)
canned beans, low-sodium
    *(black beans, cannellini,
    garbanzo, kidney, pinto)*
chipotle chiles in adobo sauce
chunk light tuna
lentils *(brown and green)*
tomatoes, diced and fire roasted
    (a popular brand is Muir Glen)
tomatoes, low-sodium
    (diced, whole, sauce, paste)

GRAINS AND FLOUR

Barilla Plus pasta or
    whole-wheat pasta
buckwheat flour
bulgur wheat *(coarse and fine)*
oatmeal *(old-fashioned
    and/or steel-cut oats)*
pearl barley
polenta
quinoa
rice *(brown, wild, brown basmati,
    and more)*
unbleached all-purpose flour
whole-wheat bread crumbs
whole-wheat couscous
whole-wheat flour

whole-wheat pastry flour
whole-wheat tortillas, corn tortillas

OILS AND VINEGARS

canola oil
extra-virgin olive oil
    *(splurge on an especially great-
    tasting one to be drizzled as
    a flavor booster; cook with an
    average-priced oil)*
toasted sesame oil
nonstick cooking spray
balsamic vinegar
cider vinegar
red wine vinegar
rice vinegar
sherry vinegar
white wine vinegar
    *(a favorite of mine is muscatel
    sweet wine vinegar)*
flavored sea salts

CONDIMENTS AND SONOMA FLAVOR BOOSTERS

canned green chiles
canola mayonnaise
capers
coarse-ground black pepper or
    peppercorns to grind
feta or goat cheese
hot sauce

inexpensive cooking wine
    (red: Burgundy, cabernet
    sauvignon, zinfandel;
    white: Chablis, chardonnay,
    sauvignon blanc)
kosher salt
low-sodium soy sauce
olives *(kalamata or nicoise)*
parmesan cheese
prepared hummus
prepared mustards
    (Dijon, whole-grain)
prepared pesto
roasted red peppers
salsa
sun-dried tomatoes

SPICES AND DRIED HERBS

bay leaves
chili powder
coriander seed
cumin seed
curry powder
dried mint
dried oregano
dried thyme
fennel seeds
ground allspice
ground cinnamon
paprika *(try smoked sweet paprika)*
whole nutmeg
your favorite spice
    (also herb rubs or pastes)

NUTS, DRIED FRUITS, AND SEEDS

applesauce *(for baking)*
dried fruit *(apples, apricots,*
    cherries, cranberries, dark
    raisins, golden raisins, pears)

nut butters *(almond, peanut)*
shelled, unsalted nuts
    (an assortment of almonds,
    hazelnuts, peanuts, pine nuts,
    pistachios, walnuts)
shelled, unsalted seeds
    (pumpkin seeds, sesame seeds,
    sunflower seeds)

SWEETENERS

agave syrup
brown sugar
dark chocolate
    (at least 60% cocoa solids)
honey
maple syrup
sugar
unsulfured molasses
unsweetened cocoa powder

PERISHABLES

basil
cilantro
garlic
Italian parsley
lemons
onions
shallots
eggs
buttermilk
milk *(low-fat or 2%)*
plain nonfat yogurt

IN THE FREEZER

edamame, shelled
fruit *(berries and peaches)*
vegetables *(artichoke hearts, corn,*
    lima beans, peas, spinach,
    squash, pureed squash)
shrimp

What people are saying about Sonoma . . .

"My weight loss has just started with 11 pounds, but I'll take it! I like being able to look in my cupboards and fridge knowing that I can eat anything that I have in them. Having your kitchen 'Sonoma ready' takes away temptation and saves time when preparing meals. I'm surprised that the grain choices are my favorite because they are new to my eating habits, and, although it may sound a little boring, I eat vegetables at every meal."

—Jean, lost 11 pounds

TAKE SOME TIME, LOSE SOME POUNDS

A logical way to plan your purchases is to follow the suggested meals for the ten days of Wave 1 on page 207. After the suggestions you'll find all the recipes you'll need, starting on page 212.

Of course, you may not intend to follow the meal guide exactly. That's fine. You don't need to as long as you stick to the given proportions of food types. But it still makes for a handy guide for estimating what you'll need to have on hand for the first ten days.

Once your pantry's stocked, you'll want to start thinking about how you'll be cooking. I'll be helping you all along the way, but there's one thing to keep in mind right now: Preparing wholesome, home-cooked meals takes about ten minutes longer, on average, than serving processed or ready-made food. That's about the best ten-minute investment you'll ever make for yourself. And even those extra ten minutes disappear if you make enough for leftovers and follow our Sonoma recipe guidelines for Cook Once/Eat Twice meals. You'll actually save time in the long run.

For the best way to reap the benefits of your Sonoma Diet recipes, keep the following tips in mind:

- Refer to portion sizes and total yield of the recipes.

- When shopping, look for seasonal variations in fruits and vegetables, to expand your menus into year-long healthy and flavorful eating.

- Keep your pantry organized.

> **· TIME-SAVING COOKING ·**
> THE SONOMA WAY
>
> ▶ **Cook Once/Eat Twice:** Creative recipes for pre-planned leftovers
> ▶ **Sonoma Express meals:** Twenty minutes or less, with fewer than ten ingredients ... and all the flavor and health you expect from Sonoma meals
> ▶ **Culinary variations:** Interesting facts and ideas for delicious new possibilities

SALT SAVVY

The beginning of Wave 1 is a good time to start thinking about salt. Do you keep the salt shaker on the table? Or do you eat most of your meals away from home? Or out of a package? If you do, you're an average American who likely consumes about 4,000 milligrams of sodium a day. That's too much.

The U.S. Dietary Guidelines for adults under fifty call for 2,300 milligrams of sodium per day (1 teaspoon of salt). For people between fifty and seventy, it's 1,500 milligrams per day, and for those over seventy, it's 1,200 milligrams. When you eat Sonoma-style, you'll get down to those recommended amounts of salt, which will help both your weight loss efforts and your overall health. For example, studies show that consuming the recommended amounts of sodium and eating more than five daily servings of fruits and vegetables—which you will do on The Sonoma Diet—lower blood pressure.

Chances are, if you "love" salt, it's more out of habit than true desire. You'll find that cutting down on salt is easy, since most of the sodium Americans consume each day, about 80%, comes from processed foods. When shopping for your pantry and preparing meals, consider how much sodium you're adding to your diet. Check nutrition labels for "low sodium," meaning that a single serving contains no more than 140 milligrams of sodium. Be aware that "reduced" or "less" sodium may not be a significant reduction. It only means the product has 25% less salt than the regular version. That could still be too high.

But don't get rid of all the salt in your cooking. Used correctly, salt has an important role to play. The phrase "salt to taste" refers to bringing out the natural flavors of herbs and spices, the bright flavors of citrus, and the rich flavors of vegetables, and not the salty flavor alone.

For many Sonoma chefs, a favorite is kosher salt—a flaked salt that offers less sodium and more flavor than equal amounts of iodized salt. Gourmet salts such as sel gris, fleur de sel, and pink or black salts can be used as finishing touches to infuse flavor without a lot of sodium. Small amounts of salty foods, such as brined olives, cheese, or soy sauce, can be using sparingly to add a burst of flavor.

ADD FLAVOR, NOT SALT

Try these ingredients to flavor your food without salt:

caramelized onions
flavored vinegars
herbs and spices
roasted vegetables
a squeeze of citrus
toasted nuts and grains

TAKE IT EASY— AT LEAST ONCE A DAY

The secret to weight loss is not just what you eat and how much, but in what manner. There's good evidence that people gain more weight by eating on the run or standing in front of a refrigerator than by sitting down to enjoy a sumptuous full meal.

There's even better evidence that people who eat fast are prone to overeat, since they're still bolting down the food while the stomach is sending a message to the brain that it's had enough. Fast eating also causes the same glucose-control problems with your metabolism that are such a major cause of excess body fat.

Stress-free, pleasurable eating is at the heart of The Sonoma Diet. You want to savor your meal, taste, and appreciate each bite of the delicious foods you're eating. You can't do that in a hurry. You need to slow down and make your meals a leisurely part of your life.

I know that's not always easy to do in today's fast-paced world. Your goal is to do it anyway. During Wave 1, start off by vowing to make at least one meal a day a Sonoma Diet–style meal—slow, stress-free, and pleasure-oriented. No rushing to eat, no eating on the run or standing up, no eating while talking on the phone or watching television. Make an effort to eat with your family. Kids who eat with their parents are less likely to consume junk food, less likely to overeat, and less likely to be overweight.

One slow meal a day should be possible. Try it. Plan for it. Make the time for it. Slow eating is something you can get used to and love. It will help your weight loss efforts.

AND GET MOVING

While one or more of your meals should be leisurely, Wave 1 is also the time to think about exercising. If you already exercise regularly, great. If you don't, here are some things to consider.

The Sonoma Diet is not a low-carbohydrate diet. You're eating grains and lots of vegetables from the get-go, plus getting carbs in dairy foods. The first and best use of a consumed carbohydrate is to be burned as energy. The second and worst use is to be stored as fat.

More physical activity means that you're using more energy. Using more energy means that you're burning more carbohydrate and body fat and therefore storing less as body fat. That may be a rather simple way of putting it, but it's basically why exercise helps you lose weight.

WHY EXERCISE?

To increase your energy

To boost your mood

To motivate yourself

To improve your sleep

To enhance your
immune system

To control arthritis

To protect against
some cancers

To lower your risk of
heart disease

To ward off depression

To reduce muscular tension

To strengthen your bones

To lower your stress levels

To accelerate weight loss

To maintain your
best weight

Calories are nothing but energy units. Burn as many calories as you consume, and your weight stays put. Burn more than you consume, and you lose weight. The Sonoma Diet takes care of providing just enough calories for you to be able to lose weight without feeling unsatisfied. Your contribution will be to burn more of those calories through exercise to lose weight even quicker.

EXERCISE FOR HEALTH, TOO

Like everything else in the Sonoma lifestyle, the weight loss benefits of exercise go hand in hand with the well-documented overall health benefits. The heart-protective effect of regular cardiovascular exercise, for example, fits in perfectly with the heart-protective Sonoma foods. Much of the longevity and low incidence of heart disease among the peoples of the Mediterranean is attributed to their active lifestyles as well as their healthy diet. The same applies to Sonoma.

Exercise improves circulation and therefore oxygen delivery throughout the body. It alters your brain chemistry for the better by boosting the activity of mood-enhancing neurotransmitters, such as dopamine and serotonin. Physical activity also triggers the release of endorphins, which are responsible for that feel-good sensation you get after exercise. It even makes cells more responsive to hunger-decreasing leptin. All exercise, be it aerobic conditioning, strength training, yoga, or tai chi, is good for your body and your mind. For more information on exercise, check out pages 132–135.

A PLATE (AND BOWL) OF YOUR OWN

After you've filled your kitchen with a generous supply of Sonoma Diet foods, you'll need to check the size of your family's plates and bowls. You need to know how much of the plate to cover and how much of the bowl to fill.

One of the best ways to lose the extra pounds around your waistline and improve your health is to downsize your plates. Nutrition research has found that simply switching from a twelve-inch plate to a smaller plate, such as nine or ten inches, leads to your eating about 20% fewer calories. After one month, that would mean a savings of about 5,000 calories—or two pounds of body fat!

There's no need to purchase new plates and bowls when you downsize. Use the same plates and bowls as the rest of your family; just measure the sizes and keep those dimensions in mind throughout your stay on The Sonoma Diet—that is, through Waves 1 and 2. Once you get to Wave 3, you'll know portion sizes so well, you'll be able to make any size plate work.

WAVE 1

BREAKFAST

OPTION 1

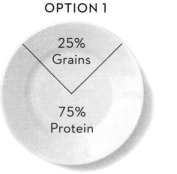

25%
Grains

OR

75%
Protein

7-INCH PLATE

OPTION 2

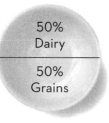

50%
Dairy

50%
Grains

2-CUP BOWL

LUNCH

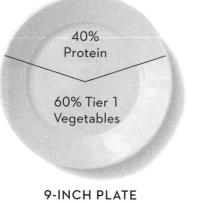

40%
Protein

60% Tier 1
Vegetables

9-INCH PLATE

DINNER

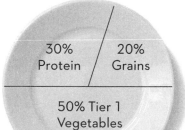

30%
Protein

20%
Grains

50% Tier 1
Vegetables

9-INCH PLATE

For breakfast, you'll need to pay attention to a circle seven inches in diameter. Your breakfast bowl (for cereals with milk or whatever else won't stay on a plate) must hold two cups of liquid—if it holds more, know where the two-cup fill line is. For lunch and dinner, you'll use a circle nine inches in diameter.

Remember, that's diameter—not radius or circumference. Take a ruler, bisect the plate with it, and see what it measures from edge to edge. If it's seven inches or nine inches, you have one of your plates. If it's larger, note where the seven- and nine-inch marks are and use only that much of the plate. For the bowl, use a one-cup liquid measuring cup to pour two cups of water into it. If that amount fills it, you've got your bowl. If the bowl could hold more, pay attention to how much of the bowl is filled by exactly two liquid cups of water. Keep in mind that plate styles differ— many have an extra-wide rim that adds one to two inches to the diameter. If the center of the plate is seven or nine inches, just ignore the rim when you place food on the plate.

You probably already have plates and bowls of those sizes in your collection somewhere. If so, fine. If not and you're afraid you'll overload your plate, cut a paper plate to the correct size. Place it over your regular plate before each meal to help you remember how much of your plate to use and how much to leave empty.

The reason for these picky plate-size requirements is portion control. You'll be eating the right amount of food at each meal because only the right amount will fit on your plate. The recipes and food choices are carefully designed to match your plate size. So to eat right, you don't count calories or grams or anything else. You just fill your plate or bowl with the foods recommended in the meal plans.

What people are saying about Sonoma...

"This is a whole new way to think about food. You name the diet, I have done it. The Sonoma Diet is different—no more being hungry on a 'diet,' and the information is not complicated. Discovering new flavors, especially the many different ways to enjoy whole grains, has been one of my highlights. Learning how to plan meals was key to my success. My four sisters are now Sonoma success stories as well. We love how we look and feel."

—Marty, lost 55 pounds

THE WAY OF WAVE 1

To repeat, the purpose of Wave 1 is to naturally recalibrate the body, to get you going with your new, healthy eating habits, to expose you to the pleasures of delicious whole-food recipes, and to reintroduce you to reasonable portion sizes.

That's a tall order, but it's all going to happen within ten days. That's how fast the transition is. It won't be gradual. You're going to leave behind your old habits and start losing weight on Day 1.

For that to happen, Wave 1 has to be more restrictive than Wave 2. Your portion sizes will be the same, but they'll contain fewer calories than Wave 2 portions. This is by far the most effective way to cure you of your overeating habit. Baby steps simply don't work.

The most important transition, though, will be to get you off the refined flour/white bread/sugar caravan that has wreaked so much havoc with your metabolism. You may have a common habit to break—cravings for breads, cakes, and other sweets.

Not that it will be a miserable experience by any means. Unlike low-carb and other diets, you'll still be eating bread and cereal even during Wave 1. But the slower-absorbing whole-grain versions will help wean you off the white bread habit.

You will stop eating refined sugar immediately. The sugar habit has to be totally eliminated or you'll continue to crave sweets and you won't lose weight. I know how hard it is to cut out all the sugar and sweets you've been consuming since childhood. Just remember: The more you give in to your cravings, the less likely you are to overcome them.

Most artificial-sugar sweets are not recommended in Wave 1, even though they don't have the same effect on your metabolism as sugar does. There's a good reason for this. You won't lose your cravings if you continue to satisfy them, even with sugarless, artificially sweetened substitutes. Scientific studies suggest that even diet drinks or artificially sweetened drinks stimulate the appetite. So it's best to avoid sugar (real or artificial) completely in the first ten days. But if you absolutely can't give up your diet soda, limit it to one can per day. Same goes for sweeteners—use just one packet of noncalorie sweetener per day.

Limiting yourself may be tough, but it's worth it. You'll be pleasantly surprised at how quickly you lose your cravings for white bread and sugary

SOME SUGAR ALTERNATIVES

Aspartame (Nutrasweet, Equal): Aspartame is a combination of two amino acids—phenylalanine and aspartic acid. It's not to be used if you have a condition known as phenylketonuria, since you cannot digest it. It may have a bitter aftertaste.

Stevia (Sweetleaf Stevia Plus): This is a concentrated powder made by extracting a sweet-tasting compound from the leaves of the stevia plant. It has 300 times the sweetening power of sugar. It's not a great option for baking.

Sucralose (Splenda): This is a compound that combines table sugar (sucrose) with three chlorine molecules. The body does not digest the calories. It is heat stable and has 600 times the sweetening power of sugar. It may leave a metallic aftertaste.

Sugar alcohols: These include xylitol (Xylosweet) and erythritol (ZSweet). These generally have acceptable flavors.

sweets. Remember, your taste buds can be taught to appreciate new and subtler flavors in fruits, grains, nuts, and vegetables, though it could take up to two weeks. The effort you put into Wave 1 will pay off throughout Waves 2 and 3 and for the rest of your life.

You'll notice one Wave 1 restriction that doesn't appear in Wave 2: wine. I encourage a glass of wine with one meal for those who enjoy it, for reasons I'll explain later. But not during Wave 1. There are two reasons for the delay. One is that wine, made from grapes, has its own form of sugar. The other is that the lower calorie count of Wave 1 meals, designed for a quick start to your weight loss, simply doesn't leave room for wine. So hold off for ten days. The pleasure will be there soon.

Your vegetable choices are also more limited in Wave 1. Only Tier 1 vegetables are allowed. That's because the vegetables in the higher tiers have less fiber and more natural sugars than their Tier 1 counterparts. That's not a terrible trait by any means, but it doesn't help your system get off the metabolic merry-go-round that's the top priority in Wave 1.

And one vegetable is out for the length of the diet. White potatoes have their charms and benefits, but their starchy nature makes them behave just like white bread. You're going to have to forget about potatoes until you weigh what you want to weigh, and even then you'll want to limit how often you eat them.

WHAT TO DRINK

What you drink can be just as important as what you eat for health. Unfortunately, for many of us, regularly sweetened beverages and soft drinks are the main source of daily hydration. A 2009 study found that consumption of beverages with added sweeteners, such as soda, sports drinks, sweet tea, and other pre-sweetened drinks, has dramatically increased in the past two decades. Previous research linked these sugary beverages to the nation's obesity epidemic and the rising incidence of type 2 diabetes.

Obviously, that kind of consumption will change for you on The Sonoma Diet. And why shouldn't it? There are so many tasty and refreshing beverages out there that quench your thirst while helping your health and weight loss effort that it makes no sense to ignore them. Water, tea, and coffee are perfect options. So are *agua frescas,* refreshing fruit-infused waters that render the essence of fruit flavors without extra sugar and calories.

In truth, The Sonoma Diet is not big on mealtime beverages (though I do recommend drinking eight 8-ounce glasses of water per day). A feeling of satisfaction from eating is of primary importance, and liquids don't provide that. On Wave 1, you can drink water, coffee, and teas such as green tea (one of the most heart-healthy of all the teas), black tea, and herbal tea (chamomile, hibiscus). You'll drink a glass of wine if you wish with one meal per day when you reach Wave 2. Sugar-free sodas are also allowed—but limit yourself to one can per day.

Why not fruit juices? Because they deliver extra calories from the natural sugars of fruits without the fiber. Drinking fruit juice doesn't address your psychological need to chew the way eating whole fruits does. When you drink fruit juices, you're ingesting calories without the "mouth" satisfaction that comes from chewing and swallowing.

Instead, try taking favorite fruit juices, like orange juice, pomegranate juice, or Concord grape juice, and mixing one part juice with three parts still (tap) or sparkling water (seltzer). Add a twist of lime or one of your favorite fresh herbs, like mint, lemon verbena, or even basil, and you'll have a refreshing and quenching spritzer. One of my favorite *agua fresca* combinations is infusing water (still or sparkling) with sliced green apples, lemons, halved grapes, and fresh lemon verbena. Other interesting combinations: cut cantaloupe, fresh basil, and a squeeze of lemon, or Concord grape juice, sparkling water, fresh mint, and a squeeze of lemon juice. Keep your favorite recipe in a clear glass pitcher and it's as appealing as refreshing.

The health benefits of tea—from black, green, and white teas to herbal infusions such as chamomile, hibiscus, lemongrass, and rooibos—range from protective antioxidants for cancer prevention to weight control. Studies show that compared to non-tea drinkers, tea drinkers generally have stronger bones, lower cholesterol levels, and lower rates of heart disease, inflammation, diabetes, and certain cancers.

And there's great news if you're a coffee lover: Besides being virtually calorie-free, it's good for you. The latest research confirms that drinking coffee regularly is associated with a lower risk of Parkinson's disease, colon cancer, liver cirrhosis, and gallstones. Plus, Harvard researchers followed 126,000 people for as long as eighteen years and found that coffee's protective antioxidants and other beneficial nutrients, such as magnesium, reduce diabetes risk. Drinking one to two cups of coffee has also been found to boost athletic performance—just what you need to hear on those days when you don't feel like getting to the gym.

So coffee is fine on The Sonoma Diet. Just keep in mind that all the extras, like whipped cream, chocolate flavoring, and syrups can turn a zero-calorie drink into an unhealthy meal with 600 or more calories.

A suggestion: Next time you enjoy a cup of java, choose a high-quality variety with rich, aromatic natural flavors. Try it black or with nonfat milk. If you must, use less than a teaspoon of sugar or one serving of a noncaloric sweetener.

HOW TO FILL YOUR PLATE

The actual food instructions for The Sonoma Diet are so simple that we can run through them in no time. Simply look at the plate diagrams on page 93 and fill your plate or bowl accordingly.

In Wave 1, you have three breakfast options. The first is to fill your seven-inch plate (remember, the nine-inch plate is only for lunch and dinner) with 75% protein and 25% whole grain. What might fit nicely, for example, is a two-egg omelet with a little diced ham for the 75% protein space and a piece of whole-wheat toast (no butter) for the 25% whole-grain area. You can also have 100% protein—a mushroom omelet, for example. The third Wave 1 breakfast option allows you to fill your bowl with half dairy and half whole grains. The most obvious way to do that is to have some whole-grain cereal, such as Kellogg's All-Bran, with nonfat milk. It's that simple.

As long as you don't pile the food high on your plate or go back for seconds, you've eaten according to Wave 1 recommendations.

For lunch and dinner, the choices are more substantial. You can see in the diagrams that there are two ways to fill your nine-inch plate. One is for lunch and the other is for dinner. It doesn't matter which is which, but it should never be two of the same (because that would throw the overall proportions out of balance).

Let's say you pick for lunch the combination calling for 40% protein and 60% vegetables (only Tier 1 vegetables, because you're in Wave 1). You might want to split your 60% vegetable space between a green salad with red tomatoes and steamed broccoli. The 40% of the plate to be filled with protein might be dedicated to sliced white turkey meat.

By the way, don't be intimidated by the preciseness of the percentages. You can interpret 60% as a little more than half and 40% as a little less than half. Once you eyeball the measurements, there's no rule against spreading the turkey over the salad greens and calling it a turkey salad.

Because you chose the 60–40 ratio for your lunch, the charts indicate that your dinner plate will be filled with 30% protein, 20% grains, and 50% Tier 1 vegetables. How about roasted vegetables on half of your plate, wild rice on 20%, and a grilled four-ounce cut of lean beef tenderloin for the 30% protein?

WHERE'S THE FAT?

There are no percentages of the plate designated for added fats. Instead, you are allotted three servings of fat a day to use as you see fit. A fat serving is a teaspoon of olive oil, eleven almonds, fourteen peanuts, ten pecan halves, or seven walnut halves.

A possible use of fats for one day might be a teaspoon of extra-virgin olive oil drizzled over a spinach salad, another teaspoon of olive oil per serving of roast vegetables, and some almonds sprinkled over the salad or as a snack.

SNACKS? OF COURSE

Letting yourself get too hungry between meals is counterproductive to your weight loss efforts. You'll simply be tempted to overeat when mealtime comes. Smart snacks can keep your energy up throughout the day and help you stay on track with making the best food choices.

That's why The Sonoma Diet allows snacking. But like most things, snacking is more restricted during Wave 1 than it is for the rest of the diet.

Between lunch and dinner, or between breakfast and lunch, you may have a small snack to tide you over. Always try to include a small amount of protein, such as nuts, dairy, seeds, or even lean meats; they will help satisfy hunger.

If you're a big man, or if you are a woman or man who leads a very physically active life with plenty of exercise, you can expand your snack menu a bit. Here are some possibilities:

- ½ cup low-fat cottage cheese with Tier 1 raw veggies or one serving of Tier 1 fruits
- 3 ounces of hummus, either homemade or store-bought, with veggies
- Low-fat cheese stick with carrots or celery
- 1 ounce of nuts
- 1 slice of whole-grain bread with one tablespoon of peanut butter and one serving of Tier 1 fruits
- 2 ounces cooked chicken breast or turkey deli meat

When you reach Wave 2, those choices and many others will be available. For now, though, keep snacking quick and simple—try a cup of raw bell pepper strips, some raw broccoli, or a sliced tomato with dried basil and other herbs.

AN ADDED BOOST

It's hard to get all the nutrients you need in one day on any diet, but especially on a weight loss plan. That's why you may choose to take a multivitamin a day that is specifically designed for women or men. Talk to your doctor about your specific needs.

CHOOSE OR FOLLOW

At the beginning of the recipe section, on page 212, you'll find a meal guide that offers exact food choices for each part of your plate and for every meal throughout the ten-day Wave 1. This has the obvious advantage of taking the guesswork out of the process. You're also guaranteed to eat delicious and healthy meals perfectly planned for weight loss. Each recommendation refers you to a Sonoma-inspired recipe in the book for bringing it to your plate.

You're not obligated to follow this meal guide. If you prefer to pick and choose your own meals according to your own taste, please do so. As long as you stick to the percentages and choose foods appropriate for Wave 1, you'll be eating The Sonoma Diet way. And you'll notice weight loss right away.

That's it. Enjoy. Your Sonoma Diet has now begun. ■

WAVE 1

SONOMA TIER 1 VEGETABLES

Unlimited

asparagus

bagged salad blend *(any type)*

bamboo shoots

beans *(green snap beans, yellow wax beans)*

bell peppers *(green, red, yellow)*

bok choy

broccoli, raw or cooked

Brussels sprouts, cooked

cabbage, raw or cooked

cauliflower, raw or cooked

celery

chayote

collard greens, cooked

cucumber

eggplant, cooked

fennel

Hubbard squash, cooked

jicama

kohlrabi

leek, cooked

lettuce *(romaine, beet greens, mustard greens, turnip greens, Swiss chard, kale or other dark green leafy lettuce, amaranth, arugula, celtuce, endive, rapini)*

mushrooms, raw or cooked

napa cabbage

okra, cooked

onion, raw or cooked

radicchio

radish

scallions

snow peas

spinach, raw or cooked

sprouts *(alfalfa, kidney bean, mung bean, radish seed)*

summer squash

tomato, raw

watercress

zucchini

SONOMA TIER 1 FRUITS

apple

apricot

blackberry

blueberry

boysenberry

canteloupe

cherry

cherimoya

cloudberry

gooseberry *(raw)*

grape

grapefruit

honeydew melon

huckleberry

java plum *(jambolan)*

kiwifruit

kumquat

lemon

lime

mulberry

orange

papaya

pineapple

plum

prickly pear

pummelo (Chinese grapefruit)

quince

raspberry

rhubarb

salmonberry

star fruit

strawberry

tangerine

ugli fruit

watermelon

SONOMA PROTEINS AND DAIRY

PROTEIN

beans and legumes: limit to half a cup per day in Wave 1 (black beans, black-eyed peas, chickpeas, lentils, pinto beans, soybeans such as edamame and tofu)

beef: lean cuts (beef round, chuck arm pot roast, eye of round, round tip, tenderloin, top loin, top sirloin)

eggs: 1 whole egg = 2 whites

fish: lean cuts (cod, flounder, grouper, haddock, halibut, monkfish, northern pike, orange roughy, perch, pike, walleye)

fish: moderate-fat: (catfish, sea bass, snapper, striped bass, swordfish, tuna, whitefish)

fish: high-fat (mackerel, salmon, trout)

game meats (bison, deer, elk)

lamb (arm, foreshank, leg, loin, shank half, shoulder, stew meat)

peanut butter: 2 tablespoons per serving for main-dish protein, 1 tablespoon as a snack

pork: lean cuts (Canadian bacon; ham, boiled or cured; canned ham; center cut loin chop; pork loin; pork sirloin chop and roast; pork tenderloin; top loin)

poultry: white meat, no skin; turkey bacon; turkey sausage

shellfish (clams, crab, lobster, mussels, oysters, scallops, shrimp)

soy substitutes: vegetarian (soy) burger or other soy "meats"

veal (arm, ground, leg, loin, shoulder, sirloin, top round)

DAIRY

low-fat cheese: 1 ounce (grated parmesan, mozzarella)

low-fat cottage cheese

fat-free (skim) milk: up to 1 cup on cereal

Sonoma Grains

½ cup = 1 serving
Barilla Plus pasta, cooked
barley, cooked
bread, whole-grain: 1 slice
  (2 or more grams of fiber per slice)
bulgur, cooked
cereal, whole grain: 8 grams fiber
  per serving or higher
  *(e.g., Kashi Golean, Kellogg's
  All Bran, Post Shredded Wheat)*
oats *(oat bran, oat groats, rolled
  oats, steel-cut oats)*
pasta, whole-grain, cooked
popcorn, air-popped, no butter*
quinoa, cooked
rice, cooked *(brown, red, or black)*
soba noodles, cooked
wheat, cooked *(bulgur, cracked
  wheat, groats, wheat berries)*
wild rice
** intended for a snack,
  not to go on the plate*

Sonoma Beverages

coffee: black or with 1 packet
  non-caloric sweetener and
  maximum 1 tablespoon
  heavy cream
tea *(black, green, herbal)*: plain
  or with 1 packet noncaloric
  sweetener and maximum
  1 tablespoon heavy cream
water *(plain or sparkling)*

Sonoma Fats

*Up to 3 servings per day;
1 teaspoon = 1 serving*
avocado: ¼ avocado = 1 serving
canola oil
olive oil

Nuts

Almonds: 11
Peanuts: 14
Pecans: 10 halves
Walnuts: 7 halves

Sonoma Flavor Boosters

Unlimited
herbs *(basil, chive, cilantro, dill,
  fennel, marjoram, mint, oregano,
  rosemary, sage, tarragon,
  thyme)*
spices *(caraway, cardamom,
  cayenne, celery seed, chili
  powder, cinnamon, clove, cumin,
  curry, nutmeg, pepper, saffron,
  turmeric)*
chile pepper
garlic
ginger, gingerroot
horseradish
lemon or lime juice or zest
lemongrass
mustard *(all types)*
vanilla
vinegar *(rice wine, balsamic)*

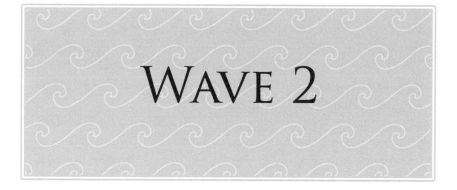

WAVE 2

Welcome to Wave 2, the major part of your Sonoma eating plan. This is the wave you'll stay with until you reach your target weight.

While Wave 1 helped you through a transition period of rapid weight loss, Wave 2 keeps the weight loss going. The loss isn't as fast as in Wave 1, but it's steady, healthy, and noticeable. It's the kind of weight loss that lasts a lifetime. By now, you're weaning your body off sweets and starting to feel the rewards—more energy, greater mental clarity, better-fitting clothes.

With Wave 2 comes your full enjoyment of the Sonoma lifestyle. That means pleasurable eating, a heightened appreciation of fresh, wholesome foods, and a new, energetic physical health you can feel all day long. So it's very important that you continue to make at least one daily meal a long and leisurely affair where you take your time to savor every bite. And keep with whatever exercise you've chosen to do.

More than anything else, Wave 2 is about variety. I've been stressing the importance of variety since the beginning of this book—not only because it brings extra zest to meals but also for its role in health and weight loss. Now you'll take variety to the next level. Your food choices multiply significantly in Wave 2, and so do the suggested recipes.

You have a much wider variety of fruits to choose from now. Two new tiers of vegetables join the lineup as well. You now have literally scores of fruits and vegetables to choose from. Eat plenty of them!

Fat-free yogurt (plain) is a new dairy choice. You're allowed some sugar-free sweets, if you still want them. Maybe even a piece of dark chocolate on occasion. Honey is allowed too and will prove particularly useful for sweetening up some of The Sonoma Diet recipes. A glass of wine can now be part of one of your daily meals. Snacks, too, can be a little more varied and substantive.

The grains list stays the same in Wave 2, because it already includes most of the whole grains you'll be able to find easily. Your fat allotment remains at three servings a day in the form of extra-virgin olive oil or canola oil, walnuts, almonds, peanuts, pecans, and avocados. (Remember, though, that these are in addition to the fats found in your protein sources and other foods.)

All in all, you'll find Wave 2 much easier than Wave 1. That's because it's designed for the long haul. Plus there's that big boost in variety. Extra satisfaction and extra variety make for a pretty good one-two punch for your confidence. And it's very much in keeping with the Sonoma approach of achieving weight loss by eating pleasing portions of delicious, healthy foods.

You may reach your target weight in a few weeks, a few months, or longer. But because of its emphasis on rich flavors and nutrient-rich meals, Wave 2 should never feel like drudgery or sacrifice, no matter how long it takes. Think of it as new adventures in eating rather than a diet. The pounds will vanish either way.

Your Wave 2 Eating Guide

The instructions for Wave 2 are even simpler than Wave 1. You don't have to overhaul your kitchen again, but do stock up on some of the new fruits and vegetables you're now encouraged to eat.

And, oh yes, choose a few bottles of decent, modestly priced wine. To save what you don't drink right away, you can invest in a hand pump designed to remove air from open bottles and plastic stoppers to seal the bottles after you pump. A newer approach uses argon to preserve the wine. You can see some options for wine preservation at the Wine Enthusiast (wineenthusiast.com).

WAVE 2

BREAKFAST

OPTION 1   **OPTION 2**

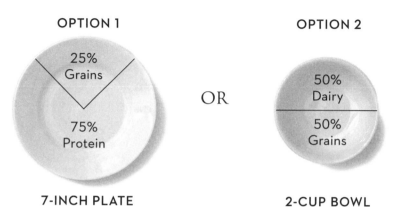

OR

7-INCH PLATE   **2-CUP BOWL**

LUNCH AND DINNER

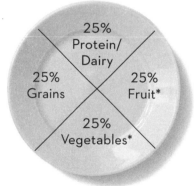

9-INCH PLATE

* Choose from Tiers 1, 2, or 3

You'll be using exactly the same plates and bowls. As you look at the plate illustrations on page 107, you'll see that your breakfast options are basically the same. But there's also a new choice not illustrated—a bowl of pure dairy. What that essentially comes down to is a breakfast of plain fat-free yogurt. That's a great option if you love yogurt. Otherwise, you'll want to go with the milk-and-cereal choice, or the 75% protein plate (with 25% grains, probably as a piece of whole grain bread or toast), or the 100% protein option. The protein plate, of course, offers the most possibilities. Remember that eggs go with protein, not dairy.

For lunch and dinner, you'll use the same plate proportions, though you'll want to choose different foods. You're really just dividing your plate into four parts and filling one part with grains, one with vegetables, one with fruit, and one with either a protein choice or dairy (which might be low-fat cheese or cottage cheese).

That's it. Use your same three fat allotments as in Wave 1—a sprinkling of nuts or a little olive oil either to cook with or to wake up greens or other vegetables as part of a dressing.

There are plenty of recipes to guide you. Remember that the tastiest and most beneficial food combinations are built into these recipes, so take advantage of them.

You also have the option of following the food guide, which tells you exactly what to have at each meal. The guide will take you through two weeks of different meal plans. If that two-week stretch doesn't get you to your target weight (and it probably won't unless you were just a tad overweight to start with), simply run through the cycle again.

THE FIBER CONNECTION

There's another reason Wave 2 will seem easier. By now you've reduced your cravings for sugar and refined white flour. You may have even eliminated those cravings completely. If you haven't, don't despair. You will soon.

Using Wave 1 to get rid of the white bread and sweets habit will pay big dividends in Wave 2. And make no mistake about it: "habit" is the right way to put it. Is there a better word to describe your daily candy bar and soft drink from the vending machine? Or the bag of crackers that disappears while you're watching television or riding the bus?

In Wave 2, you continue to avoid refined sugar. Now, however, you can replace it with sweet Power Food fruits such as blueberries and strawberries. You've already replaced white flour products with whole grains. Those two substitutions alone are a big part of what makes Wave 2 work.

But the most relevant benefit of these two smart switches is their effect on your metabolism, or the way your system processes food as potential energy. To repeat, sugar and refined flour convert to blood sugar (glucose) and then to body fat very quickly. Whole grains and most fruits and vegetables go through the digestion process more slowly and are less likely to be converted to body fat. Fiber, the undigested part of plant carbohydrates that eases waste and toxins out of your body, is the major reason for this difference. Eating fiber-rich foods is also a natural way to curb hunger. Over time, you'll notice the benefits of the slower pace when you stand on your bathroom scale.

FIBER IN YOUR FAVOR

Fiber is most abundant in whole grains, legumes, vegetables, and fruits. Not coincidentally, those are Sonoma staples. Fiber's mere presence is why you can eat so many fruits and vegetables in Wave 2 even though they do contain natural sugars. Fiber is also a big reason why whole grains are acceptable while fiber-depleted refined grains are taboo.

There are actually two kinds of dietary fiber. One dissolves in water; the other doesn't. Generally speaking (and with some key exceptions), whole grains and vegetables contain insoluble fiber. Nuts, seeds, legumes, and fruits contain soluble fiber.

For your weight loss purposes, this is mostly a distinction without a difference. Each kind of fiber slows blood sugar release. And because you'll be eating plant foods in an abundant variety, you'll get plenty of both in Wave 2 anyway. That puts you well ahead of typical Americans, who get about half the amount of fiber they need each day. Remember to make sure that every slice of whole-grain bread you eat has at least 2 grams of fiber in it and that every bowl of whole-grain cereal has at least 8 grams of fiber.

FIBER FOR HEALTH

Like just about anything you eat on The Sonoma Diet, fiber works complementarily as a weight loss aid and health protector. There's an obvious link between high-fiber diets and diabetes prevention because diabetes is characterized by an inability to properly process blood sugar levels. The weight loss that fiber encourages, especially from your waist, lowers your diabetes risk. There's also evidence that diets rich in high-fiber whole grains also reduce your chances of getting diabetes, whether you need to lose weight or not.

The abundant fiber in the Sonoma way of eating also protects you against heart disease. According to a Harvard study of 40,000 people eating the Sonoma-like Mediterranean diet, consuming lots of fiber is associated with a 40 percent lower risk of heart disease compared to low-fiber intake.

Soluble fibers especially lower blood cholesterol levels. That's one reason why oatmeal is such a fine breakfast choice; it's one of the few grains with more soluble than insoluble fiber. So it can reduce cholesterol, slow digestion, and boost energy—all at the same time.

And don't overlook fiber's gastrointestinal benefits. It helps you avoid intestinal inflammation and is well known for its ability to relieve or prevent constipation. Again, grain fiber, especially wheat bran and oat bran, seems to work the best. But a high-fiber diet in general is the surest way to get all these health benefits.

GOING GLYCEMIC

Choosing the best types of carbohydrate—such as whole grains, vegetables, and legumes—over processed, refined ones is a healthier (and easier!) way to lose weight than trying to eliminate whole categories of carbohydrates, such as all breads. Because you're already eating the best carbs, you're feeling more energy, experiencing better moods, and getting more satisfaction from your meals. And you'll find in Wave 2 that losing those extra pounds around your waist gets easier. At the same time, those wholesome carbohydrates are decreasing your risk for inflammation, heart disease, diabetes, Alzheimer's, and macular degeneration (which can lead to blindness).

A useful tool I used in creating the Sonoma meal plans is the glycemic index (GI), which was developed to help people identify foods that could ultimately influence better control of their blood sugar. The glycemic index ranks foods according to how much they raise blood sugar levels. Foods that are high on the GI (more than 70)—such as white bread or white potatoes—get digested and absorbed quickly. That means they raise blood sugar levels quickly. It also means they tend to make you hungry again soon.

On the other hand, foods farther down the GI (lower than 55) are metabolized more slowly, keeping your appetite on a more even keel. In other words, low glycemic foods are better at providing a slow energy release throughout the day. There are experts who believe that by tempering blood sugar surges, these foods may even help prevent the damage to cells caused by high blood sugar levels.

**BENEFITS OF
LOW GI MEALS**

- Help weight loss, especially around the waist

- Reduce the risk of diabetes

- Reduce the risk for heart disease

- Improve blood cholesterol levels

- Decrease inflammation inside the body

- Reduce hunger and keep you satisfied longer

- Maintain energy levels and promote physical endurance

One of the exciting added features of this version of The Sonoma Diet is a greater emphasis on foods that trickle glucose into your blood stream slowly, thereby keeping your energy levels up and your hunger under control. Needless to say, those are two welcome factors for shedding those extra pounds, especially around your waist. The glycemic index helps make that happen.

Of course, the glycemic index is far from the only factor in designing a meal plan for healthy weight loss. One drawback of relying only on the glycemic index is that it is based on a standard portion of food and not necessarily the amount you would actually be eating. That's why your Sonoma meals have also been evaluated by an even more recent standard, called the glycemic load. This is a more practical way to consider the body's blood sugar response because it considers the actual amount of the food you are eating, not just a standard portion.

STAMP OF APPROVAL

The GI symbol is based on more than twenty-five years of scientific research. (If you'd like to know more about the glycemic index, go to glycemicindex.com.

But as useful as the glycemic index and the estimated glycemic load can be, you don't need to calculate either one on The Sonoma Diet. From the beginning, you've been spared the calorie counts, gram counts, point counts, and any other kind of count. You haven't needed to worry much about weighing your food portions. You're certainly not going to be burdened with having to assign a glycemic index number to the foods you put on your plate. Your plate concept guidelines and the different tiered levels of foods have automatically ranked them for you and arranged them into smart and delicious menus using the best combinations of natural wholesome foods with the low glycemic responses in mind.

SUGAR GONE WILD

How much sugar is too much? Women should consume no more than six teaspoons of added sugar a day. "Added" refers to sugar introduced through processing or that are put in tea or coffee. This does not include natural sugars contained in fruits. For men, no more than nine added teaspoons of sugar. But the average American downs twenty-two teaspoons! Sonoma eating keeps your sugar intake in bounds, because you're avoiding the hidden sugars (usually noted as sucrose or high-fructose corn syrup) in processed foods, sweetened drinks, some yogurts, crackers, and even salad dressings. To stay sugar savvy, look for how many grams of sugar per serving are listed in any food you buy. Divide that number by four and that's how many teaspoons are in each serving (one teaspoon of sugar is approximately four grams).

MIX AND MATCH

For all the well-deserved attention that healthy food choices get, the truth is we usually eat food in combinations, especially at the main meal of the day. That's why it's so important to be aware of how different foods behave in combination when putting together recipes and meal plans. The Sonoma Diet is defined by that awareness. Careful food partnering for maximum health and taste, as well as quicker weight loss, is a major key to the Sonoma plan's success.

Let me give you just a few simple examples. Extra-virgin olive oil is such a star food on the diet not just because of its heart-healthy action but also because of its unique ability (among oils) to add to and bring out the nutrients and flavor of other foods. With cooked tomatoes, olive oil helps your body absorb more of the disease-preventing lycopenes. With spinach and other dark leafy greens, it brings out the phytonutrients while mellowing that hint of bitterness in the leaves.

Or consider the Barilla Plus pasta you'll probably be enjoying from time to time. It doesn't have all that high a GI number to start with. But the number goes down sharply when it's prepared according to The Sonoma Diet recipes. So pasta provides a clear case of the Sonoma approach to health and weight loss. A potential problem food—pasta—turns into a healthy weight loss food when you

- eat the whole grain version,

- prepare it with other ingredients such as lean protein, nuts, and seeds that slow its blood sugar release, limit the use of saturated fats, such as those found in high-fat cheeses, by using low-fat cheeses such as parmesan and mozzarella instead, andeat it slowly in reasonable portions.

So when you see unfamiliar foods or food combinations in the recipes, rest assured that they're there for a reason. Much planning has gone into the mixes and matches to bring out the maximum benefits. From something as simple as nuts over a salad to more involved plans such as mixing lean beef and a citrus vinaigrette into a vegetable stir-fry, all the combinations are the result of expert nutritionists at work with your weight loss in mind.

FRUITS, VEGETABLES, AND WINE

You did eat fruits in Wave 1, of course, but in limited amounts, so a listing wasn't needed. Now, however, you'll be eating more fruit—two fruit servings per day in Wave 2. So now you need to pay attention to tiers of fruit. There are two, based on their content of calories and natural sugars. You'll find a list of Tier 2 fruits on page 120 and a list of Tier 3 fruits on page 121. What's the difference? Tier 3 fruits (such as bananas, figs, mangoes, and peaches) have more sugar and/or less water, so they pack fewer nutrients per calorie. In Wave 2, one of your daily servings can come from the Tier 3 group, but the other (or both) must come from Tier 2. What's a serving? For typically sized fruits, such as apples, oranges, and peaches, a serving is about one piece. For bigger fruits, such as papayas and pineapples, and for small berries and grapes and the like, a serving is how much fruit, sliced, will fit into a half-cup measure.

· APPLES ·
A POWER FOOD ALTERNATIVE

Use apples as an alternative Top Twelve Sonoma Diet Power Food. When you bite into a cool, crisp apple, you're treating yourself to a cornucopia of disease-fighting antioxidants. Among fruits, only berries and prunes have more. You're also getting a double dose of fiber. A typical apple will deliver at least three grams of fiber.

Even if you stick to Tier 2 fruits in Wave 2, you'll have lots of variety. Three fruits—blueberries, strawberries, and grapes—deserve special attention because of their Power Food status. They're also examples of how the fruit on your dinner plate can serve as dessert. Though those three take top honors, they're hardly alone among power fruits. Each fruit on The Sonoma Diet Fruits lists has its own health-imparting chemical makeup, and most are heart protective. These fruits have helpful phytonutrients that rival the Top Twelve Sonoma Diet Power Foods.

One point to remember is the synergistic nature of each fruit's nutrients—that is, how they work together to strengthen your heart and otherwise make you healthier. That's why buying whole, fresh, ripe fruits is ideal in most cases. You want to get every ounce of benefit from what you eat.

Be careful with canned fruits. They almost always have added sugar, which is a no-no. They're also often peeled or otherwise diminished. Stick to fresh fruits from the market. Fruits that freeze well, however, such as berries, can be bought frozen. And as far as fruit juices—as I've mentioned before, juices alone are a concentrated source of sugar. If you want some juice, try combining one ounce juice with four ounces of water for a refreshing infused water with just a hint of flavor.

YOUR VEGETABLE BIN GROWS

With Wave 2, the full panoply of Sonoma vegetables is now available to you. In addition to the Tier 1 vegetables you ate in Wave 1, you can now enjoy Tier 2 and Tier 3 vegetables.

The higher tiers simply reflect a higher sugar and calorie level. At the highest tier (Tier 3) you'll find squashes, peas, corn, and sweet potatoes. These vegetables are fine, but make sure you choose only one serving a day from this list. And remember, one serving is not necessarily an entire yam—it's a half-cup of yams or whatever other Tier 3 vegetable you choose.

During Wave 2, choose one Tier 2 vegetable and one Tier 3 vegetable per day. Remember, as in Wave 1, you can still enjoy unlimited amounts of the Tier 1 vegetables throughout the day with meals or as snacks.

WAVE 2 SWEETS

If you still crave sweets, don't have any. That may sound backward, but eliminating those cravings is still your goal. Now that you're in Wave 2, you have the option of satisfying your sweet tooth with such fruits as berries or mangoes. You'll be surprised at how satisfyingly sweet they can be. Fruit is your dessert of choice. Try using your lunch and/or dinner fruit serving (25% of the plate) to satisfy that end-of-meal-sweet desire.

For those once-in-a-while times when you absolutely must have a special dessert treat, try dark, bittersweet chocolate. It's allowed in small amounts as an occasional treat—one bite-size piece a day, no more than three days a week.

A LITTLE WINE WITH THAT?

When you think about a family in southern France or Italy sitting down to a meal, you assume there's wine on the table. That's the Mediterranean way. It's the Sonoma way as well. Sonoma County and neighboring Napa County constitute one of the most important winemaking regions in the world. Locally grown wine is a way of life in Sonoma as much as in France, Spain, or Italy. It's a fixture on the dinner table.

Wine was put on hold during Wave 1, partly because of the sugar and partly because Wave 1 was more calorie-stingy than Wave 2. But that's over now. Wave 2 is wine time. From now on, you are encouraged to accompany one daily meal (presumably dinner) with a glass of red or white wine. I say "encouraged" rather than "allowed" because moderate wine consumption delivers health benefits perfectly in keeping with The Sonoma Diet philosophy. For a modest amount of calories, a daily glass of wine has been clearly shown in recent years to reduce your risk of heart disease. There is hardly any doubt left about this among cardiologists and nutritionists.

At the same time, wine imparts a mealtime sense of relaxation and enjoyment that is essential to your new weight loss lifestyle. Besides the obvious gustatory delight that a good glass of wine adds to food enjoyment, the very act of choosing wine, opening it, pouring it, and drinking it slows down the whole eating process—which is just what you want.

The wine ritual focuses your attention on the sensuous quality of the occasion and away from any urge to simply stuff food in your mouth. Wine reminds us that mealtime is about pleasure, not just filling up. Savor the wine and taste the food. You reawaken senses and food experiences that perhaps have been forgotten. You eat slower and you're satisfied with less. You lose weight and gain insight on how to eat for pleasure.

Note, however, that though I didn't use the word "allowed" above, I didn't use the word "obligated" either. If there's any medical or health reason why you shouldn't drink wine, by all means don't touch it. If you don't like wine, don't drink it. If you give it a try with a little help from a wine-loving friend and still don't like it, don't drink it.

But if you're used to enjoying wine, make it a part of one daily meal. Keep it to one glass and make it last. Wine isn't there to quench your thirst. It's there to enhance your pleasure.

WAVE 2 SNACKS

Snacks are to keep you from being uncomfortably hungry between meals. The best choice is still a Tier 1 vegetable, prepared however you like it. The trick with snacking between meals is to walk the line—you want to calm hunger so you won't be starving come mealtime. But you don't want to use that as an excuse to overeat, slowing down your weight loss progress.

But now that you're in Wave 2, you have more choices—if you need them. Some of the following will look familiar; they were permitted to men and physically active women in Wave 1.

- a Tier 2 fruit, keeping to the ½ cup serving size
- a spoonful or two of cottage cheese with a little sliced Tier 2 fruit
- half a bag of light microwave-popped popcorn. Plain—no oil or butter
- a piece of mozzarella cheese or a slice of lean lunch meat
- ½ cup low-fat cottage cheese with Tier 1 raw veggies
- 3 ounces of hummus, either homemade or store-bought, with veggies
- low-fat cheese stick with carrots or celery
- 1 slice of whole-grain bread with one tablespoon of peanut butter
- 2 ounces cooked chicken breast or turkey deli meat
- 1 serving of nuts (remember, you've used up a fat serving this way)

WINE AND YOUR HEALTH

There's been compelling evidence for some time now that drinking wine goes hand in hand with a healthy lifestyle and is a powerful means of preventing heart disease. In fact, it seems like a new study comes out every week verifying the health benefits of moderate wine consumption.

And it's not just the risk of heart disease that goes down with moderate wine consumption. Solid recent research is providing a clearer understanding of how wine may help prevent or relieve the effects of dementia, Alzheimer's disease, diabetes, and even osteoporosis. So the question is no longer whether moderate consumption of wine is healthy. It is. The questions is…why?

One possible explanation is that wine drinkers tend to eat healthier diets, smoke less, and exercise more than other people. Research supports that. But research also suggests that there's something in wine that has a protective health effect. Which leads to another question…what?

Wine contains polyphenols—antioxidants that include the varieties of flavonols, tannins, and anthocyanins, to name a few. It could very well be that the *combination* (there's that word again!) of these phytonutrients stimulates greater health benefits than any one of them could do alone.

What people are saying about Sonoma…

"I have never wanted to DIET or live by a diet—this is a lifestyle that has helped me to be more aware of how and what I eat, exercise, and more importantly recognize how great I feel. I went from 245 pounds to 185 pounds and have proudly kept the weight off for two years. There are times when the weight begins to creep back, but exercise and planning for meals always works. For me, I can say that The Sonoma Diet plan is easy and delicious. Having a glass of wine with meals makes it even more enjoyable. My new lifestyle does not feel like a diet!"

—Mark, lost 60 pounds

There's plenty of evidence that alcohol itself, in moderation, has cardiovascular benefits. But wine's heart-protective effect clearly goes beyond the alcohol (ethanol) in it. It's the result of a huge array of the phytonutrients I just mentioned, along with an amazing compound called resveratrol. You met resveratrol when I introduced table grapes as a Power Food. Its heart-protective antioxidant action is even stronger in wine than in grapes.

Because of these special nutrients, many scientific studies have concluded that wine consumption is much more strongly correlated with reduced risk of death from heart disease than drinking alcohol in general. In these studies, "moderate consumption" is defined as one to three glasses of wine per day. Of course, you're on a tight budget when it comes to calories, so follow the one 6-ounce glass per day guideline during Wave 2.

And remember, since many of the beneficial effects of wine are transient—meaning they last about twenty-four hours—the best pattern is to drink moderately each day, rather than saving your weekly wine allotment for the weekend. And have it with a meal. Wine consumed with food has favorable effects on the body's absorption of antioxidants from the food and wine, as well as the metabolism of dietary fats in the body. ■

WINE, THE SONOMA WAY

Enjoying wine doesn't require a degree in winemaking. Good wine is wine you enjoy drinking. Period. Try different varieties to figure out what types of wine are appealing to you and experiment by drinking different wines with foods to find combinations you enjoy. You've already learned about smart food combinations for health and flavor—such as a fresh squeeze of lemon juice on seafood or a drizzle of olive oil over dark leafy greens. Wine plays a similar role by enhancing these flavors in food. In general, pair light-bodied wines with lighter foods that use delicate preparations. Full-bodied wines go better with heartier, more intense flavors. Your Wave 2 meal plans offer some recommendations for a variety of wines to accompany your evening meals. Here are some ideas for pairing wine with food:

WHITE WINES

- chardonnay: seafood, chicken, ham, veal
- sauvignon blanc: oysters, salmon, goat cheese, salads, pastas
- Riesling: mild cheeses, pork, tandoori chicken, shellfish
- sparkling white wines: Asian, Thai, curry, chile pepper spices

RED WINES

- cabernet sauvignon: duck, spicy beef and poultry, richer foods in general
- pinot noir: braised chicken, turkey, lamb, mushrooms, earthy flavors
- merlot: braised chicken, roasted beef, lamb, game meats
- burgundy: salmon, tuna, roast chicken
- Chianti: pasta with tomato sauce, pizza

WAVE 2

SONOMA TIER 1 VEGETABLES

Unlimited; see the Wave 1 listing on page 102

SONOMA TIER 2 FRUITS AND VEGETABLES

Limit to 1 fruit and 1 vegetable from this list per day;
1 serving = ½ cup or 1 whole small piece of fruit

FRUITS

apple
apricot
blackberry
blueberry
boysenberry
cantaloupe
cherimoya
cherry, sour only
cloudberry
gooseberry, raw
grape
grapefruit
honeydew melon
huckleberry
java plum *(jambolan)*
kiwifruit
kumquat
lemon
lime
mulberry
orange
papaya
pineapple
plum
prickly pear
pummelo *(Chinese grapefruit)*
quince
raspberry
rhubarb
salmonberry
star fruit
strawberry
tangerine
ugli fruit
watermelon

VEGETABLES

artichoke
beet, cooked
carrot, raw or cooked
celeriac, raw or cooked
chile pepper
Jerusalem artichoke/sunchoke
pumpkin, raw or cooked
rutabaga, cooked
spaghetti squash
water chestnut

Sonoma Tier 3 Fruits and Vegetables

Limit to one fruit and one vegetable from this list per day; 1 serving = ½ cup or 1 whole small piece of fruit

FRUIT

banana
elderberry
fig
guava
jackfruit
jujube
mango
nectarine
passion fruit
peach
pear
persimmon
plantain
pomegranate

VEGETABLES

acorn squash
butternut squash
corn
parsnip
pea, cooked
pea pod, raw or cooked
pea sprout
sugar snap pea
sweet potato, cooked
taro, cooked
wasabi root
yam

Note: Whole fruits and vegetables are measured by cutting into slices or wedges.

Sonoma Proteins and Dairy

PROTEINS

beans and legumes *(black beans, black-eyed peas, chickpeas, lentils, pinto beans, soybeans such as edamame and tofu)*
beef: lean cuts *(beef round, chuck arm pot roast, eye of round, round tip, tenderloin, top loin, top sirloin)*
eggs: 1 whole egg = 2 whites
fish: lean cuts *(cod, flounder, grouper, halibut, haddock, monkfish, northern pike, orange roughy, perch, pike, walleye)*
fish: moderate-fat *(catfish, sea bass, snapper, striped bass, swordfish, tuna, whitefish)*
fish: high-fat *(mackerel, salmon, trout)*
game meats *(bison, deer, elk)*
lamb: *(arm, foreshank, leg, loin, shank half, shoulder, stew meat)*
peanut butter: 2 tablespoons per serving for main-dish protein, 1 tablespoon as a snack
pork: lean cuts (Canadian bacon; ham, boiled or cured; canned ham; center cut loin chop; pork loin; pork sirloin chop and roast; pork tenderloin; top loin)

poultry: white meat, no skin; turkey bacon; turkey sausage

shellfish (clams, crab, lobster, mussels, oysters, scallops, shrimp)

soy substitutes: vegetarian (soy) crumble, vegetarian (soy) burger

veal (arm, ground, leg, loin, shoulder, sirloin, top round)

DAIRY

low-fat cheese: 1 ounce (grated parmesan, mozzarella)

low-fat cottage cheese

fat-free (skim) milk: 1 cup

fat-free plain yogurt: 1 cup

Sonoma Grains

1 serving = ½ cup

Barilla Plus pasta, cooked

barley, cooked

bread, whole-grain: 1 slice (2 or more grams of fiber per slice)

bulgur, cooked

cereal, whole grain (8 grams fiber per serving or higher)

oats (oat bran, oat groats, rolled oats, steel-cut oats)

pasta, whole-grain, cooked

popcorn, air-popped, no butter*

quinoa, cooked

rice, cooked (brown, red, or black)

soba noodles, cooked

wheat, cooked (bulgur, cracked wheat, groats, wheat berries)

wild rice

* intended for a snack, not to go on the plate

Sonoma Beverages

coffee: black or with up to a maximum 1 tablespoon heavy cream and 1 packet of noncaloric sweetener

tea: no cream or sugar (black, green, herbal)

water (plain or sparkling)

wine (red or white): 6 ounces per day

Sonoma Fats

Up to 3 servings per day;
1 teaspoon = 1 serving

avocado: ¼ avocado = 1 serving

canola oil

olive oil

Nuts

almonds: 11

peanuts: 14

pecans: 10 halves

walnuts: 7 halves

Sonoma Flavor Boosters

Unlimited

herbs *(basil, chive, cilantro, dill, fennel, marjoram, mint, oregano, rosemary, sage, tarragon, thyme)*

spices *(caraway, cardamom, cayenne, celery seed, chili powder, cinnamon, clove, cumin, curry, nutmeg, pepper, saffron, turmeric)*

chile pepper

garlic

ginger, gingerroot

horseradish

lemon or lime juice or zest

lemongrass

mustard *(all types)*

vanilla

vinegar *(rice wine, balsamic)*

FAST-TRACK
YOUR WEIGHT LOSS

You have a special advantage when you follow the Sonoma plan: You feel great.

You feel great while you're eating a Sonoma meal because it's always a pleasurable celebration of delicious, flavorful foods. You feel great afterward because you're satisfied. And you feel great as the days and weeks go by because you're experiencing the energy and positive outlook that are the happy results of losing pounds and gaining health.

Because you feel great, it's easier to keep making smart choices, to stay motivated, and to continue to enjoy the pleasures of the Sonoma way of life. That's a wonderful advantage.

But there's also this disadvantage: The Sonoma Diet takes place in the real world. And in the real world, nothing is easy all the time.

In the real world, you can get impatient at what seems like too slow a weight loss pace. You can understand the eating guidelines down to the last detail but sometimes find them hard to follow. Or you can sense your enthusiasm slipping away, and you don't understand why.

Even worse, cravings lurk in the real world. So do lapses, temptations, and mistakes. Incidents occur, sometimes involving entire pints of ice cream. Frustration might set in. Seemingly for no reason, you hit plateaus when a week or more goes by without an ounce of weight lost.

And sometimes, well, you just don't care how good The Sonoma Diet food is. You want bad food, you want a lot of it, and you want it right now.

Sound familiar? All these distractions are to be expected. They are totally normal. That's why it's called the "real world."

In this book so far, I've tried to explain to you what to do and why you're doing it. Now I'm going to tell you *how* to do it—and how to keep on doing it when times get tough. You'll see that the real-world problems are part of any diet and that there are simple ways to overcome any rough patch you stumble across on the road to your ideal weight.

Make no mistake about it: you *will* get past the pitfalls, great or small. Your body wants to be at its best weight. All you're doing is helping it along.

You're Not Alone

The first thing to realize is that everybody struggles at times when they change their eating patterns for the better. They all fight cravings. They all give into temptation once in a while. And they all go through periods when they feel like giving up. You're not alone. Others have been through exactly what you're going through. And they came out the other side slimmer, healthier, and happier.

What's happening is that your body and mind are resisting change. It doesn't matter that the change is for the better or that it mostly feels good. It's still change, and your brain is hardwired to resist change. Or at least to be very cautious about accepting it.

Think about how many new habits you've been adopting. You're eating less. You're eating more slowly. You're eating healthier foods in a greater variety. You've kicked what was probably a lifelong habit of loading up on refined flour and sugar. You've changed the kind of dietary fat you're consuming.

Your body thanks you every day for these changes. At the same time, though, your brain is wondering what happened to all that other stuff you used to love so much. Occasionally your brain will remind you about those lost treats.

That's what cravings and temptations are—reminders of change. They're just thoughts. And you can deal with thoughts.

GET IT OUT, WRITE IT DOWN

The way to deal with those thoughts is openly and directly. Cravings and other diet pitfalls aren't vague annoyances that might go away. They are specific reactions to specific situations—which means they can be isolated, confronted, and understood. That's what you need to do to get them to go away. I encourage you to deal with these problems as methodically as you do with the eating part of the Sonoma plan.

Look at it this way: To get down to your target weight, you knew it

QUICK TIPS FOR QUICKER WEIGHT LOSS

If you could lose weight even faster than at the typical Sonoma Diet pace, would you do it? Here are some simple ways to speed up the process, without sacrificing the health benefits.

- Choose more of your vegetables from Tier 1, retaining just enough Tier 2 and 3 vegetables to maintain variety. Tier 1 vegetables are richer in nutrients, with fewer calories. They also have the lowest impact on your blood sugar levels. This impact is measured by the glycemic load, listed with the nutrient facts in the recipes.

- Likewise, choose most of your fruits from Tier 2, leaving Tier 3 fruits for special occasions. Tier 2 fruits have less natural sugar,

a lower impact on your blood sugar, and fewer calories.

- Eat even more slowly. The longer you take at a meal, the less you're likely to eat and the more satisfied you'll feel. Find ways to slow down at all three meals, not just the one very leisurely meal of the day.

- Eat more fish for protein.

- Skimp on your plate filling. There's no rule saying you have to load it up to the edges. Portions just a tiny bit smaller will pay off over the long run.

- Keep your snacking at Wave 1 level. That means nothing more than a Tier 1 vegetable. If that's enough to tide you over until the next meal, why have more?

wouldn't be enough to simply decide to eat a little less or try to cut down on "fattening" foods. Instead, you chose to follow the Sonoma meal plans and eat according to the Sonoma guidelines. It's the same with your cravings. It's not enough to resolve to "be strong" or to wait for them to eventually disappear. You need a plan.

The plan that works is getting the problems out in the open so you can understand where they're coming from and then deal with them. A very successful strategy for doing that is a food journal. Just the act of writing things down every day serves to focus your attention on eating right.

But a journal does more than that. Over the weeks it starts to clarify for you the whole confusing interplay of hunger, food, cravings, moods, and all the other things you feel and think and do in the course of a day. Pretty soon, the problems you're having start making sense.

Now, if you loathe the very idea of any kind of journal, breathe easy. A food journal is not obligatory on the new Sonoma Diet. But bear with me. A food journal is a proven tool for losing weight faster and easier. If it works, why not go for it?

THE POWER OF THE PEN

Here's how you keep your food journal: Every day, write down what you eat, what time you ate it, how much of it you ate, where you were eating it (family table, restaurant, car, desk), and whether you liked it or not.

- Drink your snack. Try having a cup of hot tea or a tall glass of water instead of your usual snack. You may be more thirsty than hungry, and as long as you're not reaching your next meal in starvation mode, those uneaten calories will pay off.

- Buy food instead of packages. Challenge yourself to buy only fresh food for a week—meat and fish from the butcher, fruit and vegetables from the produce section, whole grains from the health food store bins. When you buy "food" instead of "packages," you're eliminating any chance of unwanted processing, refined grains, added hydrogenated fats, and mysterious chemicals sneaking into your diet.

- If you haven't been exercising, start. If you have been exercising, push up the intensity a notch.

Note how hungry you felt as you began to eat and what else you were feeling (bored, indifferent, excited). This goes for snacks and meals, as well as whatever little extras find their way into your mouth.

Also jot down throughout the day any thoughts, feelings, or activities worth noting and what time they occurred. Feeling stressed? Write down when and (if you know) why. A special meeting or appointment? Write it down and how you feel about it, before and after. A craving? Write down when and for what.

I know this sounds like a lot of writing, but you'll soon find short-hand ways of getting these things down quickly and effortlessly. After all, you're the only one who needs to decipher your scribblings. The main goal, obviously, is to be honest and thorough; you can't deal with, say, extra snacking if you pretend it's not happening.

After a few days of journal keeping, you can start looking for patterns that might shed some light on the problems you've been having with the diet. Do you tend to eat late at night as you watch television? Do you get cravings when you're stressed or bored? Do you often overeat when specific foods are on the plate? Do your cravings seem to come a few hours after certain kinds of meals? Do you yearn for sugar on Mondays?

The connections between cravings and specific moods or habits might be quite clear. Or they might be very subtle. Either way, seeing the patterns demystifies the cravings and makes them much easier to conquer. Trust me.

You'll also find that your food journal will help pin down other reasons you're not losing weight as fast as you'd like. For example, your journal might reveal that you're eating more than you thought you were or that your snacks are regularly too generous. You might see that you're not getting enough variety in your plant foods or protein sources. Maybe you've been eating vegetables from the three tiers in the wrong proportions. All of this is worth knowing. The knowledge will help you lose weight more quickly and efficiently.

CRAVE BUSTERS

Using a food journal to notice your craving patterns helps you conquer them. Now you can take action to keep yourself from falling into the same trap time and again.

Much of the time, your course of action is obvious. If you used to mindlessly snack while watching late-night television, don't watch it. It's highly recommended that you don't have meals in front of the TV anyway. If you've realized that you never resist the bagels with cream cheese that your coworkers bring in every Friday morning, make yourself scarce at bagel time. You can't say you weren't warned.

When you feel a craving coming on, take proactive measures. Change the subject in your mind. Go for a walk immediately. Go brush your teeth. Pop some gum in your mouth. If you can get your mind off the craving for just a while, it will often go away.

You can also try taking preemptive strikes. If you find yourself regularly craving sweets at 10 p.m., shift one of your daily snacks from mid-afternoon to 8:30 p.m. If need be, have one of your allowable dark chocolate bites at that time. Savor the taste and make it last longer than the later craving pleaser ever would. It's better to indulge slowly in a small square of dark bittersweet chocolate at 8:30 than devour a candy bar at 10.

> ### MEET IT HALFWAY
>
> A good temporary measure for stopping excessive snacking is to treat yourself to a smaller, healthier version of the food you're craving. If you think you need a bag of potato chips, slice a quarter of a sweet potato instead. Brush the slices with a little olive oil and sprinkle salt or an herb over them. Bake the slices in an oven at 375 degrees until they're crisp. Satisfaction guaranteed.

THE STRESS FACTOR

Can stress dictate hunger and put extra pounds around your waist? The answer is yes, and then some. Stress is an eating trigger. It's one of the major causes of eating poorly and eating excessively, so it can be directly related to extra pounds. And it's a red flag for risk factors associated with inflammation, heart disease, and diabetes. Finding ways to manage your stress is essential to healthy weight loss.

All of us tend to overeat in times of stress; it's a natural biological response. What happens is a vicious cycle. Stress stimulates the release of

BETTER BEDTIME

A good night's sleep is not a luxury—it's a health imperative. Sleeping less than five hours a night not only produces inflammatory compounds linked to heart disease, but also hinders your weight loss effort. Studies are finding consistent data to suggest that people who sleep well have better overall health and live longer than those who don't. Try these tips for sounder sleep:

- Dim the lights an hour before bedtime.
- Sleep in total darkness.
- Stick to a regular sleep routine.
- Avoid napping during the day.
- Limit caffeine and alcohol within four hours of bedtime.
- Exercise during the day, but not just before bed.

high amounts of insulin and cortisol, which increase your appetite and cravings for sweets and fats. The resulting extra pounds around your waist lead to the release of more inflammatory compounds, and the cycle continues to feed itself until a larger problem—diabetes or insulin resistance—results.

Extreme dieting can put you into stress mode. Healthy Sonoma eating helps get you out of it. Whole grains, a Sonoma Power Food, promote the production of serotonin, a feel-good brain messenger chemical. The magnesium abundant in whole grains and almonds (another Power Food) promotes muscle relaxation. Emphasizing B vitamins from whole grains and vegetables is also very important for repairing the negative effects of stress.

There are lots of things you can do to help manage your stress levels and avoid the food cravings that stress can cause. Sleeping well and getting exercise are two of them. Eating well and focusing on the Top Twelve Sonoma Diet Power Foods are two more that I don't need to tell you about. Breathing techniques work, and they can be as simple as taking ten long deep breaths when your mind gets ahead of you. "Go with the flow" activities, such as meditation, listening to relaxing music, or gardening, are good options, as is a massage. Talking things out, expressing your feelings with friends and family, cutting down on your screen time (television, computers, cell phones), and using time management strategies, such as prioritizing your daily activities, are effective de-stressors. Also, monitor your caffeine and alcohol intake.

WHEN THE SCALE WON'T BUDGE

Just as every dieter fights cravings, every dieter gets stuck on plateaus from time to time as well. Your body doesn't always behave the way you want it to. So even though you're following the diet guidelines to a T (or believe you are), you may sometimes hit periods when the scale needle simply refuses to move. It doesn't seem fair, but it happens.

Your first and best reaction is to wait it out. Stick to your good eating habits and don't let yourself get frustrated. It's usually a matter of days before you start dropping the pounds again.

Plateaus are often easily explainable. The most likely plateau period is the shift from Wave 1 to Wave 2. Remember, you're actually adding calories to your diet at this point (compared to Wave 1), as well as a number of new foods. Water retention, an adjustment in blood sugar metabolism, and other factors could conspire against weight loss as you settle into Wave 2. Ride it out.

But if the plateau drags on for a week or if you're actually gaining weight, it's time to take a look at what's going on. Adjustments may be needed.

The first thing you need to do is make sure you're following the Sonoma Diet guidelines correctly. It's not uncommon to be firmly convinced that you're adhering faithfully to the rules, only to discover upon closer examination that something's out of kilter. This is where a food journal can help you figure it out. But whether you keep a journal or not, take a close inventory of your eating habits to see where you may be going wrong.

Are you following the plate proportions fairly closely? Are you heaping the portions into something resembling the Egyptian pyramids? Are you using a plate that's the wrong size?

Are you pulling fruits and vegetables off the wrong tier lists? Has your snacking gotten out of hand? (Remember, a Tier 1 vegetable is the best snack unless you really need something more.) Are you choosing cuts of red meat that aren't as lean as they should be?

Are your breads and cereals 100% whole grain or are refined grains also included? Check those labels! Are you cheating on the sweets? Are extra fat portions sneaking into your meals or snacks?

Go through your entire eating regimen, looking for lapses. Pledge anew to be a real stickler about the rules, at least until your weight starts dropping again. Chances are you'll see some movement soon. The Sonoma Diet will always work—but only if you follow it.

BACK ON TRACK

Another time that you might hit a plateau and stop losing weight is during Wave 2. One option you can consider is going back through Wave 1 again. This is probably your best bet if your self-inspection confirms that you're indeed meeting the diet guidelines. In that case, another ten days of Wave 1 will surely get you back on track for the simple reason that fewer calories are built into the meal plans.

You should also consider going back through Wave 1 if you suspect that your failure to continue losing weight has something to do with sugar cravings or white bread cravings. You know best, of course, whether you've been eating sugared sweets or any kinds of grains that aren't whole. Either of these transgressions on a regular basis will stop your weight loss every time.

If that's the case, a rerun of Wave 1 is called for because you still need to kick your addiction to sugar and refined white flour. Your blood sugar metabolism hasn't adjusted to a better diet yet. Your body simply isn't ready for the higher calorie consumption of Wave 2.

Another ten days of Wave 1 should do the trick. Not only will you be eating fewer calories, you'll also consume very little sugar. You'll need to redouble your efforts to stay sugar-free and refined-flour-free for those ten days. That means no bread, crackers, or pasta of any kind that isn't whole-grain—and even less of the whole-grain versions than on Wave 2.

GET MOVING

A high priority for keeping your weight loss going at full clip is to increase your physical activity. As I mentioned earlier during Wave 1, some kind of exercise that you enjoy is vital for efficient weight loss and optimum health.

Here are some specific exercise recommendations:

1. *Exercise for an hour a day, five days per week.* That's the most effective schedule. But if you've never done five minutes of exercise in your life, or if it's been years since you've been physically active, you'll have to build up to it.

2. *Start off easy.* At the beginning, what or how much you do matters a lot less than simply doing something regularly. Take a walk around the block after lunch or dinner. Play tag with your kids. Shoot some baskets. The important thing is to get in the habit of doing something physical every day. Then you can gradually work your way up to a half hour of sustained activity a few days a week and eventually to the recommended hour a day for five days.

3. *Do what you like.* Choose forms of physical activity that you enjoy, rather than what somebody else tells you is "the best." If exercise is drudgery for you or something you dread, you're not going to stick with it.

4. *Enjoy it.* The main thing is to approach exercise as something fun. You may feel a little awkward at first, no matter what you do. But if you smile your way through it and are persistent, your body will let you know how much it appreciates the chance to move. You'll feel better and lose weight faster.

5. *Do all three pillars of exercise.* These are cardiovascular (or aerobic) exercise, strength training, and flexibility work:

> *Cardiovascular exercise.* Also called aerobic exercise, this is a calorie-burner par excellence and one of the best things you can do for your heart and lungs. Jogging, biking, swimming, rowing, stair-stepping, or even brisk walking—do it indoors or outdoors, with machines or the real thing, at home or in a health club.

> *Strength training.* You can start out with a simple pair of light dumbbells to work with at home, or you can join a gym and take advantage of the full range of weights and machines built for easy use. Even regular gardening will help tone your muscles, as anyone who's ever weeded or spaded soil will testify.

Flexibility. You increase your flexibility with stretching exercises, which offer the added attraction of a meditation break, a way to relax as you listen to your body. Start with about ten minutes of stretching each day, and gradually add minutes so you'll have time to stretch muscles in your upper body (arms, shoulders, neck), back, and lower body (thighs, calves, ankles).

Here are some simple stretches that will help your weight loss program. Remember to warm up your muscles with a short walk or light exercise before you stretch. Breathe while you stretch; don't hold your breath. You want a slow, smooth, and controlled movement, with no bouncing. Stretch to the point of resistance, not pain.

FOR YOUR UPPER BODY

These are especially helpful if you sit at a desk all day, need to work on your posture, or carry tension in your upper body.

1. Place your hands on the back of your head and gently push it forward with your chin tucked in. Hold for five seconds.

2. Now place the heels of your hands on your chin, fingers pointing toward your ears. Gently push your head back. Hold for five seconds.

3. Reset your right hand on the top of your head and gently press your right ear toward your right shoulder. Hold for five seconds. Repeat on the other side.

4. Raise your arms and clasp your hands above your head. Imagine lifting and lengthening your spine. As you bend to the left, release your hands. Grasp your right elbow with your left hand and pull it to the left. Hold for five seconds. Come back to the center and repeat on the right side.

FOR YOUR BACK

1. Lie on your stomach, legs straight and feet shoulder-width apart.

2. Place your hands on the floor under your shoulders and slowly lift your chest up; hold for five seconds.

3. Come to a standing position with your feet shoulder-width apart and rotate your body so that both feet are pointed to the right. (Your left foot will be at about a 45-degree angle.) Lift the toes of your right foot off the ground, bend at the hip, and fold your body over. Hold for ten seconds.

4. Come back to a standing position and repeat on the left side with your feet pointing to the left.

FOR YOUR LOWER BODY

1. Sit on the floor with your legs straight out in front of you.

2. Lift your right leg off the floor, holding it with both hands. Flex your foot and hold for five seconds. Lower and switch legs.

3. While still seated, bend your right knee and lift your leg. Pull your knee to your chest. Flex your foot and hold for five seconds. Lower your right leg and repeat with the left. ■

WAVE 3
THE NEW SONOMA DIET
LIFESTYLE

At the very beginning, I described The Sonoma Diet as a lifestyle. In Wave 3, which starts the day you reach your target weight, you're now living that Sonoma lifestyle.

That doesn't mean you're a different person. You're still you, and you always will be. It's just that now you're a revitalized, more energetic you, a you who sleeps better, has a more positive outlook on life, is nourished both mentally and physically, and is motivated to continue this new way of thinking about and enjoying food.

YOUR SONOMA DIET SUCCESS

The fact is, you've accomplished much more than a healthy, happy (and great-looking) body weight. By following through on Waves 1 and 2 of The Sonoma Diet, you've changed your entire approach to eating—for the better.

You've rid your body and mind of any thoughts of white bread, rolls, crackers, and other bakery foods made from refined flour. You've replaced them with satisfying amounts of fiber-laden and richer-tasting whole-grain breads and cereals.

You've eliminated sugar cravings so that sugar-sweetened items are back to being what they're meant to be—occasional treats. By breaking yourself of the sugar habit, you've rediscovered that the wholesome natural sweetness of fresh ripe fruits and berries makes for as rewarding a dessert experience as you could ever want.

You've banned harmful partially hydrogenated fats from your diet and learned to keep saturated fats down to the bare minimum. At the same time, you haven't succumbed to an irrational fear of fat; instead, you've taken advantage of reasonable amounts of the healthy and weight-friendly dietary fats in olive oil, nuts, avocados, and fish.

Most important, you've made the three-way connection between eating for pleasure, eating for health, and eating to stay at your best weight. You no longer see life as a choice between enjoying food and staying slim. On the contrary, you've discovered for yourself that the most efficient way to reach your ideal body weight is to revel in the pleasure that the healthiest and most naturally delicious foods have to offer.

You didn't just learn these lessons. You put them into practice. It wasn't always easy, especially at first. But by now you should have the results to show for your efforts—an ideal weight, the slimmer body you've always wanted, a healthier heart, clothes that fit right, oodles more energy, a boosted sense of self-esteem, and a heartfelt appreciation of the almost spiritual joy that you can experience by slowly savoring a delicious, healthy meal with family or friends.

REAP THE REWARDS

Wave 3 is the time for you to reap the rewards of The Sonoma Diet lifestyle. The biggest reward is something you probably never thought about when you first opened up this book. It's a kind of liberation.

It comes down to being able to enjoy food and all the other good things life has to offer without worrying about being overweight. By eating mindfully, by mastering strategies for making smart choices, you have, by Wave 3, adopted a wholesome approach to food that will make maintaining your best weight and best health effortless, simply part of your everyday way of eating.

That's the difference between a "diet" and the Sonoma way of living.

Enjoy it to the hilt. Keep finding new sources of variety. Foods from all over the world are finding their way into every nook and cranny of

North America. You will find an endless supply of healthy world flavors from the Mediterranean, Asia, and Latin America that offers you a culinary adventure true to the spirit of the Sonoma Diet way of eating.

Keep pushing that health-and-pleasure connection. Now that weight loss is no longer the main factor in your meal planning, the satisfaction you'll get from enjoying reasonable portions of healthy, wholesome foods will actually increase. You're now eating well for its own sake. And that feels great.

What people are saying about Sonoma...

> *"In Wave 3, I'm motivated to keep healthy because I feel so good! After fifteen months on The Sonoma Diet, I love the 'new' me, and I know I will never go back to my old habits. I've learned what to eat and the right portion sizes. Even when I'm away from home, it's easy to find healthy choices with The Sonoma Diet. In fact, I just returned from a trip to New Orleans with a friend—we wined and dined our way through some of the best restaurants. I just paid attention to what I was eating, and I never felt deprived (I even had some of those evil beignets!). When I got home, I discovered I had actually lost two pounds! It's just a natural way to eat for me. I feel good, people say I look good, and I have tons of energy. Thank you, thank you, thank you!"*
>
> —Carol, lost 43 pounds

YOUR PERFECT WEIGHT FOR LIFE

Your first order of business for Wave 3, of course, is to stay at your ideal weight. This is what's often called "maintenance" in diet circles. But that's not the word of choice here.

There's nothing technically wrong with the term—you are, after all, seeking to "maintain" a certain weight. But "maintenance" sounds like something for airplane engines, not human beings. What you really want to do in Wave 3 is enhance the benefits of The Sonoma Diet lifestyle. Do that, and your weight maintenance will take care of itself.

For example, you've made the effort to turn at least one of your daily meals into a long and leisurely affair in which you eat slowly and savor every bite. You know that this elementary step not only turns mealtime into a soul-satisfying, sociable experience, but also works wonders for weight control by helping you eat less and digest better.

In Wave 3, you can work on turning the other two meals into similar experiences. True, for most of us lunchtime isn't as conducive to a leisurely pace as dinner. But chances are it can be considerably more leisurely than what you've been accustomed to.

Same for breakfast. Yes, you're rushed. Everybody's rushed in the morning. But do you really have to be rushed to the point of semi-panic? Connoisseurs of the Sonoma lifestyle will wake up fifteen minutes to a half hour earlier in the morning than they used to and use the time to slow down at breakfast. Enjoy your coffee or tea. Take it easy. Every extra second you take during any meal makes it that much easier to keep your weight down.

YOUR SATISFYING RESULTS

The reason Wave 3 is easier on The New Sonoma Diet than equivalent "maintenance" phases on other diets is that the eating plan for the bulk of the diet (Wave 2) was essentially designed to be sustainable for life. Most Sonoma dieters enjoy meals more during Wave 2 of the diet than they did before the diet started. You've been eating satisfying and well-balanced meals the whole time, so there's no eagerness to get back to the old ways once you've reached your weight goal.

With low-carb or low-fat diets, on the other hand, any weight loss you achieve is from sticking to an eating plan based on artificially reduced amounts of needed foods. So naturally you and your body are ready and eager to make up for lost nutrition, so to speak, and overeat carbs or fat to compensate. That's where the infamous yo-yo effect or "rebounding" comes in.

On The Sonoma Diet, you haven't been "depriving" yourself of white bread and sweets, waiting for the day you can have them again. Rather, you've kicked the white bread and sweets habit and replaced them with better alternatives. That's not a sacrifice. That's a positive change for life.

Still, you do have more slack on Wave 3 of The Sonoma Diet. That makes sense. Up to now your priority was to lose weight. Well, you've lost the weight by Wave 3 and you don't need to lose any more. If you continue to eat exactly as you did on Wave 2, you'll keep losing weight. You don't want that. You want to stay where you are. That means you can implement some subtle changes.

But it doesn't mean you should start eating refined flour products again, or sweets, or fatty meats. It does not mean you can ignore the proportions you've been following or the portion sizes. The guidelines hold. All you want to do is tweak them in healthy ways.

SONOMA SECRETS

There are lots of simple things you can do to keep your life humming along delightfully as you enjoy your higher health and slimmer waistline. Here's a review of some of the suggestions for better living in this book—small changes that add up.

Eat breakfast ... one that includes colorful fruits, nourishing whole grains, satisfying nuts, and lean proteins—in other words, a nutrient-rich breakfast. Include a good-quality tea rich in antioxidants.

Go to sleep earlier ... so you can wake up fifteen minutes earlier and have a few minutes of quiet time to appreciate the quiet morning, to reflect on the day ahead and the choices you'll be making.

Savor your meals. Taste, eat slowly, chew, and don't get distracted by the television, the phone, the computer, or anything else that's not at the table. Eat mindfully.

Take a breather ... literally. Practice slow, deep breathing for at least one minute a day, every day, to reduce stress.

Exercise. It helps keep you slim, energetic, and self-confident. Develop your core midsection muscles to support your spine.

Seek silence. Take time out for tranquility. It soothes stressed nerves and brains.

Be thankful ... for having been able to accomplish what you have. Many people don't get the opportunity.

HEALTHY ADJUSTMENTS

By far the most recommended tweak is to boost your servings of fruits and vegetables. This obeys the most basic bylaw of the Sonoma way of eating—get the maximum amount of nutrients for the minimum number of calories. More fruits and vegetables mean better overall health. You'll probably find you can add several servings per day and stay at your best weight. Try this strategy first.

Another surprisingly effective weight maintenance technique is to allow yourself a "nontypical" food choice once in a while—like trying the birthday cake at a friend's party you otherwise would have declined. There are actually a number of object lessons connected with going nontypical. One is that many, perhaps most, Sonoma eaters who reach Wave 3 find that these foods have lost their attraction. They may want to be a good sport at a birthday party, but that's it. And even those who still consider a sugary sweet a treat are making a choice, not succumbing to a craving. They can just as easily choose to pass on that dessert the next time.

You can now eat the occasional nontypical foods—like a sugary dessert, potatoes, smoothies, juices, pretzels—because your metabolism has changed for the better. This is one of the vital and great advantages of being on Wave 3 after shedding pounds the healthy way on The Sonoma Diet. Let's take a look at what it means.

FOOD FOR THOUGHT

Only 20% of American children and 32% of adults eat the recommended servings of fruits and vegetables. And much of what they do eat is, to varying extents, depleted of nutrients. Could it be, as some researchers believe, that this mild malnutrition status leaves the body and mind in search of more food as a way to make up for missed nutrients? Could that explain why such a large percentage of the population is overweight?

If so, this notion suggests what The Sonoma Diet stresses— that quality is more important than quantity when it comes to satisfying meals that promote whole health. The better the food quality, the less of it you need to eat in order to feel satisfied.

It may have occurred to you that for all their healthy dietary habits, many French, Italian, and other Mediterranean people do eat their share of white bread, pasta, and sweets. How do they get away with it?

Well, they don't all get away with it, of course. Somewhere in Italy, or in Sonoma, there's someone trying to lose extra weight, perhaps the result of too much refined flour and sugar.

But most do get away with it because they eat nontypical food in small amounts, and it's offset by a lifetime of olive oil, fruits, vegetables, wine, whole grains, and other dietary pluses that mark the Mediterranean and Sonoma diets. And since they don't carry a spare tire around their waists, their metabolism is able to deal with the metabolic effects of eating sugar and refined flour.

DESKTOP LUNCHES

If you must have lunch at your desk, at least turn off the computer and stay off the phone while you're eating. Better yet, take it somewhere else—the lunchroom, a park bench, anywhere you can dedicate yourself to enjoying your meal rather than putting food in your mouth while doing something else.

Your situation was probably quite the opposite when you first picked up this book. You were likely overweight, and you probably ate sweets and refined flour products habitually. So you were spinning in a vicious cycle. That's why, you'll recall, the sugar and white-flour prohibition was so strict from Day 1 of the diet. You simply had to get off that merry-go-round.

And at Wave 3 you are indeed off it. And you're no longer overweight. So your metabolism is in much better condition to deal with blood sugar rushes brought on by occasional forays into white bread and sugar territory. As long as they really are *occasional*, you can handle it.

EXERCISE

Another way to intensify your Sonoma Diet lifestyle is by seeking more ways to have fun through physical activity. By Wave 3, whatever exercise plan you've chosen should have become a habit—that is, it's by now such a routine part of your day that you feel uncomfortable any time you miss a walk, a jog, or whatever workout you had scheduled.

You'll continue, of course, to do your regular exercise. Your heart and your weight won't have it any other way. But for Wave 3, you'll want to look for opportunities to challenge yourself physically, doing things that have nothing to do with exercise as a routine. In Sonoma County, for example, biking and hiking are as normal for most people as breathing and sleeping are for people elsewhere.

Wherever you live, get used to taking a walk after dinner instead of flipping on the television. Or go bowling or hiking instead of to the movies on a weekend. Just for the heck of it, take the stairs instead of the escalator or elevator. Spend some time puttering in the garden on a regular basis.

These are little things, to be sure, but they help keep the weight off and your energy up. And, conveniently, having the weight off makes these little activities more appealing. They also accumulate to create an active lifestyle. Your life will be richer, healthier, and a lot more fun.

GUIDELINES FOR LIFE

Whichever of the suggested tweaks and adjustments you implement, they will come in the context of your newly adopted mindful eating habits that have made the Sonoma guidelines second nature and good choices a matter of course.

You know, for example, that white bread and other refined flour products are an open invitation to weight gain and metabolic problems. You realize that saturated and hydrogenated fats are just as unhealthy for people at their best weight as they are for overweight people. You won't eat them.

The Sonoma way of life also includes the plate proportions you became used to in Wave 2. For lunch and dinner, that means equal parts grains, fruit, vegetables, and either protein or dairy. You're used to reasonable portion sizes now as well, and you should stick with them—though you can eyeball the amounts instead of using the same seven- and nine-inch plates. (You may have already switched to estimates long ago; that's fine as long as you're hitting the sizes and proportions accurately.)

You'll also want to keep your kitchen stocked with Sonoma-pantry foods. There's no need to keep unhealthy foods in your cabinets. And chances are you don't want to see them there anyway.

The food lists you've been using are still operative and always will be. Continue to eat more of the Tier 1 vegetables and the Tier 2 fruits and vegetables than those on Tier 3. Continue to avoid the foods you've been avoiding since day 1—fatty meats, potatoes, full-fat dairy products, hydrogenated fats, refined grains, and sugared sweets.

These are guidelines you've been following from the get-go. Again, they're lifestyle choices. The only difference now is that you're following them for health and weight maintenance reasons, and no longer for weight loss. They're just as important as ever.

What people are saying about Sonoma...

> *"I love the Sonoma way of life; I believe in it and plan to live it! I have done some walking in the past but now it is so much easier after the weight loss. I now walk every day and have even introduced some running. I will complete my first 5K next year!"*
>
> —Donna, lost 38 pounds

IF THINGS GO WRONG

What happens if your weight starts to creep up again? First of all, understand that there's no shame in this, and it's certainly nothing to panic about. In fact, it's likely to happen to even the most dedicated devotees of The Sonoma Diet lifestyle at some point in their lives. Things can happen. And this is exactly why Wave 3 exists. It's a built-in safety net.

The most obvious reason for the new weight gain is that you've over-tweaked. In other words, your adjustment from weight loss to maintenance went a little too far, and it's showing on the scale.

You may have added too much in the way of extra fruits or breads, or let your portions edge up a little bit extra, or overdone it with the "occasional" treats. Take it back a notch. Go easier on the extra fruits and breads, watch your portions, and add some extra days between those treats. Make sure you're not oversnacking too.

It's possible that retweaking won't get your weight back down fast enough for your satisfaction. That's okay too. The solution is to simply go back to Wave 2 until you're back to your ideal weight. You're an old hand at this, after all, so it's simply a question of sticking to the Wave 2 guidelines again. That's what they're there for, and you may be reverting to them more than once over the years. Good health is a lifetime commitment.

The most drastic action you'll have to take in Wave 3 comes only if you find yourself not just regaining weight but slipping into the old sugar and white flour habits. And even this action isn't all that drastic. But you do have to nip this relapse in the bud, and the way to do that is to revert not to Wave 2 but all the way back to Wave 1.

Remember that Wave 1 is characterized by a total ban on sweets, even sugarless sweets. Stick to all the guidelines of Wave 1, including limiting yourself to Tier 1 vegetables and using the Wave 1 plate percentages.

After ten days, move to Wave 3 if you're back at your target weight. If not, go on to Wave 2 and stay there until your weight is where it needs to be.

MINDFUL LIVING

I've talked about mindful eating several times in this book. I didn't invent the term, but it's at the core of the Sonoma approach to food and eating. The easiest way to define the term is simply to think of its opposite—mindless eating.

When you eat mindfully, you take yourself off automatic pilot to actually pay attention to the food you're eating. Mindful eaters are truly aware of what they're buying when they buy food, of what they're doing to it when they cook it, and of what it tastes and feels like as they eat it. By being mindful rather than impulsive, you develop a new relationship with food and eating, one that's healthier and more enjoyable.

You've already done that as you followed the Sonoma food guides and meal plans in Waves 1 and 2. You were being mindful when you made an effort to include a variety of colors in your fruit and vegetable servings. You were being mindful when you chose whole grains like brown rice over processed grains like white bread. You were being mindful when you began focusing on whole, fresh foods instead of foods that have been processed and packaged. And you were being mindful when you began savoring every bite of your meals instead of rushing through them with the television on.

You will, of course, continue those good, mindful habits in Wave 3. I also suggest that you use Wave 3 to deepen your mindfulness in a way that will take your new healthy lifestyle to a new level. In Wave 3 you can start focusing on the big picture, on what it really takes to be healthy and happy in life, instead of just "managing" your "diet." There are lots of things you can do to open the door to that kind of mindful living.

For example, check out your local farmers' market if you haven't already, and become a regular if you have. Here is where you can really know about the food you're buying, where you can ask for recipe suggestions, and sample new or heirloom varieties. You can talk personally to the growers about what if any fertilizers and pesticides they use. It's the perfect place to develop a more "personal" relationship with the food you eat. (Visit localharvest.org for more information.)

You can try to buy local as much as possible. Food that isn't processed to travel long distances is more likely to be richer in nutrients. Buy local eggs, local produce from the farmers' market, and local bread from artisan bakers.

You can pay attention to the seasons. The fruits and vegetables you eat certainly do. By eating produce in season, you're not only getting better quality, you're connecting to something about that fruit or vegetable that is lost when you eat it any time of year. Again, your local farmers' market is a good place to find out exactly what is in season when. When local produce is in season, you can buy in bulk and freeze, pickle, or preserve the extra.

And you can find ways to eat the entire food, down to the last bit. That was standard practice in North America until the twentieth century. The stems of cauliflower, broccoli, and herbs, the inner leaves of celery, the fronds of fennel, and the greens of beets (to give a few examples) are all edible. They make tasty additions to soups, sauces, stocks, and even salads.

WHAT ABOUT ORGANIC?

Eating organic is more than just a trend. There is growing evidence that organic foods may be better for you than conventionally grown foods.

What is organic? U.S. government standards require foods to be produced without the use of most conventional pesticides and without synthetic fertilizers if they are to be labeled organic. They cannot have been genetically modified, irradiated to kill bacteria, or fertilized with sewage sludge from wastewater treatment plants. Organic meat, poultry, eggs, and dairy products must come from animals that are given organic feed without antibiotics or growth hormones.

Because of those standards, you're taking in a lot less pesticides and artificial preservatives when you eat organic. You're probably also getting less in the way of artificial ingredients, sodium, and partially hydrogenated oils (trans fats). And most people think organic food tastes better.

The drawback, as you probably know, is that organic foods tend to cost more than nonorganic. That's why it's difficult for me to recommend that you eat 100% organic. Another reason is priority. Overall, the health benefits of wholesome, nutrient-rich foods that are part of a balanced diet outweigh the sole concept of eating organic.

Still, if possible, you could easily consider eating a portion of fruits, vegetables, meats, dairy, and even whole grains from organic sources to make the most of your everyday meals. This would be a particularly good decision when buying those fruits and vegetables that tend to have the highest levels of pesticide residues. ▪

SMART SHOPPING FOR ORGANICS

This chart shows which fruits and vegetables are the least and the most contaminated by pesticides.

MOST CONTAMINATED

apples	bell peppers	cherries
imported grapes	lettuce	nectarines
peaches	pears	potatoes
spinach	strawberries	

LEAST CONTAMINATED

asparagus	avocado	bananas
broccoli	mango	pineapple
	sweet corn	

EATING OUT
· on The New Sonoma Diet ·

Enjoying meals at restaurants is a way of life in Sonoma County—and a true pleasure everywhere. The Sonoma Diet is designed so that you can eat out without missing a beat in your weight loss program.

But you do have to take action to stick with your Sonoma Diet meal plans and portion sizes when you're eating away from home. Your mission is to make sure that your restaurant meals are adjusted to your diet, not the other way around.

It's easier than you think. Most restaurants are happy to accommodate you. Even those places with more rigid menus, such as chains or fast-food restaurants, have options that fit in with your meal plans.

ON THE ROAD, ON THE PLAN

If you eat out a lot, you have several options. When staying out of town, seek out big supermarkets, health food stores, and farmers' markets. They're as easy to find as any restaurant. And they always have available Sonoma Diet-style food. Some markets even offer fresh foods prepared and ready to eat.

At restaurants, at home or away, simply order according to the food guidelines and eat controlled amounts that correspond to the plate percentages (usually 25% each of protein, whole grain, fruit, and vegetables). Rare is the restaurant that doesn't offer options that fit into The Sonoma Diet.

Even fast-food places have salads with low-calorie dressings, grilled chicken breasts, lean turkey, and vegetable broth–based soups. At regular restaurants, it's easy to order a chicken or fish dish or a lean cut of red meat. Fruits and vegetables are always there for the asking. Don't be a slave to the way things are presented on the menu; order exactly what you want.

You will have to make a few special requests. Wave away the breadbasket, hold the butter and creamy sauces, and skip any cheese, croutons, or the like. Get your entrée without white rice or potato; if the restaurant offers brown rice, order that. If not, ask for a whole-wheat roll for your whole grain. Many restaurants will make individual salads that contain lean cuts of protein with a vinaigrette. Take some ideas from The Sonoma Diet salads; they're made with ingredients that most restaurants stock. Describe a specific Sonoma Diet salad and see if they'll prepare it.

Most waiters are used to special requests, and any restaurant worth eating at will gladly accommodate you. Always remember that you're there to eat what you want and enjoy yourself. You'll be surprised at how easy and fun it is to eat out and still stick to The Sonoma Diet guidelines.

TIPS FOR DINING OUT

- *Research appropriate restaurants* online at Healthy Dining Finder (http://healthydiningfinder.com). This dietician-approved site can locate healthy dining choices across the country and in any price range.

- *Check out the menu online.* Many restaurants have a website that lists the menu. If you can get an advance look at the menu, you can avoid any confusion or discomfort that might come from making a last-minute decision about what to request.

- *Phone ahead.* The surest way to know ahead of time if a restaurant will work with your food preferences is to ask. Call during nonpeak hours, explain very briefly what your general needs are, and see what response you get.

- *Engage the waiter.* Ask questions about how a dish is prepared if the menu is not clear. For example, is it cooked with animal fat or vegetable oil? How big is the portion? Any minimally competent server will be glad to answer or find out if he or she doesn't know.

- *Seize control of your salad dressing.* Ask for extra-virgin olive oil and vinegar or reduced-fat or fat-free dressing. And order the salad dressing on the side so you can control how much you eat.

- *Have plenty of water.* Drink a glass before, during, and after your meal.

- *Watch your portion sizes.* Visualize the 2-cup bowl and the 7- or 9-inch plate as you're served. Arrange the food on the plate as you would at home to follow the prescribed proportions for the wave you're on. If decorum prevents you from doing this physically, do it in your mind. This gives you an idea of how much to eat.

- *Eat only The Sonoma Diet portion.* If you're served more than that, put the excess in a to-go box before you start eating. Or share with your dining partner.

- *Order for two.* If you know in advance that the portions will be too large, consider splitting a meal with your dining partner.

- *Order what you want.* Don't be a slave to the menu. If it indicates that white rice comes with the salmon, ask for brown or wild rice instead. If that can't be done, ask the waiter to substitute vegetables for the rice. Manipulate your order to approximate the grains/protein/vegetable/fruit proportions appropriate for The Sonoma Diet wave you're on. Focus on choosing nutrient-rich foods.

- *Eat slowly and mindfully.* Slow, pleasure-oriented dining is always a must on The Sonoma Diet. Taste and savor your meal and enjoy the conversation that goes with it.

- *Watch the 3 Bs.* Butter, refined-wheat bread, and high-calorie beverages are an easy temptation at a restaurant. Try to avoid them. If you do have bread, ask for whole-wheat and some olive oil for dipping.

- *Pass on the salt shaker.* Look for other ways to flavor your food, such as herbs or a squeeze of fresh lemon.

RESTAURANT RECOMMENDATIONS

FAST-FOOD BURGER CHAINS (BURGER KING, MCDONALD'S, WENDY'S, ETC.)

- Garden side salads with reduced-fat or fat-free salad dressing. Remove the crackers and cheese.
- Skinless, boneless chicken breast, grilled or charbroiled. Remove the bun. Eat it with a salad or use it to top your salad.

FAST-FOOD SANDWICH CHAINS (BRUEGGER'S, PANERA, SUBWAY, ETC.)

- Low-carb, whole-wheat tortilla filled with chicken or turkey breast, lean ham, or lean roast beef. Include cucumber, onion, pepper, spinach, tomato, or any other vegetables that are appropriate for your current diet wave.
- Add Dijon mustard or a reduced-fat or fat-free Italian salad dressing or a small amount of oil and vinegar for flavor.
- Add a tablespoon of feta cheese or parmesan cheese.

CHINESE RESTAURANTS

- Stir-fried skinless, boneless chicken breast, fish, scallops, shrimp, lean beef, or lean pork. Ask the chef to leave the breading off the meat.
- Stir-fried vegetables, such as asparagus, bok choy, broccoli, cabbage, cauliflower, green beans, zucchini, and/or other appropriate vegetables.
- Stir-fried tofu, once you reach Wave 2. Make sure there's no breading.
- Brown rice, and watch the portion size; estimate about ½ cup.

ITALIAN RESTAURANTS

- Grilled or broiled skinless, boneless chicken breast, lean beef, lean pork, fish, lobster, mussels, scallops, shrimp, and/or other shellfish flavored with herbs and not breaded.

- Avoid creamy sauces.

- Ask for sautéed fresh vegetables tossed with a little olive oil.

- Avoid pasta unless whole-wheat pasta is available. Watch the portion size.

- Choose a side salad with dark, leafy greens. Ask for fresh vegetables to top the salad. Drizzle a little extra-virgin olive oil and flavored vinegar or reduced-fat or fat-free salad dressing over the salad.

WATCH THE WORDS

When you're reading a menu, here are some words describing cooking methods and ingredients that usually lead to lower fat and calories. They're most likely to conform to The Sonoma Diet guidelines. And in the second column are red-flag terms that indicate a food you should avoid.

LOOK FOR	AVOID
broiled	au gratin
en papillote	basted
garden-fresh	braised
grain medley	buttered/buttery
grilled	casserole
in its own juice	creamed/cream sauce
nut-coated	crispy
plank roasted/	escalloped
oven roasted/	fried
brick roasted	hash
poached with wine/	hollandaise
herbs	in butter sauce
seared	in cheese sauce
steamed	in its own gravy
stir-fry	marinated in oil
	pan-fried
	pot pie
	prime

MEXICAN RESTAURANTS

- Choose skinless, boneless chicken breast, lean beef, lean pork, scallops, or shrimp.

- Choose black beans or whole-bean soup instead of refried beans. Avoid the rice unless brown rice is available.

- Ask for a fresh guacamole or guacamole that is not prepared with added fat such as sour cream.

- Top meat with salsa, lettuce, and/or tomatoes; leave off the sour cream.

BUFFETS

- Sit as far away from the buffet table as possible.

- Fill your plate once, approximating the portion sizes and the proportions of proteins, whole grains, and vegetables appropriate for your wave.

- Eat slowly—keep a little food on your plate until the last person at your table is finished eating to avoid the temptation of accompanying your tablemates to the buffet for their second trip. ■

BUILD A SMARTER SALAD

In the buffet line or any time you eat out, you can create a great-tasting, healthy salad if you focus on these ingredients:

dark greens
nuts and seeds
vegetables and herbs
beans and legumes
small amounts
of flavorful cheese
dry fruits
plant oils
vinegars

Many restaurants are now offering calorie counts for menu selections. This information can be used in addition to Sonoma dining tips for making the best choices. Try to keep your meals under 600 calories with less than 20 grams of fat, less than 8 grams of saturated fat, and less than 700 milligrams of sodium. Keep in mind that a three-and-a-half-ounce glass of wine is 80 calories.

WHAT ABOUT WORK?

Don't worry that workplace cafeterias might throw you off. There's not much on The Sonoma Diet that can't be prepared at home and brought to work for either microwaving or eating straight from the carrying container. Specifically, bagged salad blends are good. Try different ones for variety. Top them with cooked chicken breasts, tuna, lean lunchmeat, or hard-cooked eggs. Add a fruit and a whole-wheat roll and you have something pretty close to the usual lunch food proportions.

OTHER IDEAS: Bring leftover lean steaks, chicken breasts, or fish to heat up at work. Look for Sonoma Express recipes for easy-to-make wraps using a variety of ingredients. You can always bring frozen fruits or vegetables to microwave or just open. Cubed chicken, pork, or ham with a raw vegetable, an apple, and a whole-grain roll or whole-grain crackers will give you an easy and complete lunch. With a little creativity and some planning, you can pretty much have any lunch you want at work.

FAQS

· About The New Sonoma Diet ·

By now you know the ins and outs of The Sonoma Diet. Still, you might have some questions that the book hasn't answered so far. Here are some of the frequently asked questions about the diet, with answers that will keep you on track for living the whole-health Sonoma lifestyle.

Let's start with solutions for the direst of emergencies. Then I'll run down strategies for dealing with less urgent problems.

CRISIS QUESTIONS

I'm absolutely craving something sweet on Wave 1. Can't I have even a little of a noncaloric sweetener?

It's true that even noncaloric sweets are discouraged in Wave 1 to help you overcome your sugar addiction. Be strong, and you'll find you can do without sugary sweets by the end of Wave 1. And it's definitely worth it, because you can't eat sugar and lose weight at the same time. Plus, the natural goodness of fruits and vegetables comes out more when you're cured of the sugar habit.

Just when you think you're ready to give in, go one more day before you call it an emergency situation. That one day often makes the difference! Then, if you really can't make it ten days without something sweet, allow yourself some sugar-free gelatin or a noncaloric sweetener in your tea or coffee. That's a lot better than breaking down and eating an entire cheesecake! But it's still a stopgap. Try to have a sweetless day the day after each of these indulgences.

If you can just hang on for ten days until Wave 2, you'll have several nonsugar sweet options. Ideally, you'll want them less by that time, but they'll be available.

Why have I stopped losing weight completely on Wave 2?

Make sure you're following the guidelines faithfully. Here's a checklist:

☐ My plates and bowls are the right size.

☐ I'm filling the plate with the right percentages of grains, protein, fruits, vegetables, and dairy.

☐ I'm not heaping the portions.

☐ I'm not surpassing my three daily fat servings.

☐ The red meat I'm choosing is very lean.

☐ I'm not eating the dark meat of poultry, and I'm getting rid of the chicken skin.

☐ I'm not eating extra servings of Tier 2 or 3 vegetables.

☐ I'm snacking just enough to satisfy between-meal hunger.

☐ The breads and cereals I'm eating are truly 100% whole grain.

☐ No sugar is sneaking into my diet.

I still can't get used to doing without white bread and a sugared dessert. So naturally I'm not losing weight anymore now that I'm on Wave 2. Any suggestions?

You need to go through Wave 1 again. That will solve both your problems. You'll start losing weight again, because the calorie count is lower on Wave 1. Also, you need ten more days of no sweets—not even sugarless sweets—to kick your sugar and white-flour habit. Once you do, Wave 2 will be more enjoyable and more efficient. You'll lose weight without craving sweets and white flour.

My weight loss is going way too slow. I'll never have the patience to keep it up at this rate. What can I do?

Your best bet is to take up exercise if you haven't already done so. Even a minimum amount of physical activity—walking for half an hour a day, for example—will help you burn off calories. Refer to the information on pages 132–135 for more exercise suggestions.

Also, choose vegetables only from Tier 1 and fruits only from Tier 2. Don't fill your plate to the edges; just that slight decrease in portion size will pay off as days go by (and you'll still be eating more calories than on Wave 1). Choose skinless chicken and fish more often than red meat as your protein serving. Eat even slower; you'll eat less that way.

I still crave some foods like crazy. Sometimes I'll give in and down a ton of salty snacks like potato chips or devour enough candy bars for a week. How do I drop the bad-food bingeing habit?

As soon as you feel a craving coming on, go do something else that doesn't involve food. Go for a walk. Take a shower. Call a friend on the phone—and not a cell or wireless you can carry into the kitchen with you. Cravings are often temporary. Stall them.

- Or put something else in your mouth, such as gum or a sugar-free drop.

- Distract yourself from the craving by eating something acceptable—a Tier 1 vegetable or some other allowable snack.

- Drink a huge glass of water. Sometimes what's triggering your craving is really thirst.

- Eat a "light" version of the food you're craving. A square of dark, bittersweet chocolate is an allowed occasional sweet. Have one if a chocolate craving hits, but distance yourself from the rest of your chocolate stash. Instead of giving into potato-chip cravings, bake some salted slices of a sweet potato, sprayed with a little olive oil.

OTHER CONCERNS

Now that we've got the major crises taken care of, what about all the other nagging questions that come to you as you work your way through the diet? Every Sonoma dieter experiences doubts or confusion. In fact, the same topics seem to pop up over and over. Here are some of them, grouped by categories.

FOOD ISSUES

What do I do with recipes that have different food types in them—such as a grain-and-vegetable medley? How do I apply that to the percentages?

You can tell from the ingredients in the recipe how much of each food type is in there. Then adjust accordingly. For example, if a dish consists of equal parts whole grains, protein, and vegetables, your task is easy. Simply spoon it out to fill three quarters of your plate and add a fruit to fill the last quarter. You now have the 25-25-25-25 ratio that most Wave 2 meals call for.

If the recipe dish is, say, mostly protein with some vegetables, consider it a protein dish. Use it to fill a tad more than the 25% of the plate reserved for protein and make up the missing vegetables with another vegetable.

As you can see, this is not a precise science. But you can come pretty close to the right percentages by using a little bit of eyeballing, some basic math, and a good dose of common sense. And it gets easier as you progress in the diet and get used to the plate and the percentages.

Are canned and frozen vegetables okay?

Yes. Fresh is best, of course, but frozen is fine too. Canned is your third choice. Check the ingredient list to make sure that no sauces, sugar, or oils have been added to the canned foods.

How do I get enough protein if I don't want to eat eggs or meat?

If you eat fish, you're in fine shape. Fish is a great protein source with the added benefit of healthy omega-3 fats. If you don't want to eat fish either, you'll find other protein sources on The Sonoma Diet Proteins and Dairy lists (page 103 for Wave 1; page 121 for Wave 2). They include beans and soy products, dairy, soy, quinoa, combinations of beans with grains, and Barilla Plus pasta.

Can I eat nut butters?

Try all-natural nut butters with no added sugar or partially hydrogenated fats. Dab a tablespoon on a piece of whole-wheat bread or a fruit—the fats and protein in the nut butters slow the blood sugar release of the carbohydrates in the bread or fruit and really satisfy hunger.

Can I use butter?

In Wave 3, you can use butter as an occasional treat. Butter, whether it's in spray or stick form, is loaded with saturated fat. Margarine is not a substitute—it contains trans fats. Whenever possible, use olive oil.

What if I find a vegetable that's not on any list?

If it's starchy, such as a root vegetable, consider it Tier 3. If it's watery, such as a cucumber, it's probably low in calories and fiber rich. So you can treat it as a Tier 1 vegetable. In between the two? It's probably a Tier 2.

I like to snack all day instead of eating three big meals. Can I spread my meals out throughout the day?

The Sonoma Diet is based on three meals a day—breakfast, lunch, and dinner. There are two reasons for this. One is that three squares is the way almost everybody eats. The other is that, at each meal, the three-a-day system gives you the beneficial food combinations described earlier in the book.

If spreading out your meals is important to you, you can try it. You'll have to do the math so that you're eating the same amount of food in the same percentages as you would on a three-a-day plan. But keep in mind that you'll be sacrificing the full benefit of the food combinations that are an important part of The Sonoma Diet—and the benefits of leisurely, shared meals.

What should I look for on food labels regarding carbs and sugar?

Carbs are too general a concept to deal with. Instead, choose baked goods and breads that contain whole grains as the primary ingredients. Avoid buying foods that contain sugar, especially as one of the first five ingredients. Sugar is also called sucrose, fructose, dextrose, or high-fructose corn syrup. You can estimate how many teaspoons per serving are contained in the product by dividing the grams of sugar per serving by four. You'll be surprised how much sugar is added to everyday foods. A good rule is to look at fiber levels for whole-wheat breads. If there isn't any fiber, don't buy it. Generally, whole-wheat breads have at least two grams of fiber per slice, and cereals can start at five grams per serving.

All I want when I wake up in the morning is a steaming mug of coffee loaded with cream and sugar. Is this a no-no?

Yes and no. If you can't stand the thought of rolling out of bed unless there's a trip to the coffeepot in the near future, don't despair. You can drink two cups of black coffee per day—then switch to tea. When it comes to sugar, however, you're out of luck. Although noncaloric sweeteners are okay in small amounts, sugar is not. Try some of the premium coffees on the market now; you may find them good enough to enjoy without cream. If you absolutely cannot drink black coffee, you can add up to one tablespoon of heavy cream to your drink as long as you limit yourself to one mug per day instead of two. More involved coffee drinks, such as mochas, are to be avoided. They contain too many calories with little to no nutrients to show for them.

TIME AND MONEY ISSUES

This diet is too expensive with all the protein, fruits, and vegetables. Is there a cheaper version?

The Sonoma Diet can push your grocery bill up a bit with its emphasis on fresh, wholesome foods. On the other hand, you'll be buying few or no processed foods, which often have added costs due to labor, transportation, marketing, and so on.

You can stock up on frozen and canned fruits and vegetables (as long as they have no added sugar). Some fresh vegetables are cheaper than others; if economy is a factor, let that decide which you buy. Fresh fruits and vegetables in season cost less. Some, such as berries, you can buy a lot of when the price is down and freeze them for later use. Check out farmers' markets; there are bargains, especially locally grown produce in season.

Look for what's on sale and make the diet work around that. For example, if chicken prices are way down this week (as they sometimes are), stock up and make chicken your protein for several days. Freeze the rest.

Look for bargains in bulk. That's often the case with beans and grains.

No Excuses

Are you an expert at finding reasons to fudge the diet guidelines? That puts you in the company of a large percentage of dieters. There's always a good excuse for eating a candy bar just this once, or for piling up the pork loin so it overflows the plate, or for going with white rice instead of brown. You're in a hurry, the pork would have been wasted otherwise, and the store was out of brown rice. And so forth.

Excuses sabotage your diet. Deal with them. Get a piece of paper and a pen and write down all the excuses you use to eat what you shouldn't. Keep the paper and pen handy because you'll surely come up with new ones as the days go by.

Then, alongside each excuse list a way to address it that makes sense for the way you live. If your excuse for eating a toaster waffle in the morning instead of the prescribed Sonoma Diet breakfast is that you don't have time, write next to that excuse, "Get up fifteen minutes earlier." If your excuse for adding sugar to your coffee is that that's what you're used to, write down "Get used to noncaloric sweetener or unsweetened coffee."

True, writing down solutions is no guarantee you'll carry them out. But when you see in black-and-white how easy it can be to overcome your excuses, the solutions are harder to ignore. Try it.

Cooking for myself takes too long. How can I cut down on the time I spend?

Take shortcuts. Most of the actual work time is spent chopping and preparing. So buy precut meats and vegetables when you can. For the rest, devote one hour at the beginning of the week to chop and prepare all the ingredients for a week's worth of meals. Then at mealtime it's just a question of putting them together and throwing them on the stove or in the oven.

Also, you can make, say, eight to ten servings of grains at a time and just reheat the amount you will be eating for lunch or dinner each day for a week. Cook up lots of steel-cut oatmeal at the beginning of the week and reheat it for breakfast every day. Or you can make any of the pancakes batters, such as the Buckwheat Pancakes recipe on page 212, up to two days ahead of time and keep it in the refrigerator.

You'll find you have more time than you thought once you realize how good and helpful the Sonoma recipes are. They feature some great ideas for saving time and money. Look for the quick and easy Sonoma Express recipes and the Cook Once/Eat Twice recipes, which help turn one meal into another without too much effort. And with your Sonoma pantry guidelines, many of your meals can be no-shop or no-cook meals.

Commit to preparing just two of the recipes in a week, even if it's just a side dish such as a grain or salad. Work your way up to four. Gradually, you'll be able to free up the time for preparing good meals. Remember, the recipes are there to give you variety so you aren't bored with your diet. They're also there to expose you to The Sonoma Diet way of cooking and the delicious possibilities of healthy food. That's worth making time for.

FAMILY ISSUES

What can I do when others in my family insist on keeping non-Sonoma Diet food in the kitchen?

Keep nutrient-rich choices like ready-cut veggies, fruits, whole grains, nut butters, and yogurts available and the not-so-great foods out of sight or out of the house. Let the family see that a healthy kitchen is no deprivation.

How can I get others in my family to accept some of the unfamiliar foods I'm now eating?

There's nothing odd about the food on The Sonoma Diet. Anyone can eat it and enjoy it. There's no reason why the meal you prepare for yourself can't be for everyone. Perhaps your family can eat a little more than you, but that should be the only difference.

Give them a challenge. Ask them to try The Sonoma Diet meals for a week. Serve your favorite recipes from the diet. See what happens. If they refuse to try the recipes, you can always serve them the meat dish that coincides with The Sonoma Diet recipe you're eating that night, and they can have their own side. They can have it their way, you'll have it your way, and the conflict will at least be minimized. Anything that can be done to help all of you enjoy a slow meal together is beneficial for everybody.

How do I deal with food pushers like Aunt Agnes at family gatherings?

If the family gathering is once a year at Thanksgiving, go ahead and accept what she insists on serving—but eat very slowly and talk a lot. You can keep the damage to a minimum and make Aunt Agnes happy at the same time.

If the family meals are more frequent, take the offensive. Briefly explain that you're trying a new style of eating and that some foods just don't fit into your new eating plan. Ask your relatives to help by not insisting you eat what you'd prefer to avoid. Then no matter what Agnes or anyone else says or does, eat what you'd planned on eating and no more. Your family will get the picture … eventually.

WINE AND ALCOHOL

I like the idea of a glass of wine at a meal, but I'm confused by it. How do I know what wines are appropriate and what goes with what?

Forget about all that. On the first day, decide how much money you can spend on a bottle of wine and buy one with a name you like. If you enjoy the wine, buy it again. If you don't, try another one. Or try one a friend recommends. The only wine rule that matters is to drink what you like and don't drink what you don't like. The way to find out what you like is to try different wines.

Can I drink some kind of alcohol besides wine?

Not until you reach your target weight. Research has revealed some health benefits from alcohol in general, but only wine packs enough healthy nutrients to make the extra calories worth it. Also, among alcoholic beverages only wine contributes to the slow, leisurely, pleasurable pace of a meal.

OTHER MATTERS

Where do I find the plates?

It's interesting how many people learn they don't have a seven- or nine-inch plate in the house once they start The Sonoma Diet. If you don't want to buy a whole set of plates at the right size, you can always go to a secondhand shop, buy just enough unmatched, interesting plates for your family, and use them for the duration of the diet. If you have plates you know are too big, check back to pages 92–94 in Wave 1 for some tips on getting the plates that work.

Will this diet affect any medications I'm on?

Possibly. But almost any change in lifestyle—including changes in eating, exercise, and weight—can. Or the medications may affect the diet. That's one reason why you must see your doctor before starting The Sonoma Diet. ■

SONOMA MADE SIMPLE

Located at the top of many of the recipes are several tabs to help you save time in the kitchen. The `SONOMA EXPRESS` tab indicates the quickest and easiest recipes, and `GLUTEN FREE` indicates recipes made without gluten flour. The `COOK 1X · EAT 2X` tab identifies those recipes that you may want to prepare extra amounts of that can then be used in other recipes, which are indicated by `COOK 1X · EAT 2X` in a Culinary Note. Think of them as delicious planned meals that are far from your everyday leftovers.

For example: If you use the Roast Chicken recipe on page 325, the tab reminds you to select a large chicken so the remaining chicken can be used in the Simple Chicken Tacos on page 329 or the Sonoma Salad with Tomatoes & Feta on page 330.

· *Part Two* ·
MEAL PLANS
& RECIPES

The Sonoma Diet was designed to be two things above all else—simple and flavorful.

I promised you at the very beginning that I would do all the thinking and figuring for you. Simply said, I wanted to keep the science behind the scenes so that the general idea or broad strokes of what it takes to eat healthfully makes sense as opposed to having you micromanage your diet. In this final section of the book, you'll reap the benefit. Here you'll find the recipes, meal plans, and food lists that will guide you through your weight loss program one day at a time.

Flexibility is the key. You can follow the menu plans for each meal for the duration of The Sonoma Diet, or you can use the information to improvise your own meals within the diet's guidelines. It's your choice.

The bulk of this part of the book is recipes—dozens of them. They consist of easy-to-follow, step-by-step instructions for preparing mouth-watering dishes that will keep you satisfied as you shed pounds.

The recipes are nothing like what most people think of as "diet food." They feature international flavors inspired by Sonoma County's adventurous culinary style. Your taste buds will never be bored.

The recipes are divided into two sections. First come those that conform to the food choices for Wave 1 of your diet. Then you'll find the more varied Wave 2 recipes. You have the comfort of knowing that the recipe you choose will be 100% appropriate for your stage of The Sonoma Diet.

The meal plans for Waves 1 and 2 offer daily menus to guide you through your eating plan. Simply by preparing and eating the suggested dishes for each meal of the day, you can progress through The Sonoma Diet on automatic pilot, with every meal planned out for you.

But if you want to improvise a bit—either to save time or add variety—you'll find plenty of suggestions. For example, you always have the choice of substituting grilled or roasted chicken (skinless, of course), extra-lean cuts of beef, or fish for any main dish. That gives you the time-saving option of preparing several days' worth of chicken breasts for the protein part of your plate. Use the Seasonings section to add flavor to your meal by choosing one of the rubs, marinades, or sauces for your chicken. If you're in the mood for a quick yet refreshing meal, create your own Sonoma Express wrap or Sonoma Express salad following the guidelines below. For those times when you're too busy to prepare anything, I've made it easy for you to choose ready-made meals or snacks from the brand list provided on page 172. And if you want to or need to go gluten free, it's easy to prepare gluten-free meals. Look for suggestions in the recipes and variations.

· SAVE TIME ·
TRY SONOMA EXPRESS

When you need a quick lunch or dinner, make it easy on yourself by replacing any of the menu items in Wave 1 or 2 with a Sonoma Express wrap, Sonoma Express salad, or Sonoma Express protein dish (see guidelines). Be sure to choose Wave-appropriate fruits and vegetables based on where you are on the diet. If you're on Wave 2, be sure to include a serving of fruit with any of these meal substitutes. The recipes feature time-saving **Cook Once/Eat Twice** tips, variations, seasonal substitutions to make favorite recipes more versatile, and culinary tips with interesting information.

Sonoma Express Wrap

These make quick and easy meal substitutes when you're in a hurry or on the go. Fill your wrap with your choice of Sonoma-friendly ingredients or follow one of our recipe ideas (see pages 232, 234, and 290).

FOR ONE WRAP:

Use one whole-wheat tortilla or a large lettuce leaf to wrap your ingredients.

Fill the tortilla or lettuce leaf with up to 1 tablespoon of your favorite spread.*

Add:

2   cups mixed greens or spinach leaves
1   cup vegetables (be sure to choose Wave-appropriate vegetables based on where you are on the diet)
Cooked lean protein such as chicken, pork, beef, or ham. Use 3 ounces for lunch or 4 ounces for dinner.
2   ounces (about 2 tablespoons) mozzarella cheese, low-fat cream cheese, or goat cheese *(optional)*

*Note: See the Seasonings section (starting on page 174) for full-flavored spreads such as Cilantro Pesto or Black Bean–Smoked Chile Spread. If you're feeling pressed for time, use purchased products such as roasted tomato salsa, artichoke spread, or hummus.

SONOMA EXPRESS SALAD

This salad is a simple way to use what you have on hand for lunch or dinner. If you're on Wave 2, add a serving of fruit to your meal.

FOR ONE SALAD:

2   cups mixed greens or spinach leaves
1   cup vegetables (be sure to choose Wave-appropriate vegetables based on where you are on the diet)
½   cup cooked beans (canned work well), or have 2 whole-wheat crackers with your salad.
Cooked lean protein such as chicken, pork, beef, ham, or eggs. Use 3 ounces for lunch or 4 ounces for dinner, or 2 eggs for either meal.
2   ounces (about 2 tablespoons) mozzarella cheese, low-fat cream cheese, or goat cheese (optional)
Choice of salad dressing*

*Note: See the Seasonings section for dressings such as Gazpacho Vinaigrette or Sherry Mustard Vinaigrette. Or use a purchased low-calorie salad dressing.

SONOMA EXPRESS PROTEINS

FOR ONE SERVING:

4-ounce portion of fish, lean beef, or skinless, boneless chicken breast
Choice of rub or marinade from the Seasonings section*
Prepare the proteins according to your preferred method; the easiest is to grill, bake, or broil.

*Note: The rub and marinade recipes make enough for 4 to 6 servings of meat, so it's easy to accommodate more servings. Cooking time remains the same.

Brand List

Today's marketplace provides many food products that will fit into your diet. These specific selections are distributed nationwide and are among the best for use with this diet, since they reflect top-quality, wholesome products.

WHOLE GRAINS

Ak Mak *whole-grain crackers*
Barilla *Plus pastas*
Bobs Red Mill *ground flaxseed*
Ezequiel *Breakfast cereals*
General Mills *Fiber-One cereals*
Healthy Choice, Orowheat, Brownberry, and Earthgrains *multigrain breads*
Kashi *multigrain cereals (choose varieties with more than 8 grams of fiber per serving), multigrain crackers, and oatmeal*
Kellogg's *Bran Flakes, Bran Buds*
La Tortilla Factory *whole-grain, nutrient-rich wraps and tortillas: Look for the* Smart And Delicious *line for interesting varieties*
Lundberg *rice varieties and whole-grain rice chips*
McCann's *Steel-Cut Oats*
Nature's Path *Breakfast cereals*
Near East *tabbouleh blends*
Quaker Oats *rolled oats*
Rye-Krisp *crackers*
Wasa *high-fiber crackers*

FRUITS AND VEGETABLES

Bush Beans *canned beans*
Dole or Fresh Express *salad blends with dark greens such as spinach or romaine*
Muir Glen *fire-roasted tomatoes (canned)*

SEASONINGS

Frontera *roasted salsas*
Kraft *Light Done Right salad dressings*
Newman's Own *light salad dressings*

DAIRY

Eggland's Best *omega-3 eggs*
Fage *Greek Style Yogurt, low fat to nonfat, plain*
Stonyfield Farms *yogurt*
The Laughing Cow *Mini Babybel cheese wheels or light spreadable cheese wedges*

SOUPS

Amy's *organic entrées*
Progresso *lentil and black bean varieties*

FROZEN FOOD

Lean Cuisine *Spa Cuisine meals*

SEASONINGS

As you've read over and over throughout this book, The Sonoma Diet is all about full-flavored, delicious food. This section offers you rubs and marinades for meat and poultry, spreads for wraps, and salad dressings that you can use on salads, as marinades, or as dips and spreads. Don't be afraid to get creative with flavor!

And when you need a quick, simple meal, try the following recipes for rubs, marinades, and spreads to enhance a Sonoma Express wrap, Sonoma Express salad, or Sonoma Express protein dish.

APPLE CIDER & SAGE MARINADE
FOR PORK LOIN OR CHICKEN

Start to finish: 20 minutes, plus 15 minutes for marinating
Yield: 4 servings

1   pound pork loin or chicken breast, excess fat removed

¼   cup apple cider

1   teaspoon cider vinegar

1   pinch cinnamon, ground

½   tablespoon soy sauce

1   teaspoon sage, chopped

Salt and pepper to taste

1. Season pork or chicken with salt and pepper.

2. Combine remaining ingredients and stir to mix. Place in a leakproof container or resealable bag such as a Ziploc bag; force out all the air so that the meat is in contact with the marinade. Add pork or chicken. Let sit for 15 minutes to overnight.

3. Grill or sauté the meat.

ASIAN HERB MARINADE

Start to Finish: 25 minutes, plus 4 to 24 hours for marinating
Yield: enough for 2 pounds pork, chicken, or salmon

½ cup lightly packed fresh cilantro

¼ cup fresh ginger, minced

¼ cup lightly packed fresh mint leaves

10 cloves garlic, halved

½ to 1 fresh serrano chile pepper, seeded and cut up*

1 tablespoon toasted sesame oil

1 tablespoon lime juice

1 teaspoon freshly ground black pepper

½ teaspoon kosher salt

1. In a food processor combine cilantro, ginger, mint, garlic, serrano, sesame oil, lime juice, black pepper, and kosher salt. Cover and process to a thick paste, scraping down side of bowl as necessary.

2. To use as a marinade, spread over 2 pounds pork tenderloin, chicken breast halves, or salmon steaks. Cover and chill in the refrigerator for 4 to 24 hours. Grill or roast pork; grill or broil chicken or salmon.

CULINARY NOTES

- You can place the marinade in a freezer container, seal, label, and freeze for up to three months. Thaw before using.

- * Because hot chile peppers contain oils that can burn your skin and eyes, wear rubber or plastic gloves when working with them. If your bare hands do touch the chile peppers, wash your hands well with soap and water.

CHARMOULA MARINADE

Start to Finish: 10 minutes, plus 8 to 24 hours for marinating
Yield: enough for 3 to 4 pounds fish, poultry, beef, or pork

½ cup extra-virgin olive oil

½ cup lemon juice

½ cup chopped fresh flat-leaf parsley

½ cup chopped fresh cilantro

4 cloves garlic, minced (2 teaspoons minced)

1 tablespoon paprika

2 teaspoons ground cumin

1 teaspoon kosher salt

½ teaspoon cayenne pepper

¼ teaspoon freshly ground black pepper

1. In a medium bowl whisk together oil, lemon juice, parsley, cilantro, garlic, paprika, cumin, kosher salt, cayenne pepper, and black pepper until combined.

2. To use as a marinade, place 3 to 4 pounds fish steaks, chicken breast halves, turkey breast tenderloin, beef steaks, or boneless pork chops in a self-sealing plastic bag; pour lemon juice mixture over. Seal bag; turn bag to coat fish, poultry, or meat. Marinate in the refrigerator for 8 to 24 hours. Remove from marinade, discarding marinade. Grill or broil fish, poultry, or meat.

CHIPOTLE LIME MARINADE
FOR CHICKEN OR PORK

Start to Finish: 15 minutes   Yield: ¾ cup

½ cup lime juice

3 tablespoons chipotle in adobo sauce (canned)

1 tablespoon coriander, ground

1 pinch cumin seeds

¼ cup olive oil

Salt and pepper to taste

Combine all ingredients in a blender. Blend until smooth.

CULINARY NOTES

- Adjust the heat of the marinade by using more chile than sauce if you want a hotter marinade.

- If you taste the marinade and the chile heat shows up in the back of your throat, add more salt to the marinade. Salt will tone down the heat and bring it to the center of your palate.

MEDITERRANEAN HERB MARINADE

Start to Finish: 20 minutes plus 4 to 24 hours for marinating
Yield: enough for 2 pounds pork, chicken, or salmon

½ cup lightly packed fresh flat-leaf parsley

¼ cup olive oil

3 tablespoons fresh rosemary leaves

3 tablespoons fresh thyme leaves

2 tablespoons fresh sage, coarsely chopped

2 tablespoons lemon peel, finely shredded

10 cloves garlic, halved

½ to 1 teaspoon crushed red pepper

½ teaspoon kosher salt

¼ to ½ teaspoon freshly ground black pepper

1. In a food processor combine parsley, oil, rosemary, thyme, sage, lemon peel, garlic, crushed red pepper, kosher salt, and black pepper. Cover and process to a thick paste, scraping down side of bowl as necessary.

2. To use as a marinade, spread over 2 pounds pork tenderloin, chicken breast halves, or salmon steaks. Cover and chill for 4 to 24 hours.

3. Grill or roast pork; grill or broil chicken or salmon.

CULINARY NOTE

You can place the marinade in a freezer container; seal, label, and freeze for up to 3 months. Thaw before using.

SPANISH MARINADE
FOR PORK LOIN OR CHICKEN BREASTS

Start to Finish: 25 minutes, including 15 minutes for marinating
Yield: 4 servings

1 teaspoon garlic, mashed to a paste

1 tablespoon extra-virgin olive oil

½ teaspoon ground cumin, roasted

¼ teaspoon ground coriander, roasted

1 teaspoon Spanish paprika, smoked or plain

¼ teaspoon ground ginger

¼ teaspoon turmeric

¼ teaspoon ground black pepper

1 teaspoon lemon juice and zest

salt and pepper to taste

1. Mix ingredients together.

2. Place in a leakproof container or resealable bag, such as a Ziploc bag. Add pork or chicken. Let sit for 15 minutes to overnight. Grill or sauté the meat.

SPICY CHIPOTLE BROTH
FOR POACHING FISH

Start to Finish: 30 minutes   *Yield: 4 Servings*

½ tablespoon extra-virgin olive oil

1 cup onions, sliced

2 teaspoons garlic, chopped

1 teaspoon chipotle chiles in adobo sauce, chopped

1 large pinch cumin seeds

1 cup canned tomatoes, drained, chopped

1½ cups chicken stock

1 cup chickpeas, drained; reserve ¼ cup chickpea liquid

salt and pepper to taste

1 tablespoon chopped cilantro or parsley (optional)

1 cup spinach (optional)

1 pound fish, such as salmon, cod, halibut, or sea bass

1. Heat a large sauté pan over medium heat. Add extra-virgin olive oil and onions; sauté for 4 minutes or until slightly caramelized. Add garlic, chipotle, and cumin; cook 15 seconds. Add tomatoes, chicken stock, chickpeas and their liquid. Bring to a simmer. Cook for 10 minutes or until the flavors have melded. Season with salt and pepper. Add optional herbs and spinach; cook to wilt.

2. Add fish in a single layer. Cover and simmer for 5 to 6 minutes or until fish flakes easily when tested with a fork. Using a slotted spatula, carefully transfer fish to a platter. Serve with sauce and vegetables.

Spicy Chipotle Broth Variations:

- **Spanish:** Replace the chipotle chiles with 1 teaspoon Spanish paprika. Add ¼ cup roasted red peppers when the tomatoes are added.
- **Mediterranean:** Replace the chipotle chiles, cumin, and chickpeas with white beans and basil. Serve with basil pesto on top.

Nutrition Facts per Serving: 150 calories, 7 g protein, 3 g total fat (.5 g saturated fat), 25 g carbohydrate, 5 g fiber, 0 g cholesterol, 300 mg sodium, 3.5 glycemic load

TANDOORI MARINADE
FOR CHICKEN

Start to Finish: 15 minutes, plus 4 hours for marinating
Yield: enough for 1 to 1½ pounds chicken

6 ounces plain low-fat probiotic yogurt

¼ cup lemon juice

1 tablespoon fresh ginger, grated

2 tablespoons fresh cilantro, chopped

2 cloves garlic, minced (1 teaspoon)

1 tablespoon cumin seeds, toasted and crushed

½ teaspoon kosher salt

¼ teaspoon cayenne pepper

1. In a small bowl stir together yogurt, lemon juice, ginger, cilantro, garlic, cumin seeds, kosher salt, and cayenne pepper.

2. To use as a marinade, place 1 to 1½ pounds chicken breast halves in a self-sealing plastic bag; pour yogurt mixture over chicken. Seal bag; turn bag to coat chicken. Marinate in the refrigerator for 4 hours. Remove from marinade, discarding marinade. Grill or broil chicken.

CULINARY NOTE

To toast and crush seeds, heat a small skillet over medium heat. Add seeds. Cook about 2 minutes or until toasted and aromatic, shaking skillet frequently. Place toasted seeds in a spice grinder and process until crushed.

COFFEE RUB
FOR BEEF OR PORK

Start to Finish: 20 minutes   Yield: ½ cup, enough for 4 pounds of meat

¼ cup chili powder

¼ cup coffee, finely ground

2 tablespoons
   Spanish paprika

2 tablespoons brown sugar

1 tablespoon coriander,
   ground

½ teaspoon cinnamon, ground

1 tablespoon salt

1 tablespoon black
   peppercorns, ground

¼ teaspoon cayenne

1. Combine all ingredients in a bowl.

2. Season meat with salt and pepper. Sprinkle 2 tablespoons rub evenly on 1 pound of meat. Let sit for 30 minutes prior to cooking. Sprinkle the meat with ½–1 tablespoon of oil before grilling.

Jamaican Jerk Rub

Start to Finish: 35 minutes
Yield: enough for 1 pound meat or poultry

½ cup onion, coarsely chopped	¼ teaspoon curry powder
2 tablespoons lime juice	¼ teaspoon freshly ground black pepper
1 teaspoon crushed red pepper	⅛ teaspoon dried thyme, crushed
½ teaspoon kosher salt	⅛ teaspoon ground ginger
¼ teaspoon ground allspice	2 cloves garlic, quartered

1. In a blender combine onion, lime juice, crushed red pepper, kosher salt, allspice, curry powder, black pepper, thyme, ginger, and garlic. Cover and blend until smooth.

2. Sprinkle evenly onto 1 pound boneless pork chops, chicken breast halves, or turkey breast tenderloin; rub in with your fingers. Cover and refrigerate for 30 minutes.

3. Grill or broil pork or poultry.

MUSTARD-PEPPERCORN RUB

Start to Finish: 5 minutes, plus 15 minutes to 4 hours for chilling
Yield: enough for 3 pounds meat

1 tablespoon coarse-grain brown mustard

2 teaspoons extra-virgin olive oil

2 teaspoons cracked black peppercorns

2 teaspoons chopped fresh tarragon or ½ teaspoon dried tarragon, crushed

1 teaspoon kosher salt

1. In a small bowl stir together mustard, oil, peppercorns, tarragon, and kosher salt.

2. Spread evenly onto 3 pounds boneless beef steaks, boneless pork chops, or boneless lamb chops. Refrigerate for 15 minutes to 4 hours.

3. Grill or broil meat.

BLACK BEAN GUACAMOLE

Start to Finish: 20 minutes
Yield: approximately 5 cups

5 diced avocados
3 chopped scallions
2 limes, juiced
½ cup tomatoes, chopped

1 tablespoon cilantro, chopped
1 15-ounce can black beans, drained and rinsed
Salt and black pepper to taste

1. Place avocados, scallions, and lime juice in a large bowl.

2. Mash avocados to a coarse puree.

3. Stir in tomatoes, cilantro, and beans.

4. Season with salt and pepper.

Nutrition Facts per Serving: 100 calories, 3 g protein, 8 g total fat (1 g saturated fat),
8 g carbohydrate, 5 g fiber, 0 mg cholesterol, 90 mg sodium

BLACK BEAN–
SMOKED CHILE SPREAD

Start to Finish: 25 minutes   Yield: about 1⅔ cups

½ cup onion, finely chopped
¼ cup scallions, sliced
1 teaspoon ground coriander
1 teaspoon ground cumin
1 tablespoon canola oil
¼ cup chopped fresh cilantro
1 15-ounce can black beans,
   drained and rinsed

½ cup water
1 tablespoon lime juice
1 teaspoon canned chipotle
   in adobo sauce,*
   finely chopped
¼ teaspoon kosher salt

1. In a covered small saucepan cook onion, scallions, coriander, and cumin in hot oil about 10 minutes or until very tender, stirring occasionally. Remove from heat; stir in cilantro.

2. Transfer onion mixture to a blender or food processor. Add black beans, water, lime juice, chipotle pepper, and kosher salt. Cover and blend or process until nearly smooth. Serve immediately or cover and chill for up to 3 days before serving.

CULINARY NOTE

* Because hot chile peppers contain oils that can burn your skin and eyes, wear rubber or plastic gloves when working with them. If your bare hands do touch the chile peppers, wash your hands well with soap and water.

Nutrition Facts per Serving: 18 calories, 1 g protein, 1 g total fat (0 g saturated fat), 3 g carbohydrate, 1 g fiber, 0 mg cholesterol, 61 mg sodium

HARISSA
(TUNISIAN HOT CHILE PASTE)

Start to Finish: 1 hour 25 minutes   Yield: about ½ cup

4 dried guajillo chile peppers
   (¾ ounce), stems and seeds
   removed*
5 dried ancho chile peppers
   (2½ ounces), stems and
   seeds removed*
Boiling water
2 tablespoons extra-virgin
   olive oil
2 tablespoons water
2 cloves garlic, halved

2 teaspoons caraway seeds,
   toasted and ground,
   or 2 teaspoons caraway
   seeds, finely crushed
1 teaspoon coriander seeds,
   toasted and ground,
   or ½ teaspoon ground
   coriander
¼ teaspoon kosher salt
⅛ teaspoon freshly ground
   black pepper

1. Heat a very large skillet over medium heat. Add dried chile peppers; toast for 2 minutes, turning occasionally. Place peppers in a very large bowl. Add enough boiling water to cover. Cover bowl and let stand for 1 hour. Drain well. Place peppers in a food processor; add oil, 2 tablespoons water, garlic, caraway seeds, coriander seeds, kosher salt, and black pepper. Cover and process to a nearly smooth paste. Press mixture through a coarse-mesh strainer to remove pepper skins.

2. Transfer paste to a small bowl and use in recipes as directed. Use immediately or cover and chill for up to 2 weeks before using.

> **CULINARY NOTE**
>
> * Because hot chile peppers contain oils that can burn your skin and eyes, wear rubber or plastic gloves when working with them. If your bare hands do touch the chile peppers, wash your hands well with soap and water.

Nutrition Facts per Serving: 73 calories, 2 g protein, 5 g total fat (0 g saturated fat),
7 g carbohydrate, 3 g fiber, 0 mg cholesterol, 71 mg sodium

HARISSA SAUCE

Start to Finish: 15 minutes
Yield: ¾ cup

¼ cup harissa (Tunisian Hot Chile Paste, page 187, or use purchased harissa)

¼ cup water

2 tablespoons extra-virgin olive oil

2 tablespoons lemon juice

1 teaspoon caraway seeds, toasted and ground, or 1 teaspoon caraway seeds, finely crushed

½ teaspoon coriander seeds, toasted and ground, or ¼ teaspoon ground coriander

¼ teaspoon kosher salt

⅛ teaspoon freshly ground black pepper

In a small bowl whisk together harissa, water, oil, lemon juice, caraway seeds, coriander seeds, kosher salt, and pepper until combined. Serve with meat or fish, use as dip for whole-wheat pita bread, or add to Tunisian couscous.

CULINARY NOTE

To toast and grind seeds, heat a small skillet over medium heat. Add seeds. Cook about 2 minutes or until toasted and aromatic, shaking skillet frequently. Place toasted seeds in a spice grinder and process until finely ground.

Nutrition Facts per Serving: 46 calories, 1 g protein, 4 g total fat (0 g saturated fat), 3 g carbohydrate, 1 g fiber, 0 mg cholesterol, 64 mg sodium

HUMMUS

Start to Finish: 15 minutes
Yield: 1¾ cups (2 tablespoons per serving)

1   15–16 ounce can garbanzo
    beans (chickpeas), drained
    and rinsed
¼   cup tahini
    (sesame seed paste)
3   tablespoons water
2   tablespoons lemon juice
1   tablespoon extra-virgin
    olive oil
1   clove garlic, halved

½   teaspoon kosher salt
½   teaspoon cumin seeds,
    toasted and ground, or
    ½ teaspoon ground cumin
¼   teaspoon cayenne pepper
1   tablespoon fresh flat-leaf
    parsley, chopped
Lemon juice *(optional)*
Fresh flat-leaf parsley

1. In a food processor combine garbanzo beans, tahini, water, 2 tablespoons lemon juice, olive oil, garlic, kosher salt, cumin seeds, and cayenne pepper. Cover and process until smooth. Transfer to a medium bowl.

2. Stir in the 1 tablespoon parsley. If desired, stir in additional lemon juice to taste. Garnish with additional parsley. Serve with baked pita chips or vegetable dippers, or use as a spread in a grilled vegetable sandwich.

CULINARY NOTE

To toast and grind seeds, heat a small skillet over medium heat. Add seeds. Cook about 2 minutes or until toasted and aromatic, shaking skillet frequently. Place toasted seeds in a spice grinder and process until finely ground.

Nutrition Facts per Serving: 71 calories, 2 g protein, 4 g total fat (0 g saturated fat) 8 g carbohydrate, 2 g fiber, 0 mg cholesterol, 162 mg sodium

PESTO WITH CILANTRO

Start to Finish: 20 minutes
Yield: ¾–1 cup (1 tablespoon per serving)

1 cup cilantro leaves (a little bit of stem is okay)
¼ cup parsley leaves
½ teaspoon garlic
2 tablespoons toasted blanched almonds

2 tablespoons parmesan cheese or cotija cheese, grated
2 tablespoons extra-virgin olive oil
2 tablespoons water
salt and pepper to taste

1. Fill a bowl with ice water.

2. Bring a small pot of water to a boil. Add the cilantro and parsley leaves; stir and cook for 15 seconds or until just wilted. Remove and immediately place in the ice water. Drain as soon as the herbs are cool.

3. Place all ingredients in a food processor or blender. Blend until smooth. Add more water to adjust consistency if necessary.

CULINARY NOTES

- Cooking the herbs for a few seconds in boiling water helps to set the color. The pesto should stay a nice bright green for a few days.
- Adjust the amount of garlic if you'd like. Raw garlic tends to be a bit harsh and can become hot and spicy after a day or two.

Variation:

- For basil pesto, replace the cilantro with 1½ cups basil leaves (a little bit of stem is okay) and the almonds with 2 tablespoons toasted pine nuts.

Nutrition Facts per Serving: 25 calories, 0 g protein, 2 g total fat (0 g saturated fat), 1 g. carbohydrate, 0 g fiber, 0 mg cholesterol, 10 mg sodium

SALSA VERDE
FOR MEAT OR VEGETABLES

Start to Finish: 15 minutes   Yield: ⅔ cup (1 tablespoon per serving)

½ cup flat-leaf parsley, leaves and thin stems only

¼ cup combination of oregano, basil, and mint

2 tablespoons scallions, chopped

1 tablespoon capers, rinsed and chopped

1 teaspoon lemon zest

½ teaspoon garlic, minced or mashed

1 pinch red chile flakes

2 tablespoons extra-virgin olive oil

1 tablespoon water

Salt and pepper to taste

Finely chop all herbs; place in a bowl. Add remaining ingredients and stir to combine. Let sit for 15 minutes; then adjust seasoning as necessary.

CULINARY NOTES

- Experiment with a combination of herbs in addition to the parsley: basil, chives, chervil, tarragon, cilantro, marjoram, savory, thyme, mint.

- Add lemon juice or vinegar to make the sauce zestier, but add it just prior to serving, since the acid in the lemon and vinegar will cause the herbs to discolor.

- This would be a delicious sauce to serve with a frittata or omelet. It is also a great accompaniment to grilled meats or vegetables.

Variations:

- Add 1 tablespoon chopped shallots.
- Add 1 chopped anchovy filet.
- Add 1 chopped or grated hard-cooked egg.
- Add 1 tablespoon toasted whole-wheat bread crumbs.

Nutrition Facts per Serving: 65 calories, 5 g protein, 6.8 g total fat (.95 g saturated fat), 1.5 g carbohydrate, .5 g fiber, 0 mg cholesterol, 69 mg sodium

Spicy Fruit Salsa

Start to Finish: 30 minutes, plus 15 minutes to 24 hours for chilling
Yield: 6 servings

½ cup fresh mango, peeled, seeded, and chopped

½ cup fresh papaya, peeled, seeded, and chopped

½ cup fresh pineapple, peeled, cored, and chopped

¼ cup red bell pepper, chopped

¼ cup fresh poblano chile pepper,* seeded and chopped

¼ cup chopped red onion

2 tablespoons chopped fresh cilantro

1 tablespoon lime juice

2 teaspoons extra-virgin olive oil

1 teaspoon rice vinegar

½ medium fresh jalapeño chile pepper, seeded and finely chopped*

⅛ teaspoon kosher salt

1. In a medium bowl combine mango, papaya, pineapple, bell pepper, poblano pepper, red onion, cilantro, lime juice, oil, vinegar, jalapeño pepper, and kosher salt. Stir gently to combine.

2. Cover and chill for 15 minutes to 24 hours before serving. Serve with fish, pork, beef, chicken, or turkey.

CULINARY NOTE

* Because hot chile peppers contain oils that can burn your skin and eyes, wear rubber or plastic gloves when working with them. If your bare hands do touch the chile peppers, wash your hands well with soap and water.

Nutrition Facts per Serving: 39 calories, 0 g protein, 2 g total fat (0 g saturated fat), 7 g carbohydrate, 1 g fiber, 0 mg cholesterol, 42 mg sodium

PEACH SALSA

Start to Finish: 20 minutes
Yield: 1 cup

1 cup peaches, peeled, cut in ¼-inch chunks

2 tablespoons red onion, finely chopped, rinsed

2 tablespoons red pepper, finely chopped

½ tablespoon jalapeño, chopped fine

½ tablespoon cilantro, chopped

½ tablespoon mint, chopped

1 tablespoon lime juice

Salt and pepper to taste

Combine all ingredients in a bowl. Gently mix. Let sit for 5 minutes for flavors to meld.

Variations:

- Replace jalapeño with ½ teaspoon chopped chipotle in adobo sauce.
- Replace mint with cilantro.

CULINARY NOTES

- Use ripe peaches; the skin will peel off the fruit if it is ripe.
- Rinsing the onions helps deflame them, making them less intense.

ROASTED TOMATO JALAPEÑO SALSA

Start to Finish: 20 minutes   Yield: 2 cups

2 (1 pound) ripe tomatoes
1 (1 ounce) jalapeño pepper
2 garlic cloves, unpeeled
¼ cup onion, diced small, rinsed, and drained

2 tablespoons cilantro, chopped
1 teaspoon lime juice
Salt and pepper to taste

1. Preheat oven to 450°F.

2. Place tomatoes on a sheet pan and roast until soft and blackened all over (turn halfway during the roasting process, about10 minutes). When cool enough to handle, remove skin and roughly chop tomatoes.

3. Place jalapeño and garlic in an ungreased skillet and roast in the oven until soft and slightly browned. Remove skin from garlic. Roughly chop garlic and jalapeño.

4. Combine the garlic, jalapeño, and tomatoes in a bowl. Add onion, cilantro, and lime juice to taste. Season with salt and pepper.

Variations:

- Replace the jalapeño with a serrano or habanero for a spicier version.

- Replace the tomatoes with tomatillos for a tart salsa. You may need to add a pinch of sugar if the tomatillos are sour and bitter.

CULINARY NOTES

- Roasting the tomatoes concentrates the juices and flavor, making mediocre tomatoes taste better. The tomatoes should be soft all the way through and slightly charred.

- Rinsing and draining the onions remove some of the harshness that raw onions can have.

- Add jalapeño to taste. You never know exactly how hot a chile pepper will be. It depends on how long ago it was harvested, the growing conditions, and the soil. Don't assume all chiles will have the same heat level.

CONCORD GRAPE
BALSAMIC VINAIGRETTE

Start to Finish: 25 minutes   Yield: ⅓ cup

½ cup unsweetened concord grape juice

1 tablespoon balsamic vinegar

2 tablespoons extra-virgin olive oil

Salt and pepper to taste

1. Place grape juice in a small saucepan. Reduce by half. Remove from heat and cool.

2. Stir in balsamic vinegar and whisk in extra-virgin olive oil. Season with salt and pepper.

CULINARY NOTE

Keep an eye on the reducing grape juice. It will burn if it reduces too far.

Variations:

- Use red wine vinegar in place of balsamic vinegar.
- Use lemon juice in place of vinegar.

Nutrition Facts per Serving: 80 calories, 0 g protein, 6.75 g total fat (3.7 g saturated fat), 4.5 g carbohydrate, 0 g fiber, 0 mg cholesterol, 0 mg sodium, 8.5 glycemic load

GAZPACHO VINAIGRETTE

Start to Finish: 30 minutes
Yield: ¾ cup

¼ cup green pepper, seeded and diced small

¼ cup red pepper, seeded and diced small

1 tablespoon red onion, diced small

2–3 vine-ripe tomatoes (about ¾ pound), cut in chunks

2 tablespoons chopped onion, rinsed

½ teaspoon garlic, mashed to a paste

1 cup cucumber, peeled, seeded, chopped

2 tablespoons sherry vinegar

1 teaspoon Spanish paprika, smoked or plain

2 tablespoons extra-virgin olive oil

Salt and pepper to taste

1. Combine half of the red and green peppers and the red onions in a bowl. Season with 1 teaspoon sherry vinegar, salt, and pepper.

2. Combine the tomatoes, onion, garlic, cucumber, and remaining red and green peppers in a blender. Blend until smooth. Add remaining sherry vinegar, paprika, and extra-virgin olive oil. Season with salt and pepper.

CULINARY NOTE

Gazpacho is always better the day after it is prepared, when the flavors have had time to meld.

3. Stir red onion mixture into the pureed tomato mixture. Chill well.

Variations:

- Serve with 3 ounces poached shrimp and ½ cup sliced cucumbers.
- Serve as a soup: add ¼ cup diced avocado and ¼ cup diced cucumber.

Nutrition Facts per Serving: 45 calories, 0 g protein, 3 g total fat (0 g saturated fat), 3 g carbohydrate, 1 g fiber, 0 mg cholesterol, 3 mg sodium, 0 glycemic load

GREEK VINAIGRETTE

Start to Finish: 15 minutes
Yield: about ⅓ cup

1 tablespoon red wine vinegar
1 tablespoon lemon juice
1 tablespoon red onion, finely chopped
3 tablespoons extra-virgin olive oil
1 tablespoon fresh mint, chopped
1 tablespoon fresh oregano, chopped
Dash kosher salt
Dash freshly ground black pepper

1. In a small bowl combine vinegar, lemon juice, and red onion. Let stand for 5 minutes.

2. Add oil in a thin, steady stream, whisking constantly until combined. Stir in mint, oregano, kosher salt, and pepper. Use immediately or cover and chill for up to 3 days before using. If chilled, let stand at room temperature for 30 minutes; whisk before using.

Nutrition Facts per Serving: 73 calories, 0 g protein, 8 g total fat (1 g saturated fat), 0 g carbohydrate, 0 g fiber, 0 mg cholesterol, 24 mg sodium

PESTO VINAIGRETTE

Start to Finish: 10 minutes
Yield: ¾ cup

1 cup packed fresh basil leaves
½ cup extra-virgin olive oil
2 tablespoons pine nuts or walnuts, toasted
2 cloves garlic minced (1 teaspoon)

¼ cup white wine vinegar
½ teaspoon kosher salt
¼ teaspoon freshly ground black pepper

1. In a food processor combine basil leaves, ¼ cup of the oil, nuts, and garlic. Cover and pulse to a coarse puree.

2. Transfer mixture to a small bowl. Whisk in remaining ¼ cup oil, vinegar, kosher salt, and pepper.

Nutrition Facts per Serving: 92 calories, 1 g protein, 10 g total fat (1 g saturated fat), 1 g carbohydrate, 0 g fiber, 0 mg cholesterol, 81 mg sodium

Red Wine Vinaigrette

Start to Finish: 10 minutes
Yield: about ⅓ cup

2 tablespoons red wine vinegar
1 tablespoon shallot, finely chopped
1½ teaspoons Dijon mustard
2 tablespoons extra-virgin olive oil

⅛ teaspoon kosher salt
⅛ teaspoon freshly ground black pepper

1. In a small bowl combine vinegar and shallot. Let stand for 5 minutes.

2. Whisk in mustard. Add oil in a thin, steady stream, whisking constantly until combined. Stir in kosher salt and pepper.
Use immediately or cover and chill for up to 3 days before using.

3. If chilled, let stand at room temperature about 30 minutes; whisk before using.

Nutrition Facts per Serving: 51 calories, 0 g protein, 5 g total fat (1 g saturated fat),
1 g carbohydrate, 0 g fiber, 0 mg cholesterol, 85 mg sodium

SHERRY HONEY VINAIGRETTE

Start to Finish: 5 minutes
Yield: 1 cup

½   cup sherry vinegar
¼   cup extra-virgin olive oil
¼   cup olive oil

3   tablespoons honey
Salt and pepper to taste

Whisk all ingredients together in a small bowl until the honey has dissolved.

CULINARY NOTE

Slightly heat the honey in the microwave so it will dissolve more easily.

Variations:

- Substitute red wine vinegar for the sherry vinegar.
- Substitute white wine or champagne vinegar for the sherry vinegar. You may need less honey depending on how sweet your vinegar is.
- Add 1 tablespoon Dijon mustard.
- Add 1 tablespoon chopped herbs such as chives, parsley, mint, or tarragon.

Nutrition Facts per Serving: 150 calories, 0 g protein, 13 g total fat (1.5 g saturated fat), 7 g carbohydrate, 0 g fiber, 0 mg cholesterol, 0 mg sodium, 7 glycemic load

SHERRY MUSTARD VINAIGRETTE

Start to Finish: 15 minutes
Yield: ½ cup

2   tablespoons shallot, finely diced
¼   cup sherry vinegar

1   tablespoon Dijon mustard
¼   cup extra-virgin olive oil
Salt and pepper to taste

Place shallots in a small bowl. Add vinegar and let sit for 10 minutes. Whisk in mustard and oil. Season with salt and pepper.

Variation:

- Add 1 tablespoon chopped fresh herbs such as chives, parsley, or thyme.

CULINARY NOTE

Use a good-quality sherry vinegar. It will have less of an acid bite and a richer sherry flavor than a lower-quality vinegar.

Nutrition Facts per Serving: 60 calories, 0 g protein, 6 g total fat (1 g saturated fat), 1 g carbohydrate, 0 mg cholesterol, 45 mg sodium, 0 glycemic load

SIMPLE SPICY LIME CILANTRO VINAIGRETTE

Start to Finish: 10 minutes   Yield: ½ cup

¼   cup lime juice
¼   teaspoon garlic, chopped
1   tablespoon cilantro, chopped

½   teaspoon chipotle in adobo sauce, chopped
¼   cup extra-virgin olive oil
Salt and pepper to taste

Combine all ingredients. Whisk well.

Nutrition Facts per Serving: 30 calories, 0 g protein, 3 g total fat (.5 g saturated fat), 0 g carbohydrate, 0 g fiber, 0 mg cholesterol, 32 mg sodium

SOY SESAME VINAIGRETTE

Start to Finish: 10 minutes
Yield: ½ cup

4   tablespoons soy sauce
1   tablespoon sugar
1   tablespoon rice vinegar
½   tablespoon lemon juice
½   teaspoon garlic, chopped

1   tablespoon ginger, minced
    or grated
2   teaspoons sesame oil
Salt and pepper to taste

Combine all ingredients.
Whisk well.

Variation:

- For a spicier vinaigrette,
  add ¼ teaspoon chile sauce
  (sambal oelek or chopped
  Thai bird chiles).

CULINARY NOTE

Use a microplane to grate the
ginger. It allows you to grate
the pulp from the ginger root
and leaves the stringy fibrous
core behind.

Nutrition Facts per Serving: 22 calories, 15 g protein, 1 g total fat (0 g saturated fat),
2 g carbohydrate, 0 g fiber, 0 mg cholesterol, 300 mg sodium

SONOMA CAESAR SALAD DRESSING

Start to Finish: 15 minutes   Yield: 1 cup

1   cup cannellini beans or white beans, cooked, plus liquid
4   anchovy filets
¼   cup lemon juice
1   teaspoon lemon zest
1   teaspoon garlic

1   teaspoon Dijon mustard
¼   cup parmesan cheese, grated
¼   cup extra-virgin olive oil
¼   cup olive oil
⅓   cup water
Salt and pepper to taste

Combine all ingredients in a blender. Blend until smooth.

CULINARY NOTES

- Scoop the white beans into the measuring cup and add enough bean liquid to come to the top of the beans.
- No need to chop anything because all ingredients will be placed in the blender.

Nutrition Facts per Serving: 80 calories, 2 g protein, 7 g total fat (1 g saturated fat), 3 g carbohydrate, 1 g fiber, 2 mg cholesterol, 90 mg sodium, 13 glycemic load

SIMPLE LEMON VINAIGRETTE

Start to Finish: 10 minutes   Yield: ½ cup

¼ cup lemon juice
¼ teaspoon garlic, chopped

¼ cup extra-virgin olive oil
Salt and pepper to taste

Combine all ingredients. Whisk well.

Nutrition Facts per Serving: 30 calories, 0 g protein, 3 g fat, .5 g saturated fat, 0 g carbohydrate, 0 g fiber, 0 mg cholesterol, 32 mg sodium, 0 glycemic load

BALSAMIC VINAIGRETTE

Start to Finish: 10 minutes   Yield: 1 cup

½ cup chicken stock or broth
¼ cup balsamic vinegar
1   tablespoon fresh basil, chopped, or 1 teaspoon dried basil, crushed

Dash kosher salt
¼ cup extra-virgin olive oil
Kosher salt (optional)

In a small bowl combine chicken stock, vinegar, basil, and a dash of kosher salt. Add oil in a thin, steady stream, whisking constantly until combined. If desired, season to taste with additional kosher salt. Use immediately or cover and chill for up to 1 week before using. If chilled, let stand at room temperature for 30 minutes; whisk before serving.

Nutrition Facts per Serving: 33 calories, 0 g protein, 3 g total fat (0 g saturated fat), 1 g carbohydrate, 0 g fiber, 0 mg cholesterol, 38 mg sodium

WAVE 1 MEAL PLANS

The meal plans that follow suggest exactly what to eat for breakfast, lunch, dinner, and snacks for each of the ten days of Wave 1. As you use these menus, your meals will automatically conform to the Wave 1 guidelines. You'll also enjoy delicious new dishes that will actually increase your mealtime pleasure as you lose weight.

Instructions for preparing the main dishes for each meal are given in the Wave 1 recipe section. As with everything in The Sonoma Diet, the emphasis is on simplicity. All you have to do is fill the right size plate with the Wave 1 plate-guidelines portion sizes for each of the foods given. Then eat and enjoy. Your recipes also recommend the portion amounts. Look for the new features, such as Cook Once/Eat Twice, to keep your time in the kitchen short and your grocery shopping minimal. Other features, such as gluten-free options, Culinary Tips, and my favorite, Variations, give you more than one way to prepare your favorite recipes!

Wave 1 is designed for fast initial weight loss as well as overcoming your sugar and refined-grain cravings. These menus reflect the food choices that are part of Wave 1. For example, you'll find only Tier 1 fruits and vegetables on any given day. Follow the menus closely, especially for the selections of the Tier 1 vegetables and fruits. The big plus of these menus is that they offer you tasty, satisfying meals.

But remember that these meal plans are optional. You can use them on all ten days of Wave 1, on some of the days, or on none. You might find it convenient, for example, to follow the Wave 1 menus for most meals, but substitute a Sonoma Express recipe (see pages 234 and 253) when you're pressed for time. As long as your choices conform to the plate-guidelines sizes and the Wave 1 proportions, you're home free. And throughout the day, don't forget to drink lots of water—at least eight tall glasses each day. Try the many different teas for more variety. Drinking plenty of fluids is especially important on this first part of the diet.

For even more variety, you'll also find additional Wave 1 recipes not featured in the meal plans. ▪

DAY ONE

BREAKFAST: 2 scrambled eggs with 1 slice of whole-grain toast
Green tea
½ cup blueberries

LUNCH: Minestrone Soup, page 223
Salad of 1½ cups baby spinach, 1 tablespoon sliced almonds, Sherry Vinaigrette or choice of dressing from Seasonings section, pages 195–204

DINNER: Roast Chicken with Roasted Vegetables, Mediterranean Variation, page 326
½ cup Toasted Quinoa Pilaf, page 244

SNACK:
Men: 1 mozzarella cheese stick, 1 ounce peanuts, ½ cup grape tomatoes
Women: ½ cup grape tomatoes, 1 ounce peanuts or almonds, 1 mozzarella cheese stick

DAY TWO

BREAKFAST: Sonoma Frittata with ½ cup roasted vegetables from previous meal or choice of variations, page 215
Green tea

LUNCH: Toasted Quinoa Chicken and Cucumber Dill Salad, COOK 1X · EAT 2X , page 226
2 Wasa crackers

DINNER: Herb-Marinated Flank Steak, page 254
Grilled vegetables, 1½ cups: choose from zucchini, eggplant, bell peppers, squash. Cut in 1-inch-wide strips, lengthwise.

SNACK: 1 ounce almonds, one fruit serving

DAY THREE

BREAKFAST: 1 tablespoon nut butter, 1 slice whole-wheat bread, ½ cup berries, Hot tea or coffee

LUNCH: Steak and Blue Cheese Wrap COOK 1X · EAT 2X , page 232

DINNER: Spicy Chipotle Broth for Poaching Fish, with salmon, page 180
Grilled Vegetable Rolls Stuffed with Feta Cheese, Pine Nuts, and Mint COOK 1X · EAT 2X , page 239
Or 1½ cup mixed green salad with choice of dressing in Seasonings, pages 195–204

SNACK: 1 low-fat Laughing Cow Mini Babybel cheese wheel, 1 cup raw bell pepper slices

DAY FOUR

BREAKFAST: Grilled Vegetable Frittata COOK 1X · EAT 2X , page 219
Or 2 scrambled eggs with 1 slice of whole-wheat bread
Hot tea or coffee

LUNCH: Sonoma Chopped Salmon Salad COOK 1X · EAT 2X , page 229
2 Wasa crackers or whole-grain option

DINNER: Coffee Rub for Beef, 4 ounces, page 182
Grilled Asparagus Salad, choice of variation, page 238

SNACK: 1 tablespoon peanut butter with raw celery sticks

Day Five

BREAKFAST: Mushroom Omelet, page 220
Tea or coffee
½ cup mixed berries

LUNCH: Greek Salad with Grilled Shrimp, page 227
½ whole-wheat pita

DINNER: Roast Chicken with Roasted Vegetables, Latin variation,
page 327
Sautéed Cherry Tomatoes with Basil and Garlic,
page 243
½ cup brown or wild rice

SNACK:
Men: 1 ounce almonds, 1 cup raw veggie slices,
1 ounce sliced turkey or lean ham
Women: 1 ounce almonds, 1 cup raw veggies

Day Six

BREAKFAST: 1 tablespoon of nut butter with 1 slice of
whole-wheat toast
Green tea

LUNCH: Sonoma Express wrap with chicken COOK 1X · EAT 2X ,
page 170
1 serving fruit

DINNER: Grilled Tuna with Rosemary, page 263
White Bean Ratatouille, page 247

SNACK: 1 mozzarella cheese stick, 1 cup sliced bell peppers
or cucumbers

DAY SEVEN

BREAKFAST: 2 scrambled eggs with 1 slice of whole-wheat toast
Tea or coffee

LUNCH: Wine Country Salad with Grilled Tuna `COOK 1X · EAT 2X`,
page 231
½ whole-wheat pita

DINNER: Spanish Roast Pork Tenderloin with Chickpeas and
Spinach, page 260
1 serving of fruit

SNACK: 1 low-fat Laughing Cow Mini Babybel cheese wheel,
1 cup of sliced carrots

DAY EIGHT

BREAKFAST: 1 cup whole-grain cereal with milk
½ cup blueberries or other berries
Green tea

LUNCH: Spiced Pork Wrap with White Beans and Watercress,
`COOK 1X · EAT 2X`, page 234
1 serving of fruit

DINNER: Spiced Jerk London Broil, page 255
Sautéed Broccoli Rabe, variations, pages 241–242
½ cup Toasted Quinoa Pilaf, page 244

SNACK:
Men: 2 tablespoons peanut butter with raw celery sticks
Women: 1 tablespoon peanut butter with raw celery sticks

Day Nine

BREAKFAST: Omelet with broccoli rabe and Parmesan COOK 1X· EAT 2X
or variations on page 242
Tea or coffee

LUNCH: Tomatoes Stuffed with Quinoa, Cucumber, and Feta, with
chicken or tuna GLUTEN FREE , page 224

DINNER: Cioppino Seafood en Papillote with vegetable medley,
page 261

SNACK: 1 ounce almonds, 1 cup vegetables;
select any from Tier One

Day Ten

BREAKFAST: Buckwheat Pancakes *(regular or gluten-free)*,
pages 212 or 213
½ cup berries
1 cup of tea

LUNCH: Asian Chicken Salad, page 225

DINNER: Chicken and White Bean Chile Verde with Sonoma Pesto,
page 249

SNACK:
Men: 1 cup grape tomatoes, 1 ounce peanuts
Women: ½ cup grape tomatoes, 1 ounce peanuts

BUCKWHEAT PANCAKES

Start to Finish: 45 minutes
Yield: 4 servings, 2 pancakes each

1 cup buttermilk	½ cup unbleached all-purpose flour
1 egg	
1 egg white	½ cup buckwheat flour
4 tablespoons applesauce	2 teaspoons sugar
½ teaspoon vanilla	½ teaspoon salt
½ teaspoon lemon zest	1½ teaspoons baking soda
	Nonstick cooking spray

1. Preheat pancake griddle over medium heat.

2. Combine the buttermilk, egg, egg white, applesauce, vanilla, and zest in a bowl. Mix well.

3. In another bowl, combine flours, sugar, salt, and baking soda. Mix well.

4. Gently incorporate the wet ingredients into the dry ingredients. Mix just enough to combine. Overmixing will make the pancakes tough.

5. Lightly spray the pancake griddle. Pour ¼ cupfuls of pancake batter on griddle, ¼ inch thick. Cook until golden brown and the edges start to set. Flip and cook on the other side.

> **CULINARY NOTE**
>
> The leavening agent is baking soda, so once the wet and dry ingredients are combined, the pancakes should be cooked immediately. This batter does not hold well.

Variations:

- **Blueberry Buckwheat Pancakes:** Add 1½ cup blueberries to the buttermilk mixture.

- **Banana Buckwheat Pancakes:** Omit lemon zest; add 1 cup chopped bananas and ½ teaspoon cinnamon to the buttermilk mixture.

Nutrition Facts per Serving: 160 calories, 8 g protein, 2.5 g total fat (1 g saturated fat), 29 g carbohydrate, 3 g fiber, 55 mg cholesterol, 800 mg sodium, 16 glycemic load

BUCKWHEAT BUTTERMILK PANCAKES

Start to Finish: 20 minutes   Yield: 16 silver dollar pancakes

1¼ cup buttermilk
2 tablespoons canola oil
2 tablespoons agave syrup
½ teaspoon vanilla extract
¾ cup brown rice flour
¾ cup buckwheat flour

2 teaspoons baking powder
½ teaspoons baking soda
1 pinch salt
1 egg, beaten
Nonstick cooking spray
   as needed

1. Combine buttermilk, oil, agave syrup, and vanilla in a bowl.
2. Combine flours, baking powder, baking soda, and salt in a large bowl.
3. Add egg to the buttermilk mixture; then stir into the rice flour mixture. Stir just to wet the ingredients.
4. Heat the griddle over medium-low heat and spray with nonstick cooking spray.
5. Pour heaping tablespoonfuls of batter on griddle. Spread to shape of a silver dollar, approximately ¼ inch thick. Cook until golden brown; flip and cook on the other side.
6. Serve with fresh fruit or your favorite sugar-free syrup.

> **CULINARY NOTE**
>
> For light and fluffy pancakes, do not overmix the batter. The batter should be barely mixed and will seem lumpy and coarse.

Variations:

- Add ½ cup blueberries to the buttermilk mixture.
- Add ½ cup sliced bananas and 2 tablespoon toasted almonds to the buttermilk mixture.

Nutrition Facts per Serving: 83 calories, 2.5 g protein, 2.8 g total fat (.5 g saturated fat), 12 g carbohydrate, 1 g fiber, 18 mg cholesterol, 140 mg sodium, 8 glycemic load

FLUFFY BROWN RICE PANCAKES

Start to Finish: 20 minutes
Yield: 16 silver dollar pancakes

1¼ cup buttermilk
2 tablespoons canola oil
2 tablespoons agave syrup
½ teaspoon vanilla extract
1½ cups brown rice flour

2 teaspoons baking powder
½ teaspoon baking soda
1 pinch salt
1 egg, beaten
Nonstick cooking spray as needed

1. Combine buttermilk, oil, agave syrup, and vanilla in a bowl.

2. Combine rice flour, baking powder, baking soda, and salt in a large bowl.

3. Add egg to the buttermilk mixture; then stir into the rice flour mixture. Stir just to wet the ingredients.

CULINARY NOTES

- For light and fluffy pancakes, do not overmix the batter. The batter should be barely mixed and will seem lumpy and coarse.
- This batter will cook at a slightly lower temperature than regular pancake batter.

4. Heat the pancake griddle over medium low and spray with nonstick cooking spray.

5. Pour heaping tablespoonfuls of batter on griddle. Spread to shape of a silver dollar, approximately ¼ inch thick. Cook until golden brown; flip and cook on other side.

6. Serve with fresh fruit or your favorite sugar-free syrup.

Variations:

- Add ½ cup blueberries to the buttermilk mixture.
- Add ½ cup sliced bananas and 2 tablespoons toasted almonds to the buttermilk mixture.

Nutrition Facts per Serving: 90 calories, 2 g protein, 2 g fat (5 g saturated fat), 14 g carbohydrate, .6 g fiber, 15 mg cholesterol, 140 mg sodium, 9 glycemic load

SONOMA FRITTATA

Start to Finish: 15 minutes
Yield: 1 9-inch frittata, 4 servings

4 eggs
2 teaspoon fresh herbs—
 basil, chives, or parsley
1 pinch black pepper

Filling:
¼ teaspoon chopped garlic
 or ⅛ tsp. garlic powder
1 cup cooked vegetables
 for filling
2 tablespoons cheese—
 parmesan, goat, feta,
 or ricotta
2 tablespoons scallions, sliced
Salt and pepper to taste
Nonstick cooking spray

1. In a medium bowl, whisk together eggs, herbs, and pepper.
2. Heat a small nonstick skillet over medium. Coat with nonstick
cooking spray. Add garlic and sauté 10 seconds. Add vegetables and toss
to warm. Spread the vegetables in the bottom of the skillet. Sprinkle
with cheese. Pour eggs over vegetables and cheese in skillet. Cook over
medium heat. As eggs set, run a spatula around the edge of the skillet,
lifting eggs so the uncooked portion flows underneath. Continue
cooking and lifting the edge until
eggs are almost set (surface will be
moist). Remove from heat.
3. Cover and let stand for 3 to 4
minutes or until top is set.
To serve, cut the frittata into
wedges. If desired, garnish with
tomato wedges.

CULINARY NOTES

- For lighter frittatas, add
 2 tablespoons of low-fat
 milk to the eggs.

- Use a nonstick Teflon pan
 to prepare these and a
 nonmelting silicon spatula.

Nutrition Facts per Serving: 125 calories, 9 g protein, 8 g fat (3 g saturated fat),
5 g carbohydrate, 1 g fiber, 250 mg cholesterol, 80 mg sodium, 0 glycemic load

Frittata Variations:

ROASTED PEPPERS, TOMATO, & PESTO

Yield: 1 9-inch frittata, 4 servings

1 teaspoon extra-virgin olive oil

2 tablespoons onion, sliced

½ teaspoon garlic, chopped

¼ cup bottled roasted red peppers, diced

¼ cup canned tomatoes, drained well, chopped

¼ cup canned white beans, drained

2 tablespoons parmesan cheese

1 tablespoon pesto, purchased or prepared (optional)

salt and pepper to taste

1. Heat a small nonstick sauté pan over medium-high heat; add olive oil and onion. Sauté for 1 minute. Add garlic; cook until aromatic. Add peppers, tomatoes, and beans; toss to warm through. Add cheese.
2. Add pesto (optional) to eggs mixture. Continue preparing as above.

LATIN-STYLE FILLING

Yield: 1 9-inch frittata, 4 servings

½ teaspoon garlic, chopped, or ⅛ teaspoon garlic powder

¼ cup bottled roasted red peppers, diced

2 tablespoons canned roasted green chiles, drained, diced

½ cup frozen corn, defrosted

1 pinch ground cumin

½ teaspoon dry jack cheese or Queso Fresco

½ teaspoon chipotle in adobo sauce

Salt and pepper to taste

Nonstick cooking spray

1. Heat a small nonstick skillet over medium heat. Coat with nonstick cooking spray. Add garlic and sauté 10 seconds. Add vegetables and cumin and toss to warm. Spread the vegetables in the bottom of the skillet. Sprinkle with cheese. Season with chipotle, salt, and pepper.
2. Garnish finished frittata with salsa fresco if desired.

ROASTED VEGETABLE FILLING #1

Yield: 1 9-inch frittata, 4 servings

½ teaspoon chopped garlic or ⅛ teaspoon garlic powder

¾ cup roasted vegetables

1 teaspoon Spanish paprika

2 tablespoons manchego cheese or parmesan cheese

2 tablespoons scallions, sliced

Salt and pepper to taste

Nonstick cooking spray

Heat a small nonstick skillet over medium heat. Coat with nonstick cooking spray. Add garlic and sauté 10 seconds. Add vegetables and toss to warm. Spread the vegetables in the bottom of the skillet. Sprinkle with paprika, cheese, and scallions. Season with salt and pepper.

ROASTED VEGETABLE FILLING #2

Yield: 1 9-inch frittata, 4 servings

½ teaspoon garlic, chopped, or ⅛ teaspoon garlic powder

¼ cup onions, sliced thin

1 cup roasted vegetables

½ tablespoon basil, chopped

1 tablespoon goat cheese or parmesan cheese

Salt and pepper to taste

Nonstick cooking spray

Heat a small nonstick skillet over medium. Coat with nonstick cooking spray. Add garlic and sauté 10 seconds. Add onions and cook 5 minutes. Add vegetables and toss to warm. Spread the vegetables in the bottom of the skillet. Sprinkle with basil and cheese. Season with salt and pepper.

SPRING VEGETABLE FILLING

Yield: 1 9-inch frittata, 4 servings

½ teaspoon garlic, chopped, or ⅛ teaspoon garlic powder

½ cup asparagus, cooked, cut in 1-inch pieces

¼ cup peas

2 tablespoons scallions, sliced

1 teaspoon Spanish paprika

2 tablespoons parmesan cheese

Salt and pepper to taste

Nonstick cooking spray

Heat a small nonstick skillet over medium heat. Coat with nonstick cooking spray. Add garlic and sauté 10 seconds. Add vegetables and toss to warm. Spread the vegetables in the bottom of the skillet. Sprinkle with paprika and cheese. Season with salt and pepper.

CULINARY NOTES

- Frittatas can be served warm or at room temperature.

- Prepare the frittata in mini muffin pans for bite-size souffléed appetizers or snacks. Preheat oven to 375°F. Heat mini muffin pans. Spray with nonstick cooking spray. Pour frittata filling into pans. Add eggs. Bake for 10–15 minutes or until just cooked through. Let cool slightly. Run a knife around the edge to remove the frittatas. This recipe will yield approximately 18 mini frittatas.

- Cook the frittata on medium heat so it cooks gently. This prevents the eggs from becoming tough.

- For a more tender frittata, add 3 tablespoons low-fat or nonfat milk to the eggs.

- Leftover vegetables can be COOK 1X · EAT 2X ingredients.

GRILLED VEGETABLE FRITTATA

Start to Finish: 30–40 minutes
Yield: 4 servings

8 large eggs
¾ cup low-fat milk
1 tablespoon olive oil
1 cup onions, sliced thin
1 teaspoon garlic, minced

3 cups grilled vegetables cut into ½-inch pieces
1 tablespoon mint, chopped
Salt and pepper to taste
¼ cup feta cheese, crumbled

1. Preheat oven to 325°F.
2. Beat eggs with milk, salt, and pepper to taste.
3. Heat oil in 10-inch nonstick sauté pan with nonmelting handle. Add onions; sauté 4 minute until slightly caramelized. Add garlic; cook 10 seconds until aromatic. Add vegetables and mint; toss until warm. Season with salt and pepper.
4. Reduce heat to low; add eggs and stir slightly. Crumble cheese on top. Cook 2–3 more minutes.
5. Place pan in oven and bake for 25–30 minutes or until the top is golden brown and the eggs are just set in the center. Remove from oven. Let sit for a few minutes; then slide out of pan onto a cutting board. Cut into wedges and serve warm.

CULINARY NOTES

- If the nonstick pan has a plastic handle, wrap the handle in several layers of aluminum foil.
- Cook until the center of the frittata, about the size of a dime, is still moist. The frittata will finish cooking after it is removed from the oven.

Variations:

- Use leftover grilled vegetables or roasted vegetables.
- Replace the feta with parmesan cheese or goat cheese.
- Replace the feta with ricotta or mozzarella for a mild frittata.

Nutrition Facts per Serving: 250 calories, 18 g protein, 16 g fat (5 g saturated fat), 11 g carbohydrate, 2.5 g fiber, 400 mg cholesterol, 250 mg sodium, 0 glycemic load

Mushroom Omelet

Start to Finish: 15 minutes
Yield: 1 serving

2   eggs
⅛   teaspoon kosher salt
⅛   teaspoon freshly ground
       black pepper

2   teaspoons canola oil
½   cup fresh mushrooms, sliced

1. In a small bowl, beat eggs, kosher salt, and pepper with a whisk until combined; set aside.

2. In a medium nonstick skillet with flared sides, heat 1 teaspoon of the oil over medium heat. Add mushrooms; cook until tender, stirring occasionally. Remove mushrooms from skillet; set aside.

3. Add remaining 1 teaspoon oil to same skillet. Heat over medium heat. Add eggs to skillet. Immediately begin stirring gently but continuously with a wooden or plastic spatula until egg mixture forms small pieces of cooked egg surrounded by liquid egg. Stop stirring. Cook for 30 to 60 seconds more or until egg mixture is set but shiny.

4. Sprinkle mushrooms across center of the eggs mixture. With a spatula, lift and fold an edge of the omelet about a third of the way toward the center. Fold the opposite edge toward the center; transfer to a warm plate, seam side down.

CULINARY NOTES

- Mix the eggs well when preparing omelets so there are no spots of egg white in the omelet. A pinch of salt added to the eggs helps denature the protein so the eggs mix more easily.

- It's important to use a nonstick Teflon pan when preparing omelets; otherwise the egg may stick to the pan or require the use of more oil to keep the omelet from sticking.

Nutrition Facts per Serving: 236 calories, 14 g protein, 19 g total fat (4 g saturated fat), 2 g carbohydrate, 0 g fiber, 423 mg cholesterol, 383 mg sodium

Variations:

RANCHERO OMELET

Prepare as above, except omit mushrooms and 1 teaspoon of the oil. Top cooked egg mixture with:

- 1 tablespoon red, green, or yellow bell pepper, chopped
- 1 tablespoon tomato, chopped
- 1 tablespoon shredded Monterey Jack cheese with jalapeño chile peppers, or cheddar cheese
- ½ teaspoon chopped fresh cilantro
- ¼ teaspoon seeded fresh jalapeño or serrano chile pepper,* finely chopped. Then fold as above.

Nutrition Facts per Serving: 219 calories, 15 g protein, 17 g total fat (5 g saturated fat), 2 g carbohydrate, 0 g fiber, 429 mg cholesterol, 420 mg sodium

CULINARY NOTE

* Because hot chile peppers contain oils that can burn your skin and eyes, wear rubber or plastic gloves when working with them. If your bare hands do touch the chile peppers, wash your hands well with soap and water.

ARTICHOKE & ROASTED PEPPER OMELET

Prepare as above but omit the mushrooms and 1 teaspoon of the oil. Top cooked egg mixture with ¼ cup sliced artichoke hearts (frozen or leftover), 2 tablespoon bottled roasted red peppers (diced), and 1 teaspoon chopped herbs (chives, parsley, tarragon, or oregano). Season with salt and pepper before folding.

Nutrition Facts per Serving: 215 calories, 15 g protein, 15 g fat (4 g saturated fat), 2 g carbohydrate, 1 g fiber, 420 mg cholesterol, 400 mg sodium

POACHED EGGS
IN SPICY CHIPOTLE BROTH

Start to Finish: 15 minutes   Yield: 4 servings

1 recipe Spicy Chipotle Broth
  for Poaching Fish, page 180

4 eggs

1 tablespoon nonfat
  sour cream

¼ cup salsa fresca (purchased)

1 teaspoon chopped cilantro

Salt and pepper to taste

1. Bring the spicy chipotle broth to a simmer.

2. Crack each egg separately into a bowl, making sure there are no bits of shells. Gently drop the eggs into the liquid, keeping them separate. Sprinkle tops with salt and pepper.

3. Cover the pan and simmer over medium low heat for 8–10 minutes or until the eggs are cooked. Periodically baste the top of the eggs with the broth.

4. Gently scoop each egg along with broth and vegetables into a bowl. Garnish with sour cream and salsa fresca. Sprinkle with cilantro.

Nutrition Facts per Serving: 188 calories, 11 g protein, 6 g fat (1.5 g saturated fat), 21 g carbohydrate, 4.5 g fiber, 200 mg cholesterol, 600 mg sodium, 3.5 glycemic load

MINESTRONE SOUP

Start to Finish: 1 hour, 15 minutes
Yield: 8 cups (8 servings)

2 tablespoons extra-virgin olive oil	1 pinch chile flakes
1 tablespoon garlic, sliced thin	1 14-ounce can white beans
2 cups onions, chopped	6 cups chicken stock
1 cup celery, chopped	½ cup orzo pasta
1 cup carrots, chopped	1 tablespoon extra-virgin olive oil
1 tablespoon oregano, chopped	1 cup zucchini, cut in quarters lengthwise, then ¼-inch slices crosswise
1 14-ounce can tomatoes, chopped	2 cups baby spinach
	Salt and pepper to taste

1. Place 2 tablespoons extra-virgin olive oil and garlic in a medium sauté pan. Cook over low heat until the garlic is soft, approximately 4 minutes.

2. Add onions, celery, carrots, and oregano. Cook for 10 minutes until translucent, not browned.

3. Add tomatoes, chile flakes, and white beans. Cook 5 minutes.

4. Add chicken stock. Bring to a simmer. Cook for 20 minutes.

5. Stir in pasta; cook 15 minutes, or until the pasta is cooked through.

6. Heat a sauté pan over high heat. Add 1 tablespoon olive oil and zucchini. Sauté until crisp-tender. Add to soup with the spinach. Adjust seasoning with salt and pepper.

CULINARY NOTES

- Cooking the pasta in the soup gives the soup a thicker, richer consistency because the starch from the pasta thickens the broth.

- Use bite-size pasta shapes. Ditalini or macaroni work well.

Nutrition Facts per Serving: 175 calories, 10 g protein, 2.5 g fat (1 g saturated fat), 29 g carbohydrate, 7 g fiber, 0 mg cholesterol, 300 mg sodium, 7 glycemic load

TOMATOES STUFFED
WITH QUINOA, CUCUMBER, & FETA

Start to Finish: 1 hour*   *Yield: 4 servings*

4   large tomatoes
1½ cups toasted quinoa, cooked
½   cup cucumber, peeled, seeded, cut in small dice
2   scallions, chopped

1   tablespoon parsley, chopped
¼   cup feta cheese, crumbled
1   ounce lemon juice
1   ounce extra-virgin olive oil
Salt and pepper to taste

1. Cut off the tops of the tomatoes. Using a paring knife, gently cut around the sides of the tomatoes to loosen the pulp. Gently scoop out the center of the tomatoes with a spoon or grapefruit knife, being careful not to poke through the sides. Save the pulp and juice. Season inside of the tomatoes with salt and pepper.

2. Remove the seeds from the pulp; chop up the pulp. Combine chopped tomato pulp, quinoa, cucumber, scallions, parsley, and feta cheese. Season with lemon juice, extra-virgin olive oil, salt and pepper.

3. Stuff each tomato shell with ¼ of the quinoa mixture.

Variations:

- Replace quinoa with farro, wheat berries, or bulgur.
- Replace parsley with mint.
- To make a more substantial an entrée, add 4 ounces shredded roasted chicken to the filling.

CULINARY NOTE

* Start to finish time will be only 20 minutes using leftover quinoa.

Nutrition Facts per Serving: 175 calories, 7 g protein, 9 g fat (2 g saturated fat), 19 g carbohydrate, 2 g fiber, 8 mg cholesterol, 115 mg sodium, 8 glycemic load

ASIAN CHICKEN SALAD

Start to Finish: 45 minutes
Yield: 4 servings (1½ cups each)

1   cup cucumbers, peeled, seeded, sliced thin

½   cup carrots, peeled, cut in half lengthwise, then sliced thin

½   cup snowpeas, blanched, ½ inch bias cut

1   cup chicken, cooked, shredded

1   cup jicama, peeled, julienne

½   cup bean sprouts

1   cup hearts of romaine lettuce, julienne

4   scallions, chopped

2   tablespoons cilantro, chopped

4   tablespoons Soy Sesame Vinaigrette (page 202)

2   tablespoons toasted almonds, chopped

Salt and pepper to taste

1. Place cucumbers, carrots, and snow peas in a bowl. Lightly season with salt and pepper. Let sit for 5 minutes.

2. Add chicken, jicama, bean sprouts, lettuce, scallions, and cilantro. Toss with Soy Sesame Vinaigrette. Add toasted almonds. Adjust seasoning with salt and pepper.

Optional: Add ¼ or more teaspoon chile sauce (sambal oelek or chopped Thai bird chiles).

Nutrition Facts per Serving (both vinaigrette and salad): 140 calories, 14 g protein, 4.5 g fat (.6 g saturated fat), 13 g carbohydrate, 4 g fiber, 30 mg cholesterol, 300 mg sodium, 1.5 glycemic load

TOASTED QUINOA, CHICKEN, CUCUMBER, & DILL SALAD

Start to Finish: 20 minutes   Yield: 4 servings (1½ cup each)

2 cups cucumbers, peeled, seeded, diced

1 cup radishes, cut in quarters, sliced thin

1½ cups cooked quinoa

1 cup chicken, cooked, shredded

2 scallions, chopped

2 tablespoons dill, chopped

1 tablespoon mint, chopped

5 tablespoons Simple Lemon Vinaigrette (page 204)

2 tablespoons almonds, toasted, chopped

Salt and pepper to taste

1. Place cucumbers and radishes in a bowl. Lightly season with salt and pepper. Let sit for 5 minutes.

2. Add quinoa, chicken, scallions, dill, and mint. Gently mix. Add the vinaigrette and fold in nuts. Adjust seasoning with salt and pepper.

Variations:

- Replace the dill and mint with basil.
- Replace the chicken with water-packed canned tuna
- Replace ½ cup of radishes with ½ cup peeled, sliced celery.
- Add ½ cup cooked corn; replace dill with chopped parsley.

CULINARY NOTES

- The quinoa and roast chicken can be COOK 1X · EAT 2X ingredients if you you have enough leftover from a previous meal.
- When preparing salads with grains, remember that grains and starchy ingredients will absorb seasoning and need to be reseasoned just before serving.
- This dish can be vegan if you omit the chicken and cook the quinoa in vegetable broth.

Nutrition Facts per Serving: 225 calories , 14 g protein, 9 g fat (2 g saturated fat), 28 g carbohydrate, 5 g fiber, 2 mg cholesterol, 89 mg sodium, 0 glycemic load

Greek Salad
with grilled shrimp

Start to Finish: 1 hour   Yield: 4 servings

1   pound fresh or frozen large shrimp in shells

2   cloves garlic, minced (1 teaspoon)

½   teaspoon lemon peel, finely shredded

3   cups whole fresh baby spinach leaves

3   cups torn romaine

2   medium tomatoes, cut into thin wedges

1   medium cucumber, quartered lengthwise and sliced ¼ inch thick

⅓   cup pitted kalamata olives

¼   cup red onion, chopped

¼   cup radishes, thinly sliced

¼   cup feta cheese, crumbled (1 ounce)

1   recipe Greek Vinaigrette (page 197)

2   large whole-wheat pita bread rounds, halved crosswise

4   skewers

1. Thaw shrimp, if frozen. Peel and devein shrimp, leaving tails intact if desired. Rinse shrimp; pat dry with paper towels. In a small bowl toss shrimp with garlic and lemon peel. Cover and chill for 30 minutes.

2. Meanwhile, in a large bowl combine spinach, romaine, tomatoes, cucumber, olives, red onion, and radishes; toss to combine. Set aside.

3. Thread shrimp onto four 8-inch skewers,* leaving a ¼-inch space between pieces.

4. For a charcoal grill, place skewers on the greased rack of an uncovered grill directly over medium coals. Grill for 6 to 8 minutes or until shrimp are opaque, turning once halfway through grilling. For a gas grill, preheat grill. Reduce heat to medium. Place skewers on greased grill rack over heat. Cover and grill as above.

5. To serve, divide greens among 4 dinner plates. Sprinkle with feta cheese. Top with grilled shrimp. Drizzle with Greek Vinaigrette. Serve with pita bread.

- Season the spinach-and-vegetable mixture with a pinch of salt and pepper before adding the vinaigrette. This allows the greens and vegetables to reveal their true flavor before they are coated by the oil in the vinaigrette.
- When adding dressing to the salad, add it gradually. Some people like heavily dressed salads; others like lightly dressed salads.
- Cherry tomatoes, cut in half, can be used in place of tomato wedges.
- * If using wooden skewers, soak in enough water to cover for at least 1 hour before grilling.

Variations:

- Replace shrimp with ½-inch by 3-inch strips of boneless skinless chicken breasts.
- Replace shrimp with four 4-ounce portions of salmon fillet. Leave each portion in a single piece and do not skewer. Grill or sauté until fish is approximately 130°F.
- Broiler method: Place skewers on the unheated rack of a broiler pan. Broil 4 inches from the heat for 2 to 4 minutes or until shrimp are opaque, turning once halfway through broiling.

Nutrition Facts per Serving: 369 calories, 30 g protein, 16 g total fat (3 g saturated fat), 29 g carbohydrate, 6 g fiber, 179 mg cholesterol, 571 mg sodium

SONOMA CHOPPED SALMON SALAD

Start to Finish: 35 minutes
Yield: 4 servings

Nonstick olive oil cooking spray
¾ cup smoked salmon, flaked
¼ cup scallions, thinly sliced
½ cup yellow bell pepper, coarsely chopped
1⅓ cups seeded tomatoes, chopped
¼ cup chopped onion

1 medium cucumber, coarsely chopped (2 cups)
2 tablespoons ripe olives, chopped
2 teaspoons small capers, drained
1 recipe Lemon Vinaigrette (see below)

1. Coat four 6-ounce coffee cups with nonstick cooking spray. Equally divide and layer ingredients in each cup in the following order: salmon, scallions, bell pepper, tomatoes, onion, and cucumber. Cover tops with plastic wrap and firmly press mixture into cups with a soup can or similar object slightly smaller than diameter of cup.

2. To serve, invert salads onto 4 salad plates; carefully lift off cups. Sprinkle salads with olives and capers; drizzle with Lemon Vinaigrette.

LEMON VINAIGRETTE: In a screw-top jar combine 3 tablespoons extra-virgin olive oil, 3 teaspoons finely shredded lemon peel, 3 tablespoons lemon juice, sugar substitute to equal ½ teaspoon sugar, ¼ teaspoon kosher salt, and several dashes bottled hot pepper sauce. Shake well before serving.

Nutrition Facts per Serving: 135 calories, 7 g protein, 8 g total fat (1 g saturated fat), 9 g carbohydrate, 2 g fiber, 7 mg cholesterol, 430 mg sodium

Variations:

- Place items in this order in a 12-ounce cup.
- Sprinkle each vegetable with salt and pepper.

SONOMA CAESAR SALAD

2 tablespoons Sonoma Caesar Salad Dressing (page 203)

½ cup tomatoes, chopped

¼ cup cooked chicken, shredded, or flaked fish

½ tablespoon grated parmesan

¼ cup white cannellini beans

2 tablespoons scallions, sliced

1 cup romaine lettuce, chopped

ASIAN CHOPPED SALAD

2 tablespoons Soy Sesame Vinaigrette (page 202)

¼ cup red and yellow peppers, chopped

¼ cup snow peas, blanched

¼ cup cooked chicken, shredded

¼ cup cucumber, peeled, cut in half lengthwise, seeded, and sliced thin

1 cup red leaf lettuce

1 tablespoon toasted almonds, chopped

WINE COUNTRY SALAD
WITH GRILLED TUNA

Start to Finish: 35 minutes   Yield: 4 servings

4   ounces fresh green beans
5   cups packaged European-
    style torn mixed salad greens
1   pound fresh tuna
4   medium tomatoes,
    quartered
2   hard-cooked eggs, peeled
    and quartered
½   cup chopped fresh
    flat-leaf parsley

3   scallions, cut into
    ½-inch slices
4   anchovy fillets, drained,
    rinsed, and patted dry
    (optional)
¾   cup pitted ripe olives
Salt and pepper to taste
1   recipe Niçoise Dressing
    (below)

1. Wash green beans; remove ends and strings. Leave beans whole or snap in half. In a covered medium saucepan cook green beans in a small amount of boiling lightly salted water about 5 minutes or just until tender. Drain and place in ice water until chilled; drain well. If desired, cover and chill for 2 to 24 hours.

2. Cut tuna into 4-ounce portions; season with salt and pepper. Grill over medium-high heat until medium or medium rare.

3. Line a large platter or 4 serving plates with salad greens. Arrange green beans, tuna, tomatoes, and eggs on the greens. Sprinkle with parsley and scallions. If desired, top with anchovy fillets. Top with olives. Drizzle Niçoise Dressing over all.

NIÇOISE DRESSING: In a small bowl combine 3 tablespoons extra-virgin olive oil, 1 tablespoon white wine vinegar, ½ teaspoon Dijon mustard, ¼ teaspoon kosher salt, and ⅛ teaspoon freshly ground black pepper. Whisk together until combined.

Variation:

• Replace fresh tuna with 1 6-ounce can of chunk white tuna (in water), drained and broken into chunks

Nutrition Facts per Serving: 260 calories, 16 g protein, 17 g total fat (3 g saturated fat), 12 g carbohydrate, 5 g fiber, 124 mg cholesterol, 570 mg sodium

STEAK & BLUE CHEESE WRAP

Start to Finish: 10 minutes
Yield: 1 serving

3   ounces leftover grilled Herb-Marinated Flank Steak (page 254), thinly sliced

1   cup romaine or whole fresh baby spinach leaves, shredded

¼   cup bottled roasted red bell peppers, drained and cut into thin strips

1   tablespoon crumbled blue cheese

1   8-inch whole-wheat flour tortilla

Arrange sliced beef, romaine, roasted bell pepper strips, and blue cheese on top of the tortilla. Roll up (tortilla will be very full).

CULINARY NOTES

- Heat the tortilla over medium heat for a few seconds on both sides to make it more pliable.

- Use whole-wheat flat bread or lavash to replace the tortilla.

- Plan ahead: prepare Herb-Marinated Flank Steak (page 254) for dinner, then turn leftover steak into a COOK 1X · EAT 2X ingredient of lunch the next day.

Variations:

- **Steak, Grilled Portabello, and Blue Cheese Wrap:** Add half a grilled portabello mushroom sliced ¼ inch thick.

- **Steak, Avocado, and Goat Cheese Wrap:** Replace blue cheese with goat cheese; add ¼ avocado, sliced, and ¼ tomato, sliced.

- **Portabello and Blue Cheese Wrap:** Replace steak with one grilled portabello mushroom sliced ¼ inch thick.

Nutrition Facts per Serving: 390 calories, 33 g protein, 19 g total fat (6 g saturated fat), 21 g carbohydrate, 13 g fiber, 46 mg cholesterol, 775 mg sodium

SPICED PORK WRAP
WITH WHITE BEANS & WATERCRESS

Start to Finish: 20 minutes   Yield: 4 servings

1 cup tomatoes, diced

1 cup white beans, drained

½ teaspoon garlic, mashed

2 tablespoons lemon juice

1 tablespoon extra-virgin olive oil

1 cup heart of romaine lettuce, shredded

2 cups watercress, washed, large stems removed

4 whole-wheat tortillas

1 pound leftover Indian-Spiced Pork tenderloin, cooked and sliced thin (page 256)

1. Salt and pepper to taste

2. Combine the tomatoes, white beans, garlic, and lemon juice. Season with salt and pepper. Let sit for 10 minutes. Stir in olive oil.

3. Combine the lettuce and watercress. Season with salt and pepper.

4. Heat the tortillas. Divide the lettuce mix among the tortillas. Top with the white bean mixture and sliced pork. Roll up and serve.

Variations:

- Replace pork with chicken.
- Add 2 tablespoons yogurt mint dressing to wraps.

CULINARY NOTES

- Pick the large stems of the watercress off, leaving a little of the smaller younger stem.

- Slice the pork against the grain.

- Allowing the tomatoes, white beans, garlic, and lemon juice to sit for a few minutes without the oil allows them to absorb flavors better.

- Plan ahead: prepare Pork Tenderloin with Indian-Spiced Yogurt Marinade (page 256) one day, then turn leftover pork into a COOK 1X · EAT 2X ingredient.

Nutrition Facts per Serving: 420 calories, 32 g protein, 15 g fat (2 g saturated fat), 37 g carbohydrate, 6.5 g fiber, 65 mg cholesterol, 350 mg sodium, 9.2 glycemic load

Shrimp, White Beans, Spinach, & Sun-Dried Tomatoes Salad

Start to Finish: 20 minutes   Yield: 4 servings

¼ cup Red Wine Vinaigrette (page 199)

¼ teaspoon garlic, minced

¾ pound shrimp, cooked, cut in half lengthwise

1   14–16-ounce can white beans, drained; reserve liquid

4   cups spinach, cut in 1-inch pieces, or baby spinach, packed

¼ cup sun-dried tomatoes, chopped

1   tablespoon basil, chives, parsley, or your choice of fresh herbs, chopped

Salt and pepper to taste

Combine all ingredients in a large bowl. Add 1 tablespoon liquid from the beans.

Variations:

- Add 1 tablespoon rinsed capers or chopped kalamata olives.

- Substitute canned tuna or leftover chicken for the shrimp.

CULINARY NOTES

- Use the liquid from the beans to dilute the vinaigrette and add viscosity to the salad.

- You can use frozen shrimp.

- The shrimp can be a COOK 1X · EAT 2X ingredient if you have enough leftover from a previous meal.

Nutrition Facts per Serving: 225 calories, 25 g protein, 2 g fat (.3 g saturated fat), 26 g carbohydrate, 8 g fiber, 125 mg cholesterol, 220 mg sodium, 5 glycemic load

BROCCOLI SALAD
WITH SUN-DRIED TOMATOES & PINE NUTS

Start to Finish: 20 minutes   Yield: 4 servings

1   pound broccoli,
    florets and stems
1   ounce sun-dried tomatoes,
    soft, julienned
1   ounce pine nuts, toasted
2   scallions, sliced thin
    on a bias

1   tablespoon basil, julienned
1   tablespoon capers, rinsed
5   tablespoons Red Wine
    Vinaigrette (page 199)
Salt and pepper to taste

1. Fill a 2-quart pot with water. Bring to a boil. Add 1 tablespoon salt; bring back to a boil.

2. Add the broccoli florets and cook until crisp-tender. Place in ice water to shock. Let cool for 3–5 minutes; drain well.

3. Peel and trim the broccoli stems. Cut stems in half lengthwise; then slice ⅛ inch thin on a bias.

4. Combine the broccoli florets, stems, and the remaining ingredients in a bowl. Toss well.

Variations:

- Replace broccoli with cauliflower.
- Add ½ cup cherry tomatoes cut in half.
- Add 2 ounces shaved parmesan cheese.

CULINARY NOTE

To keep the salad from discoloring, add the vinaigrette just before serving.

Nutrition Facts per Serving: 150 calories, 5 g protein, 8 g fat (.5 g saturated fat),
15 g carbohydrate, 8 g fiber, 0 mg cholesterol, 550 mg sodium, 1 glycemic load

GRAIN MEDLEY
WITH ASIAN SEASONINGS

Start to Finish: 55–85 minutes   Yield: 8 servings

2   stalks celery,
    cut into 1-inch pieces

1   large carrot,
    cut into 1-inch pieces

1   small onion,
    cut into 1-inch pieces

2   tablespoons Chinese
    black bean sauce

1   2-inch piece fresh ginger,
    sliced

2   cloves garlic, halved

8   ounces (about 1¼ cups)
    mixed grains (such as
    kamut; spelt; triticale;
    brown rice; wild rice;
    brown, French, or green
    lentils; regular barley;
    and/or quinoa),
    rinsed and drained

3   cups water

¼   teaspoon kosher salt

¼   teaspoon freshly ground
    black pepper

1. Cut a 12-inch square from a double thickness of 100% cotton cheesecloth. Place celery, carrot, onion, black bean sauce, ginger, and garlic in center of the cheesecloth square. Bring up corners and tie with 100% cotton string.

2. In a 2- to 3-quart saucepan combine desired grains, water, and cheesecloth bag. Bring to boiling; reduce heat. Cover and simmer for 30 to 60 minutes (depending upon the grains) or until grains are tender. Remove from heat. Let stand, covered, for 5 minutes. Discard cheesecloth bag, allowing any liquid to drain off. Drain any excess liquid from grains. Stir in kosher salt and pepper.

Nutrition Facts per Serving: 110 calories, 5 g protein, 1 g total fat (0 g saturated fat), 21 g carbohydrate, 4 g fiber, 0 mg cholesterol, 153 mg sodium

Variation:

GRAIN MEDLEY WITH MEXICAN SEASONINGS

Replace black bean sauce and ginger with 3 canned chipotles in adobo sauce, 1 tablespoon of the adobo sauce, and 4 sprigs of fresh Mexican oregano or regular oregano. Use 3 cloves of garlic.

Nutrition Facts per Serving: 103 calories, 4 g protein, 1 g total fat (0 g saturated fat), 20 g carbohydrate, 4 g fiber, 0 mg cholesterol, 73 mg sodium

CULINARY NOTE

You can cook kamut, spelt, triticale, brown rice, and wild rice together; they will take 45 to 60 minutes to cook. You can cook lentils, barley, and quinoa together; they will take about 30 minutes to cook. If you want to combine shorter-cooking grains with longer-cooking grains, cook the longer-cooking grains for 20 to 30 minutes and then add the shorter-cooking grains and cook about 30 minutes more or until tender.

GRILLED ASPARAGUS SALAD

Start to Finish: 20 minutes
Yield: 2 servings

12 ounces fresh asparagus (thick spears), trimmed	3 tablespoons lemon juice
1 tablespoon extra-virgin olive oil	1 tablespoon extra-virgin olive oil
¼ teaspoon kosher salt	2 hard-cooked eggs, peeled and chopped
⅛ teaspoon freshly ground black pepper	1 tablespoon shredded parmesan cheese

1. In a large bowl toss asparagus spears with 1 tablespoon olive oil. Sprinkle with kosher salt and pepper.

2. For a charcoal grill, place asparagus spears crosswise on the rack of an uncovered grill directly over medium coals. Grill for 5 to 7 minutes or until asparagus is crisp-tender and slightly charred all over, turning occasionally. For a gas grill, preheat grill. Reduce heat to medium. Place asparagus spears crosswise on grill rack over heat. Cover and grill as above.

3. To serve, transfer grilled asparagus to serving platter. Drizzle with lemon juice and 1 tablespoon olive oil. Sprinkle with chopped eggs and parmesan cheese. Serve immediately or cover and chill for up to 24 hours.

Broiler method: Place asparagus on the unheated rack of a broiler pan. Broil 4 to 5 inches from the heat for 5 to 7 minutes or until asparagus is crisp-tender, turning once halfway through broiling.

Nutrition Facts per Serving: 247 calories, 11 g protein, 20 g total fat (4 g saturated fat), 9 g carbohydrate, 4 g fiber, 214 mg cholesterol, 350 mg sodium, 0 glycemic load

GRILLED VEGETABLE ROLLS
STUFFED WITH FETA CHEESE, PINE NUTS, & MINT

Start to Finish: 45 minutes   Yield: 32 rolls (4 rolls per serving)

1	red pepper	4	ounces low-fat ricotta cheese
½	pound small zucchini or yellow squash (about 2)	1	ounce pine nuts, toasted
½	pound Japanese eggplant (about 2)	1½	tablespoons mint, chopped
½	ounce extra-virgin olive oil	½	teaspoon lemon zest
3	ounces feta cheese, crumbled	½	teaspoon lemon juice
		1	scallion, chopped
			Salt and pepper to taste

1. Preheat grill on high.

2. Place the pepper on the grill and roast until charred on all sides. Place in a bowl and cover with plastic wrap. Let steam for 15 minutes. Peel; remove stem and seeds. Cut into 1-inch-thick strips.

3. Trim ends from squashes and eggplants. Slice lengthwise into ¼-inch-thick pieces. Season with salt and pepper. Let sit for 10 minutes. Pat dry. Drizzle with olive oil and grill over high heat, cooking on both sides until crisp-tender, for 3–4 minutes. Cool on a wire rack in a single layer until ready to use. This will keep them from overcooking. The vegetables can be prepared the day before or you can use leftover grilled vegetables.

CULINARY NOTE

Zucchini, yellow squash, and eggplant that are approximately 1 inch wide and 7 inches long are ideal for this recipe.

4. Combine the feta and ricotta cheese. Stir in ½ ounce chopped nuts, 1 tablespoon mint, zest, lemon juice, and scallion. Season with salt and pepper.

5. Lay 3½-inch-long pieces of the grilled vegetables on a flat surface. Season vegetables with salt and pepper. Place 1 teaspoon of filling at the end of each vegetable. Roll the vegetable around the filling. Do not roll too tightly. Place seam side down on a platter.

6. Garnish with remaining ½ ounce pine nuts and ½ tablespoon mint.

Variations:

- Replace the mint and scallions with 1 tablespoon finely chopped sun-dried tomato and 1 tablespoon basil.
- Replace the feta cheese, mint, and scallions with 3 ounces goat cheese, 1 tablespoon chopped roasted red peppers, and 1 tablespoon basil.
- Replace feta cheese with ricotta cheese; add 1 tablespoon chopped capers and 1 tablespoon chopped olives.

Nutrition Facts per Serving: 25 calories, 1 g protein, 1.5 g fat (.7 g saturated fat), 1.5 g carbohydrate, .7 g fiber, 3.5 mg cholesterol, 37 mg sodium, 0 glycemic load

SAUTÉED BROCCOLI RABE

Start to Finish: 20 minutes
Yield: 4 servings

2 pounds broccoli rabe, thick stems trimmed, leaves and florets rinsed well

1 tablespoon garlic, minced

1 tablespoon extra-virgin olive oil

¼ teaspoon crushed red pepper flakes

1 teaspoon lemon zest

Salt and pepper to taste

1 tablespoon aged balsamic vinegar or lemon juice

1. Fill a large bowl with ice and water.

2. Bring a large pot of water to a rolling boil. Add the broccoli rabe and blanch for 3 minutes. Drain and place in ice water to cool. Drain well, gently squeezing to remove excess water.

3. Heat the garlic and oil in a sauté pan over low heat. Cook until the garlic is slightly browned. Add the red pepper flakes. Cook 5 seconds. Add the broccoli rabe and turn up the heat. Sauté for 5 minutes or until just warmed through. Add lemon zest and season with salt and pepper.

4. Just before serving, drizzle with balsamic vinegar or lemon juice.

CULINARY NOTES

- Place a lid on the pot of water as you are bringing it to a boil.
- The broccoli rabe can be blanched in advance. Return to room temperature before proceeding with the recipe.
- This recipe can be the base for several   COOK 1X · EAT 2X   dishes; see variation ideas on the following page.

Nutrition Facts per Serving: 100 calories, 8 g protein, 4 g fat (.5 g saturated fat), 12 g carbohydrate, 2 g fiber, 0 mg cholesterol, 60 mg sodium, 0 glycemic load

Variations:

- **Omelet:** Chop up broccoli rabe and use in a frittata with feta cheese and lemon zest.

- **Risotto:** Chop up broccoli rabe and stir into rice at end of cooking.

- Stir fry: Use 1 teaspoon slivered garlic and 1 teaspoon chopped ginger. Replace 1 bunch of broccoli rabe with 1 cup sliced onions, red peppers, and carrots. Season with 2 tablespoons soy sauce and 1 teaspoon of sesame oil.

- **Bruschetta:** Spread a toasted piece of whole-grain baguette with ricotta cheese filling and top with seasoned broccoli rabe.

- **Sandwich:** Use in a sandwich with fresh mozzarella, sliced tomatoes, and capers.

- **Salad:** Toss leftover broccoli rabe with ¼ cup ponzu sauce, 1 teaspoon lemon zest, and 1 teaspoon sesame oil.

SAUTÉED CHERRY TOMATOES WITH BASIL & GARLIC

Start to Finish: 10 minutes   Yield: 4 servings

1   tablespoon olive oil
2   pints cherry tomatoes
1   tablespoon garlic, chopped
1   tablespoon basil, chopped

1   teaspoon lemon zest
    (optional)
Salt and pepper to taste

1. Heat a sauté pan over high heat. Add the olive oil and tomatoes; sauté until the tomatoes are soft and skins are just beginning to wrinkle, but not exploding.

2. Add the garlic and toss until aromatic. Add basil and lemon zest and remove from heat. Season with salt and pepper. Serve immediately.

CULINARY NOTE

Use a microplane to grate the lemon zest. Do not go past the yellow surface of the lemon, since the white pithy part of the lemon will add bitterness to the dish.

Nutrition Facts per Serving: 60 calories, 2 g protein, 5.5 g fat (.5 g saturated fat), 6.5 g carbohydrate, 2 g fiber, 0 mg cholesterol, 8 mg sodium, 0 glycemic load

TOASTED QUINOA PILAF

Start to Finish: 30 minutes
Yield: 8 ½-cup servings

2 tablespoons olive oil
2 cups quinoa, rinsed, drained well
1 cup onion, diced

1 tablespoon garlic, chopped
2 teaspoons thyme, chopped
2½ cups water or stock
Salt and pepper to taste

1. Heat a small saucepan over medium heat. Add olive oil and quinoa. Stir over medium heat to toast the quinoa. It will start to pop like popcorn and have a slightly nutty aroma. Add onion, garlic, and thyme; stir until aromatic.

2. Add water; bring to a simmer. Season with salt and pepper. Reduce heat to low, cover tightly, and cook for 15 minutes.

3. Remove from heat, let sit for 4 minutes, and fluff with a fork.

CULINARY NOTES

- Quinoa has a natural coating on the outside called saposin. It is bitter, so it is important to rinse the quinoa in water, then let it drain for a few minutes before toasting. If the grain is wet, it is more difficult to toast.

- Quinoa can also be toasted by spreading it on a sheet pan and placing in a 350°F oven for 5–10 minutes, stirring periodically.

- It is important to let the grain sit for a few minutes once it is removed from the heat. This allows the grain to settle and slightly firm up. If you stir it immediately after it has finished cooking, it will mush up and become gummy.

- This recipe can be the base for COOK 1X · EAT 2X salads and wraps.

Variations:

- Add 1 cup diced roasted red peppers and 1 cup roasted corn; serve as a side vegetable.

- Add 1 cup roasted butternut squash and 1 tablespoon parsley.

- Add 1 tablespoon chopped chipotle in adobo sauce (less if you do not like spicy foods), 1 cup diced canned green chiles, and 1 cup roasted corn.

- Add 2 cups mushrooms sautéed with garlic.

- Add ¼ cup chopped sun-dried tomatoes and 1 tablespoon basil.

Nutrition Facts per Serving: 100 calories, 4 g protein, 3 g fat (1 g saturated fat), 16 g carbohydrate, 2 g fiber, 0 mg cholesterol, 10 mg sodium, 8.5 glycemic load

WHEAT BERRIES

Start to Finish: 1 hour
Yield: 3 cups

1 cup wheat berries	1 bay leaf
4 cups water	2 teaspoons extra-virgin olive oil
¼ onion, in a large piece	Salt and pepper to taste
½ carrot, peeled in one piece	

1. Combine wheat berries, water, onion, carrot, and bay leaf in a saucepan. Bring to a simmer. Cook until the wheat berries are tender but not mushy.

2. Remove and discard the vegetables and bay leaf. Drain wheat berries well. Stir in extra-virgin olive oil. Season with salt and pepper. If not using immediately, spread on a sheet pan to cool. Then store in the refrigerator.

Variations:

• This method can be used for a variety of grains, including spelt, kamut, faro, and barley (not pearled barley).

CULINARY NOTES

• Wheat berries can be stored in the refrigerator for three days or frozen for up to one month.

• Other herbs and flavoring, such as chipotle in adobo sauce or Chinese black bean sauce, can be added when cooking grains.

• This recipe can be the base for COOK 1X·EAT 2X salads and soups.

Nutrition Facts per Serving: 110 calories, 4.5 g protein, 2 g fat, 0 g saturated fat, 20 g carbohydrate, 3 g fiber, 0 mg cholesterol, 8.5 mg sodium, 6.8 glycemic load

WHITE BEAN RATATOUILLE

Start to Finish: 45 minutes
Yield: 6 servings

2 teaspoons extra-virgin olive oil

2 cups onion, diced

1 tablespoon garlic, chopped

3 cups unpeeled eggplant cut in half, then diced

2 cups zucchini cut in half, then diced

1 15.5 ounce can cannellini beans, drained; reserve ½ cup of liquid

1½ cups seeded tomatoes, diced, or low-sodium canned tomatoes

1½ tablespoons white wine vinegar

½ teaspoon sugar

¼ teaspoon salt

¼ cup fresh basil, finely chopped

1. Heat large sauté pan over high heat. Add oil and onions, sauté for 3 to 5 minutes.

2. Add garlic; sauté for 30 seconds or until aromatic, being careful not to brown it.

3. Add eggplant, zucchini, and ½ cup of bean liquid. Cover pan, bring to simmer over low to medium heat, and cook 15 minutes.

4. Add tomatoes and beans and bring back to simmer; cook 5 minutes. Set aside to cool.

5. Mix the vinegar, sugar, and salt in a small bowl and combine with the cooled ratatouille. Sprinkle with fresh basil.

Nutrition Facts per Serving: 130 calories, 6 g protein, 2.5 g fat, 0 g saturated fat, 27 g carbohydrate, 7 g fiber, 0 mg cholesterol, 280 mg sodium, 5 glycemic load

BLACK-EYED PEAS
WITH SMOKED TURKEY

Start to Finish: 1 hour   Yield: 4 cups

1 tablespoon olive oil
1 cup onion, diced
2 teaspoons garlic, chopped
8 ounces black-eyed peas,
  rinsed and drained

3 cups chicken stock
6 ounces smoked turkey leg,
  bone in
Salt and pepper to taste

1. Heat a small saucepan over low heat. Add the olive oil and onions; cook until translucent. Add the garlic; cook until aromatic. Add the black-eyed peas, chicken stock, and turkey leg. Bring to a simmer. Cook for 45 minutes or until the black-eyed peas are tender.

2. Remove the turkey leg and pull the meat from the bone. Discard the bone, chop up the meat, and stir the meat into the black-eyed peas. Adjust seasoning with salt and pepper.

CULINARY NOTES

- Do not season until the end of cooking. Salt inhibits the softening of the peas. It tends to toughen the skin coating and pea. Black-eyed peas would normally cook in 30–40 minutes, but due to the addition of the smoked turkey, they will take a little longer.

- Prepare twice the recipe and use half for Hoppin' John to accompany roast chicken or grilled barbecued chicken. To make Hoppin' John, gently stir in 2 cups cooked brown rice to an equal amount of the cooked peas.

Nutrition Facts per Serving: 260 calories, 21 g protein, 10 g fat (2 g saturated fat), 20 g carbohydrate, 5 g fiber, 40 mg cholesterol, 280 mg sodium, 4 glycemic load

CHICKEN & WHITE BEAN CHILE VERDE
WITH SONOMA PESTO

Start to Finish: 55 minutes   Yield: 6 to 8 servings

1   pound tomatillos
½   pound poblano chiles
2   teaspoons olive oil
1½ cups yellow onion,
     finely chopped
1   tablespoon garlic, minced
1   teaspoon Mexican oregano
3   cups chicken stock

2   15.5-ounce cans cannellini
     beans, with liquid
2   tablespoons chopped
     fresh cilantro
2   cups cooked, shredded
     chicken
4   cups chard, stemmed,
     cut in 1-inch-wide strips
Salt and black pepper, to taste

1. Preheat oven or toaster oven to 400°F.

2. Place tomatillos and poblano chiles on sheet pan. Roast in oven until peppers have blistered and tomatillos are soft. Remove from oven. Place tomatillos in blender. Once poblanos are cool enough to handle, remove seeds and skins. Add to blender; blend until smooth.

3. Heat olive oil in a sauté pan. Add onions and cook until caramelized, approximately 5 minutes. Add garlic and oregano; cook until aromatic.

4. Add tomatillo mixture; cook for 10 minutes until slightly thickened.

5. Add stock, beans and their liquid. Bring to simmer; cook for 20 minutes.

6. Add cilantro, chicken, and chard. Bring to a simmer; cook for 10 minutes. Adjust seasoning with salt and pepper.

Nutrition Facts per Serving: 380 calories, 24 g protein, 15 g fat (2 g saturated fat), 41 g carbohydrate, 13 g fiber, 30 mg cholesterol, 450 mg sodium, 7 glycemic load

SONOMA PESTO

Combine all pesto ingredients in a blender. Blend until smooth. Adjust seasoning with salt and pepper. Drizzle the pesto on top of the chile verde and finish with 2 tablespoons of salsa verde (purchased), as desired.

1 bunch fresh cilantro

1 serrano chile

1 tablespoon pine nuts or peanuts

1 clove garlic

2 ounces extra-virgin olive oil

1 lime, juiced, with zest

Salt and black pepper, to taste

CULINARY NOTES

- Baby spinach may be substituted for chard.

- For a less spicy chile, Anaheim peppers may be substituted for poblano peppers.

- For a special local flair, try the small tomatillo variety named Milpero. It is flavorful and fruity with a concentrated flavor of the green tomatillo.

- The chicken can be a COOK 1X· EAT 2X ingredient if you have enough leftover from a previous meal.

ROAST CHICKEN, GARBANZO BEAN, RED PEPPER, & CAPER SALAD

Start to Finish: 30 minutes   Yield: 4 servings

¼ teaspoon garlic, mashed

⅛ teaspoon ground cumin

2 teaspoons Spanish paprika

¼ cup Red Wine or Sherry Vinaigrette (pages 199, 200–201)

1 pound chicken, cooked, cut in ½-inch by 1-inch pieces

2 cups garbanzo beans, rinsed; reserve liquid

1 cup bottled roasted red pepper, cut in strips

2 cups spinach, cut in 1-inch pieces, or baby spinach

2 tablespoons capers, rinsed

Salt and pepper to taste

1. Combine garlic, cumin, paprika, and vinaigrette in a small bowl.

2. Place remaining ingredients in a large bowl. Add vinaigrette mixture and mix well.

Variations:

- Replace garbanzo beans with white beans.
- Replace chicken with roast pork.
- Replace spinach with shredded romaine lettuce or arugula.

CULINARY NOTES

- If the salad is too vinegary, add some of the canned bean liquid.
- This salad will become more delicious as it sits. You can prepare it the day before but leave out the spinach. Add the spinach just before serving.
- The chicken can be a COOK 1X · EAT 2X ingredient if you use leftovers.

Nutrition Facts per Serving: 390 calories, 36 g protein, 14 g fat (2.5 g saturated fat), 27 g carbohydrate, 8 g fiber, 85 mg cholesterol, 850 mg sodium, 4.5 glycemic load

TANDOORI CHICKEN

*Start to Finish: 30 minutes, plus 24 to 48 hours for chilling
and 1 to 3 hours for marinating   Yield: 4 servings*

½ cup plain fat-free yogurt

4 skinless, boneless chicken
breast halves
(1 to 1¼ pounds total)

⅛ teaspoon kosher salt

⅛ teaspoon freshly ground
black pepper

¼ cup lemon juice

3 cloves garlic, minced
(1½ teaspoons minced)

2 teaspoons paprika

¼ teaspoon cayenne pepper

⅛ teaspoon ground cinnamon

⅛ teaspoon ground cumin

1. To make yogurt cheese, line a yogurt strainer, sieve, or small colander with three layers of 100% cotton cheesecloth or a paper coffee filter. Suspend lined strainer over a bowl. Spoon yogurt into lined strainer. Cover with plastic wrap. Refrigerate for 24 to 48 hours. Discard liquid.

2. Sprinkle chicken with kosher salt and black pepper. Place chicken in a self-sealing plastic bag set in a shallow dish. In a small bowl combine the yogurt cheese, lemon juice, garlic, paprika, cayenne pepper, cinnamon, and cumin. Pour over chicken. Cover and marinate in the refrigerator for 1 to 3 hours.

3. Remove chicken from marinade; discard marinade. For a charcoal grill, place chicken on the rack of an uncovered grill directly over medium coals. Grill for 10 to 12 minutes or until chicken is no longer pink (170° F), turning once halfway through grilling. For a gas grill, preheat grill. Reduce heat to medium. Place chicken on grill rack over heat. Cover and grill as above.

> **CULINARY NOTES**
>
> • Be sure to use yogurt that contains no gums, gelatin, or fillers. These ingredients may prevent the curd and whey from separating to make the yogurt cheese.
>
> • COOK 1X · EAT 2X in salads, frittatas, omelets, wraps, or sandwiches.

Nutrition Facts per Serving: 152 calories, 28 g protein, 2 g total fat (0 g saturated fat), 5 g carbohydrate, 1 g fiber, 66 mg cholesterol, 144 mg sodium, 1 glycemic load

TOASTED BULGUR, CHICKEN, & ALMOND SALAD

Start to Finish: 15 minutes   Yield: 4 servings (1¼ cup each)

1½ cups cucumbers, peeled, seeded, diced

2 cups cooked coarse bulgur

1 cup chicken, cooked, shredded

1½ cups baby spinach, julienned

2 scallions, chopped

2 tablespoons parsley, chopped

4 tablespoons Simple Lemon Vinaigrette (page 204)

3 tablespoons toasted almonds, chopped

Salt and pepper to taste

1. Place cucumbers in a bowl. Lightly season with salt and pepper. Let sit for 5 minutes.

2. Add the bulgur, chicken, spinach, scallions, and parsley. Mix well. Drizzle with lemon vinaigrette. Add toasted almonds. Adjust seasoning with salt and pepper.

Variations:

- Add ½ cup diced roasted red peppers.

- Replace the bulgur with toasted cooked quinoa, spelt, barley, or farro (the quinoa substitution will make it gluten-free).

- Replace chicken with canned tuna packed in water. Leave in chunks. It will break up as it is mixed.

CULINARY NOTES

- When preparing salad with grains, remember that grains and starchy ingredients will absorb seasoning and need to be re-seasoned just before serving.

- Use leftover bulgur pilaf and leftover chicken as COOK 1X · EAT 2X ingredients.

Nutrition Facts per Serving: 250 calories, 16 g protein, 10 g fat (2 g saturated fat), 24 g carbohydrate, 7 g fiber, 30 mg cholesterol, 50 mg sodium, 6.5 glycemic load

Herb-Marinated Flank Steak

Start to Finish: 1 hour, plus 1 to 24 hours for marinating
Yield: 8 servings

1   1½- to 2-pound beef
    flank steak

¼   cup fresh rosemary,
    chopped, or 1 tablespoon
    dried rosemary, crushed

1   tablespoon fresh marjoram,
    chopped, or 1 teaspoon
    dried marjoram, crushed

1   tablespoon fresh oregano,
    chopped, or 1 teaspoon
    dried oregano, crushed

3   cloves garlic, minced
    (1½ teaspoons minced)

1½ teaspoons paprika

1   teaspoon kosher salt

1   teaspoon crushed
    red pepper

1   teaspoon freshly ground
    black pepper

3   tablespoons extra-virgin
    olive oil

1. Trim fat from meat. Score both sides of steak in a diamond pattern by making shallow cuts at 1-inch intervals; set aside. In a small bowl stir together rosemary, marjoram, oregano, garlic, paprika, kosher salt, crushed red pepper, and black pepper. Stir in the oil until combined.

> **CULINARY NOTE**
>
> Plan ahead: save leftover steak to use as a COOK 1X · EAT 2X ingredient for Steak & Blue Cheese Wrap (page 233).

2. Spoon herb mixture evenly over both sides of steak; rub in with your fingers. Place steak in a shallow dish. Cover and marinate in the refrigerator for 1 to 24 hours.

3. For a charcoal grill, place meat on the rack of an uncovered grill directly over medium coals. Grill for 17 to 21 minutes or until medium doneness (160°F), turning once halfway through grilling. For a gas grill, preheat grill. Reduce heat to medium. Place meat on grill rack over heat. Cover and grill as above.

4. Transfer grilled meat to a cutting board. Cover and let stand for 10 minutes. To serve, slice very thinly across the grain.

Nutrition Facts per Serving: 183 calories, 19 g protein, 11 g total fat (3 g saturated fat), 1 g carbohydrate, 0 g fiber, 34 mg cholesterol, 287 mg sodium, 0 glycemic load

SPICED JERK LONDON BROIL

Start to Finish: 30 minutes, plus 4 to 24 hours for marinating
Yield: 6 servings

4 scallions	3 cloves garlic
¼ cup lime juice	2 teaspoons Jamaican Jerk
1-inch piece fresh ginger, sliced	Rub (page 183)
½ Scotch bonnet chile pepper, seeded and finely chopped (optional)	1 1¼- to 1½-pound beef flank steak
2 tablespoons extra-virgin olive oil	Kosher salt (optional) Freshly ground black pepper (optional)

1. For marinade, in a blender combine scallions, lime juice, ginger, Scotch bonnet pepper (if desired), oil, garlic, and jerk rub; cover and blend until smooth. Score both sides of steak in a diamond pattern by making shallow cuts at 1-inch intervals. If desired, season steak with kosher salt and pepper. Place steak in a glass dish; spread marinade over the steak. Cover dish with plastic wrap and marinate in the refrigerator for 4 to 24 hours. Drain steak, discarding marinade.

2. For a charcoal grill, place steak on the rack of an uncovered grill directly over medium coals. Grill for 17 to 21 minutes or until medium doneness (160°F), turning once halfway through grilling. For a gas grill, preheat grill. Reduce heat to medium. Place steak on grill rack over heat. Cover and grill as above.

3. To serve, thinly slice meat diagonally across the grain.

Variations:

- Replace the Scotch bonnet with a habanero chile. If habaneros are not available, use chopped serrano chiles or red Thai bird chiles.
- Replace beef with chicken breast or legs or pork tenderloin.

> **CULINARY NOTE**
> COOK 1X·EAT 2X
> in salads, frittatas, omelets, wraps, or sandwiches.

Nutrition Facts per Serving: 189 calories, 20 g protein, 11 g total fat (3 g saturated fat), 2 g carbohydrate, 0 g fiber, 47 mg cholesterol, 161 mg sodium, 0 glycemic load

INDIAN-SPICED PORK LOIN
WITH YOGURT MARINADE

Start to Finish: 20 minutes   *Yield: 4 servings*

1 pound pork loin,
   excess fat removed
Salt and pepper to taste
¼ cup plain probiotic yogurt
¼ teaspoon turmeric
¼ teaspoon paprika

½ teaspoon ground cumin
½ teaspoon ground coriander
¼ teaspoon dried mint
Salt and pepper to taste

1. Season pork with salt and pepper.

2. Combine remaining ingredients and stir to mix. Place in a leakproof container or resealable bag such as a Ziploc bag; force out all the air so that the meat is in contact with the marinade. Add pork. Let sit for 15 minutes to overnight.

3. Grill or sauté the meat.

Variation:

- Replace pork with 1 pound chicken breast.

> **CULINARY NOTES**
>
> - Plan ahead: save leftover pork tenderloin and you'll have a COOK 1x · EAT 2x ingredient for Spiced Pork Wrap (page 233).
>
> - *15 minutes to overnight for marinating

Nutrition Facts per Serving: 155 calories, 25 g protein, 4 g total fat (1.2 g saturated fat), 1.5 g carbohydrate, .3 g fiber, 79 mg cholesterol, 78 mg sodium, 0 glycemic load

ROAST PORK LOIN
WITH VEGETABLE RATATOUILLE

Start to Finish: 1 hour 20 minutes   Yield: 4 servings

3   cloves garlic, minced
     (1½ teaspoons)

2   teaspoons fresh rosemary,
     chopped, or ½ teaspoon
     dried rosemary, crushed

2   tablespoons extra-virgin
     olive oil

1   1- to 1¼-pound pork
     tenderloin

2   tablespoons fresh oregano,
     chopped, or 2 teaspoons
     dried oregano, crushed

2   teaspoons finely shredded
     lemon peel

3   tablespoons lemon juice

1   pound small zucchini,
     halved lengthwise

1   pound small yellow summer
     squash, halved lengthwise

1   medium onion,
     sliced ½ inch thick

2   small red bell peppers,
     halved and seeded
     (8 ounces)

2   small yellow bell peppers,
     halved and seeded
     (8 ounces)

2   medium tomatoes,
     seeded and chopped

1   tablespoon capers,
     rinsed and drained

4   large fresh basil leaves,
     cut into thin strips

Kosher salt

Freshly ground black pepper

1. Preheat oven to 425°F.

2. In a small bowl combine 2 cloves of the garlic, rosemary, and
1 tablespoon of the oil. Spoon mixture evenly over pork; rub in with
your fingers.

3. In the same small bowl combine remaining clove of garlic, remaining
1 tablespoon oil, oregano, lemon peel, and lemon juice. Brush over
zucchini, yellow summer squash, onion, and bell peppers.

4. Place a rack in the center of a large shallow roasting pan. Place
tenderloin on rack. Arrange seasoned vegetables in a single layer in the
bottom of the pan, around the edge, so they roast, not steam.

(The vegetables don't need to be on the rack). Stir the vegetables periodically during the roasting period.

5. Roast for 30 to 40 minutes or until an instant-read thermometer inserted into center of tenderloin registers 155°F. Remove tenderloin from roasting pan. Cover with foil and let stand for 10 minutes before slicing. The temperature of the meat after standing should be 160°F.

6. Transfer vegetables to a very large serving bowl; add tomatoes, capers, and basil. Toss to combine. Season to taste with kosher salt and black pepper. Cover and let stand until pork is ready to serve.

7. Cut pork into ¼-inch slices. Serve pork on top of vegetables.

CULINARY NOTES

- COOK 1X·EAT 2X in salads, frittatas, omelets, wraps, or sandwiches.
- The vegetable ratatouille can also be served as a side dish for roast poultry or used as a filling in a sandwich with sliced meat.

Variations:

- Replace ¼ pound zucchini and ¼ pound yellow squash with ½ pound sliced Japanese eggplant. Use canned tomatoes in place of fresh tomatoes.

Nutrition Facts per Serving: 308 calories, 29 g protein, 11 g total fat (2 g saturated fat), 26 g carbohydrate, 7 g fiber, 73 mg cholesterol, 252 mg sodium

SPANISH ROAST PORK TENDERLOIN

Start to Finish: 15 minutes, plus 15 minutes to overnight for marinating
Yield: 4 servings

1   pound pork tenderloin, excess fat removed

1   teaspoon garlic, mashed to a paste

1   tablespoon extra-virgin olive oil

½   teaspoon ground cumin

¼   teaspoon ground coriander

1   teaspoon Spanish paprika, smoked or plain

¼   teaspoon ground ginger

¼   teaspoon turmeric

¼   teaspoon ground black pepper

1   teaspoon lemon juice and zest or red wine vinegar

Salt and pepper to taste

1. Season pork with salt and pepper.

2. Mix the mashed garlic with a pinch of salt. Add remaining ingredients and stir to mix. Spread all over the pork.

3. Let sit for 15 minutes to overnight.

4. Grill or sauté the meat.

Variation:

- Use chicken instead of pork.

CULINARY NOTE

COOK 1X · EAT 2X in salads, frittatas, omelets, wraps, or sandwiches.

SPANISH ROAST PORK TENDERLOIN
WITH CHICKPEAS AND SPINACH

Start to Finish: 1 hour   Yield: 4 servings

1 tablespoon extra-virgin olive oil

1 pound pork tenderloin in Spanish Marinade (page 179)

1 tablespoon extra-virgin olive oil

1 cup onions, chopped

1 tablespoon garlic, chopped

1½ teaspoons Spanish paprika

1 can chickpeas, drained; reserve liquid

1 cup cherry tomatoes, cut in half, or chopped tomatoes

4 cups baby spinach

Salt and pepper to taste

1. Preheat oven to 400°F.

2. Heat a sauté pan over medium heat. Add extra-virgin olive oil and pork tenderloin. Cook until lightly browned. Turn tenderloin over and move to the side of the pan.

3. Add onions to the side of the pan where the pork had browned. Add 1 tablespoon of the bean liquid. Add garlic and paprika to the onions and stir. Let pork continue to brown. Once brown, remove pork from pan. Add chickpeas to onions; stir to coat. Place pork on top of chickpeas and place in hot oven. Roast for 15–20 minutes or until the pork is 143°F (turn at 8 minutes).

4. Remove pork from pan and let rest in a warm spot. Sprinkle cherry tomatoes on top of chickpeas. Place in oven and roast for 10 minutes until slightly dried. Stir in the spinach and 1 tablespoon chickpea liquid. Adjust seasoning with salt and pepper. Slice pork ¼ inch thick on bias.

5. To serve, place 1 cup of chickpea mixture on a plate and top with 4 ounces of sliced pork.

Nutrition Facts per Serving: 450 calories, 35 g protein, 19 g fat (3.5 g saturated fat), 39 g carbohydrate, 11 g fiber, 60 mg cholesterol, 350 mg sodium, 6 glycemic load

CIOPPINO SEAFOOD EN PAPILLOTE

Start to Finish: 50 minutes   Yield: 4 servings

8 ounces fresh or frozen large shrimp in shells

8 ounces fresh or frozen sea scallops or 10 ounces fresh or frozen halibut steaks

parchment paper or foil

2 medium Roma tomatoes, seeded and chopped

1 tablespoon lemon juice

1½ teaspoons fresh basil, chopped, or ½ teaspoon dried basil, crushed

1½ teaspoons fresh thyme, chopped, or ½ teaspoon dried thyme, crushed

1 teaspoon extra-virgin olive oil

1 clove garlic, minced (½ teaspoon)

¼ teaspoon kosher salt

pinch thread saffron, crushed, or ¼ teaspoon ground turmeric

1 small zucchini, halved lengthwise and sliced ¼ inch thick

4 scallions, cut into 1-inch pieces

1. Preheat oven to 400°F.

2 Thaw shrimp and scallops or halibut, if frozen. Peel and devein shrimp. Halve any large scallops or skin, bone, and cut halibut into 1-inch pieces. Set aside.

3. Cut four 12-inch squares of parchment paper or foil. Fold each square in half to form a triangle. Unfold.

4. In a large bowl combine tomatoes, lemon juice, basil, thyme, oil, garlic, kosher salt, and saffron. Add shrimp, scallops, zucchini, and scallions; toss to coat. Divide mixture among parchment or foil squares, spooning it onto the center of one triangle-shaped side of each square. Fold the other half of the square over the mixture to re-form a triangle. To seal packets, fold each of the open sides over ½ inch, then fold over again ½ inch.

5. Place packets on a very large baking sheet. Bake for 12 to 15 minutes or until shrimp and scallops are opaque or halibut flakes easily when tested with a fork. (To test, carefully open the packets and peek.)

CULINARY NOTES

- Cooking en papillote is similar to steaming or baking in a bag. If you do not have parchment paper, use foil, but be wary of using high-acid ingredients and letting them sit in the foil for more than 1 hour.
- When using paper, be sure to seal the edges tightly so the pouches do not open up when steaming.
- Use high-moisture vegetables in the packets.

Variations:

- Use 1 pound large shrimp in shells and omit the scallops and halibut.
- Substitute fish for shrimp.
- Use 1 pound chicken and omit the scallops and halibut.
- Use cherry tomatoes cut in half instead of chopped tomatoes.
- **For a Latin version:** Replace lemon, basil, thyme, and saffron with lime juice, 2 teaspoons cilantro, 1 teaspoon Mexican oregano, and 1 teaspoon chopped jalapeño chile.

Nutrition Facts per Serving: 141 calories, 22 g protein, 3 g total fat (0 g saturated fat), 6 g carbohydrate, 1 g fiber, 105 mg cholesterol, 305 mg sodium, 1 glycemic load

GRILLED TUNA WITH ROSEMARY

Start to Finish: 20 minutes
Yield: 4 servings

1 pound fresh or frozen tuna, halibut, or salmon steaks, cut 1-inch thick	2 teaspoons fresh rosemary or tarragon, chopped, or 1 teaspoon dried rosemary or tarragon, crushed
2 teaspoons extra-virgin olive oil	
2 teaspoons lemon juice	1 tablespoon drained capers, slightly crushed
⅛ teaspoon kosher salt	Fresh rosemary sprigs (optional)
⅛ teaspoon freshly ground black pepper	
2 cloves garlic, minced (1 teaspoon minced)	

1. Thaw fish, if frozen. Rinse fish; pat dry with paper towels. Cut fish into 4 serving-size pieces. Brush both sides of fish with oil and lemon juice; sprinkle with kosher salt and pepper. Sprinkle garlic and rosemary evenly onto fish; rub in with your fingers.

> **CULINARY NOTE**
>
> COOK 1X · EAT 2X in salads, frittatas, omelets, wraps, or sandwiches.

2. For a charcoal grill, place fish on the greased rack of an uncovered grill directly over medium-hot coals. Grill for 8 to 12 minutes or until fish flakes easily when tested with a fork, turning once halfway through grilling. For a gas grill, preheat grill. Reduce heat to medium. Place fish on grill rack over heat. Cover and grill as above.

3. Top fish with capers. If desired, garnish with fresh rosemary.

Broiler method: Place fish on the greased unheated rack of a broiler pan. Broil 4 inches from the heat for 8 to 12 minutes or until fish flakes easily when tested with a fork, turning once halfway through broiling.

Nutrition Facts per Serving: 145 calories, 27 g protein, 3 g total fat (1 g saturated fat), 1 g carbohydrate, 0 g fiber, 51 mg cholesterol, 179 mg sodium, 0 glycemic load

ORANGE ROUGHY
WITH CILANTRO PESTO

Start to Finish: 30 minutes   Yield: 4 servings

1 to 1¼ pounds fresh or frozen orange roughy or cod fillets

1½ cups loosely packed fresh cilantro leaves

1 fresh jalapeño chile pepper, seeded and chopped*

1 clove garlic, halved

2 tablespoons extra-virgin olive oil

1 tablespoon lime juice

¼ teaspoon kosher salt

¼ teaspoon freshly ground black pepper

1. Thaw fish, if frozen. Rinse fish; pat dry with paper towels. Cut fish into 4 serving-size pieces, if necessary. Measure thickness of fish. Set fish aside.

2. For cilantro pesto, in a small food processor or blender combine cilantro, jalapeño pepper, garlic, 1 tablespoon of the oil, and the lime juice. Cover and process or blend with several on/off turns until almost smooth, stopping the machine and scraping the sides several times. Set aside.

3. Place fish on the greased unheated rack of a broiler pan, tucking under any thin edges. Brush with remaining 1 tablespoon oil. Sprinkle with kosher salt and pepper. Broil 4 inches from the heat until fish flakes easily when tested with a fork. Allow 4 to 6 minutes per ½-inch thickness of fish. If fish is 1 inch or more thick, turn once halfway through broiling. Serve with cilantro pesto.

CULINARY NOTES

- COOK 1X · EAT 2X in salads, frittatas, omelets, wraps, or sandwiches.

* Because hot chile peppers contain oils that can burn your skin and eyes, wear rubber or plastic gloves when working with them. If your bare hands do touch the chile peppers, wash your hands well with soap and water.

Nutrition Facts per Serving: 148 calories, 17 g protein, 8 g total fat (1 g saturated fat), 2 g carbohydrate, 1 g fiber, 22 mg cholesterol, 233 mg sodium, 0 glycemic load

WAVE 2 MEAL PLANS

For Wave 2, you have two weeks' worth of meal plans to follow. Like the Wave 1 meal plans, they suggest three complete meals for you each day, plus two snacks. Also as in Wave 1, these meal plans are optional. You can prepare the suggested meals from the menus or their recipe variations, or you can improvise your own meals following the guidelines for Wave 2 of The Sonoma Diet.

There are two ways that the Wave 2 menus differ from the Wave 1 menus. One is that there are fourteen days' worth of recipes instead of ten. Of course, you'll probably need to stay on Wave 2 for more than fourteen days before you reach your target weight. You can either keep repeating the fourteen-day cycle or eventually start choosing new dishes from the additional Wave 2 recipes and/or rearranging the combinations within the Wave 2 guidelines. Using recipes and/or menus from Wave 1 is also an option.

The other major difference is the far greater variety in the Wave 2 meal plans. That's because they take advantage of the ample food choices available to you in this main phase of The Sonoma Diet. You'll never have to worry about boring or unsatisfying meals.

You'll find preparation instructions, culinary tips, and flavor variations for the dishes in these meal plans in the Wave 2 recipe section. Though it's not obligatory, I recommend that you follow the daily meal plans as much as possible for at least the first two weeks of Wave 2. Not only do they take all the guesswork out of adhering to the guidelines, they'll also introduce you to new sources of Sonoma-style culinary pleasure, and you'll find wine-pairing recommendations (if you choose to drink wine).

For even more variety, you'll also find additional Wave 2 and Wave 3 recipes not featured in the meal plan, including some by local chefs and wineries from the Sonoma and Napa Wine Country. ■

DAY ONE

BREAKFAST: Whole-grain cereal and nonfat milk
½ cup berries
Green tea

LUNCH: Smoky White Bean and Tomato Soup, page 283
Spinach salad, 1 tablespoon nuts, mixed veggies, with choice of dressing from Seasonings section, pages 195–204

DINNER: Almond-Crusted Salmon, page 343
Roasted Zucchini, page 304
1 glass sauvignon blanc (optional)
Cherry Almond Clafoutis, page 354

SNACK:
Men: 4 ounces plain nonfat yogurt, with 1 cup fruit
Women: 4 ounces plain nonfat yogurt, with ½ cup fruit

DAY TWO

BREAKFAST: 8 ounces plain nonfat yogurt mixed with ½ cup
Sonoma Granola, page 280, and ¼ cup berries
Green tea

LUNCH: Chicken, Tomato, Basil, and Penne Salad, page 288
1 serving of fruit

DINNER: Veracruz-Style Fish, page 349
½ cup of brown rice
Romaine and Watercress Salad, Latin Style variation
(chicken omitted), page 328
1 glass of pinot noir (optional)

SNACK:
Men: 2 tablespoons hummus, 16 Kashi whole-grain crackers,
1 cup sliced raw veggies
Women: 1 tablespoon hummus, 8 Kashi whole-grain crackers,
1 cup sliced raw veggies

DAY THREE

BREAKFAST: Omelet, variations, pages 220–221
Green tea

LUNCH: Sonoma Express wrap, page 170
1 serving of fruit
or Baby Greens with Apples, Chicken, Walnuts, page 315

DINNER: Roast Chicken with Roasted Vegetables, Latin Variation,
page 327
or Broccoli Salad with Sun-Dried Tomatoes and Pine
Nuts, page 235, instead of the roasted vegetables
1 glass merlot (optional)
Grapefruit Mint Sorbet, page 363

SNACK: 4 ounces low-fat cottage cheese, ½ cup vegetables,
1 ounce nuts

DAY FOUR

BREAKFAST: 1 tablespoon nut butter, one slice whole-grain bread
½ cup of berries
Green tea

LUNCH: Asian Chopped Salad with chicken, variation of Sonoma
Chopped Salmon Salad, COOK 1X · EAT 2X , page 230
1 whole-wheat pita or 2 Wasa crackers

DINNER: Oven-Fried Pork Cutlets, page 340
Roast Cauliflower with Capers and Garlic, page 303
1 glass merlot (optional)
½ cup Toasted Quinoa Pilaf, page 244

SNACK: 1 mozzarella cheese stick, 2 Wasa Crackers,
1 serving of fruit

DAY FIVE

BREAKFAST: Baked Eggs, page 274
½ cup fruit
Green tea

LUNCH: Toasted Quinoa, Chicken, Corn, and Avocado Salad,
COOK 1X · EAT 2X , page 289

DINNER: Cuban-Style Flank Steak, page 333
2 corn tortillas with favorite salsa
1 glass cabernet sauvignon (optional)
Mango Apple Granita with Basil, page 364

SNACK: 1 mozzarella stick, 1 cup raw vegetables, 1 ounce nuts

Day Six

BREAKFAST: Sonoma Frittata, choice of variation, page 215
Green tea

LUNCH: 1 whole-wheat pita, 2 ounces sliced turkey
Nectarine, Arugula, and Goat Cheese Salad, page 286,
with Sherry Honey Vinaigrette, page 200

DINNER: Halibut and Summer Vegetables en Papillote,
choice of variations, page 344
½ cup Barilla Plus Pasta, tossed with 1 teaspoon Pesto,
page 190
1 glass chardonnay (optional)

SNACK:
Men: 1 Laughing Cow Light Cheese,
16 Kashi whole-grain crackers
Women: 1 Laughing Cow Light Cheese,
8 Kashi whole-grain crackers

Day Seven

BREAKFAST: 1 tablespoon nut butter, 1 slice whole-grain bread
1 serving fruit
Green tea

LUNCH: California Chicken Salad, page 287

DINNER: Wild Mushroom and Barley Risotto, page 312
Grilled Asparagus Salad, page 238
1 glass merlot (optional)

SNACK:
Men: 1 serving of fruit, 8 ounces plain nonfat yogurt,
1 ounce nuts
Women: 1 serving of fruit, 4 ounces plain nonfat yogurt,
1 ounce nuts

Day Eight

BREAKFAST: ½ cup steel-cut oats with nonfat milk,
1 teaspoon of agave syrup, ½ cup berries
Green tea or coffee

LUNCH: Hearty Lentil Soup, page 282
Mixed greens salad, choice of vinaigrette, pages 195–202
2 Wasa crackers

DINNER: Mediterranean White Wine Poached Fish, page 347
½ cup Toasted Quinoa Pilaf, page 244
or brown basmati rice prepared with
low-sodium chicken broth
Broccoli Salad with Dried Figs, Walnuts, and Mint,
page 296
1 glass chardonnay (optional)

SNACK:
Men: 1 mozzarella cheese stick, 1 cup raw vegetables,
8 Kashi whole grain crackers
Women: 1 mozzarella cheese stick, 1 cup raw vegetables

Day Nine

BREAKFAST: 2 eggs, 1 slice of whole-wheat bread
1 serving of fruit
Green tea or coffee

LUNCH: Sonoma Caesar Salad with 4 ounces chicken or shrimp,
page 230
½ whole-wheat pita

DINNER: Spicy Black Bean and Corn Chowder, page 307
Mixed greens salad with choice of vinaigrette,
pages 195–202
1 glass of zinfandel (optional)

SNACK: 1 ounce nuts, 4 ounces plain nonfat yogurt, 1 cup berries

DAY TEN

BREAKFAST: Baked Eggs, page 274
1 serving fruit
Green tea or coffee

LUNCH: Chicken and Black Bean Wrap, page 290

DINNER: Herb-Marinated Flank Steak, page 254, with salsa verde, page 191
Watermelon, Arugula, and Feta Salad, page 310
2 corn tortillas
1 glass of zinfandel (optional)

SNACK:
Men: 16 Kashi whole-wheat crackers,
2 tablespoons Hummus, page 189
Women: 8 Kashi whole-wheat crackers,
2 tablespoons Hummus, page 189

DAY ELEVEN

BREAKFAST: Whole-grain cereal with nonfat milk
½ cup berries, 1 ounce almonds or walnuts
Green tea

LUNCH: Grilled Beef and Hummus Whole-Wheat Pita,
COOK 1X · EAT 2X , page 291
1 cup sliced tomatoes and cucumbers, 1 teaspoon Pesto
Vinaigrette, page 198

DINNER: Sicilian Tuna Steak, page 348
Concord Grape and Arugula Salad, page 300
1 glass sangiovese (optional)

SNACK:
Men: 2 cups light popcorn, 1 ounce nuts
Women: 1 cup light popcorn, 1 ounce nuts

DAY TWELVE

BREAKFAST: Sonoma Frittata variation, page 215

LUNCH: Mediterranean Tuna and Caper Salad, COOK 1X · EAT 2X ,
page 346
1 serving of fruit

DINNER: Roast Pork Tenderloin with Grilled Peach Salsa,
page 342
Steamed Spaghetti Squash, page 308
1 glass pinot noir (optional)
Almond Cherry Biscotti, page 350
½ cup berries

SNACK:
Men: 1 cup raw veggies, 1 cup nonfat cottage cheese
Women: 1 cup raw veggies, ½ cup nonfat cottage cheese

DAY THIRTEEN

BREAKFAST: scrambled eggs, 1 slice of whole-wheat bread,
1 serving fruit
Green tea

LUNCH: Roasted Pork Tacos with Peach Salsa,
COOK 1X · EAT 2X , page 292

DINNER: Sonoma Stuffed Artichokes, optional variations,
page 305
1 glass sauvignon blanc (optional)
Nectarine Blueberry Galette, page 357

SNACK:
Men: 1 cup nonfat cottage cheese, ¼ cup baby carrots,
1 ounce almonds
Women: ½ nonfat cup cottage cheese, ½ cup baby carrots,
1 ounce almonds

Day Fourteen

BREAKFAST: ½ cup steel-cut oats, nonfat milk
½ cup berries, 1 ounce nuts
Green tea

LUNCH: 4 ounces grilled shrimp marinated in Simple Spicy Lime
Cilantro Vinaigrette, page 201
Latin-Style Sautéed Corn, page 285,
or mixed green salad with choice of dressing from
Seasonings section, pages 195–204

DINNER: Wheat Berry Chicken Paella, page 331
Mixed green salad with Gazpacho Vinaigrette, page 196
1 glass of merlot (optional)
Spiced Ginger Cookies, page 352
1 cup sliced oranges

SNACK: 1 cup raw veggies, 1 tablespoon hummus

BAKED EGGS
WITH GRILLED VEGETABLES

Start to Finish: 25 minutes   Yield: 4 servings

1   teaspoon olive oil
½   teaspoon garlic, minced
1   tablespoon basil, chopped
¼   cup mozzarella cheese, cut into ¼-inch pieces
4   cups grilled vegetables, cut into ½-inch pieces

4   slices tomato
4   large eggs
1   tablespoon parmesan cheese, grated
Salt and pepper to taste

1. Preheat oven to 325°F.

2. Lightly oil 4 four-inch-diameter oven-proof glass or ceramic dishes with olive oil.

3. Mix the garlic, basil, mozzarella cheese, and grilled vegetables; season with salt and pepper.

4. Place 1 slice of tomato in bottom of each baking dish. Divide vegetable mixture between the 4 dishes. Crack an egg into each dish. Season with salt and pepper. Sprinkle with parmesan cheese.

5. Bake for 10 minutes or until the vegetables are warm and the egg whites are cooked through. The egg yolk should be slightly runny like a poached egg.

6. Serve immediately.

Variations:

- Replace grilled vegetables with roasted vegetables.
- Replace grilled vegetables with leftover sautéed spinach and mushrooms.
- Replace mozzarella cheese with goat cheese or feta cheese

Nutrition Facts per Serving: **150** calories, **12** g protein, **9** g fat (**2.5** g saturated fat), **7** g carbohydrate, **3** g fiber, **240** mg cholesterol, **139** mg sodium, **0** glycemic load

BLUEBERRY RICOTTA PANCAKES

Start to Finish: 30 minutes
Yield: 4 servings, 2 pancakes each

½ cup buttermilk
¾ cup low-fat ricotta cheese
¼ cup applesauce
½ teaspoon vanilla
½ teaspoon lemon zest
¼ cup unbleached all-purpose flour
½ cup whole-wheat pastry flour

1 teaspoon sugar
¼ teaspoon baking soda
1 teaspoon baking powder
½ teaspoon cinnamon
1 pinch salt
2 egg whites
1½ cup blueberries
Nonstick cooking spray

1. Preheat pancake griddle over medium heat.

2. Combine the buttermilk, ricotta cheese, applesauce, vanilla, and zest in a bowl. Mix well.

3. In another bowl, combine flours, sugar, baking soda, baking powder, cinnamon, and salt. Mix well.

4. Gently incorporate the wet ingredients into the dry ingredients. Mix just enough to combine. Beat egg whites until soft peaks form. Add to pancake mixture. Gently fold blueberries into the pancake mixture. Overmixing will make the pancakes tough.

5. Lightly spray the pancake griddle. Pour ¼ cup pancake batter on griddle, ¼" thick. Let cook until golden brown and the edges start to set. Flip and cook on the other side.

Nutrition Facts per Serving: 190 calories, 11 g protein, 3 g fat (1.5 g saturated fat), 32 g carbohydrate, 4 g fiber, 16 mg cholesterol, 450 mg sodium, 12 glycemic load

CULINARY NOTES

- The leavening agent is baking soda, so once the wet and dry ingredients are combined, the pancakes should be cooked immediately. This batter does not hold well.

- Once the eggs are separated, let sit at room temperature for 30 minutes. Room temperature egg whites will whip up faster.

- Make sure the egg whites are yolk-free and that your bowl and whisk are free from any fat. The tiniest bit of fat or egg yolk interferes with the formation of the foam.

- Do not stop halfway through the process of beating the egg whites. Beating until soft peaks form means that when the beaters are lifted from the bowl, the whipped egg whites will form peaks with tips that curl over.

- When folding in the egg whites, leave a few lumps of egg whites in the batter. If the batter is completely mixed, it will most likely be overmixed.

Variations:

- **Lemon Poppy Seed Pancakes:** Omit cinnamon and blueberries. Fold in 1 tablespoon lemon juice and 1 teaspoon poppy seeds; increase lemon zest to 1 teaspoon.

- Serve with lemon agave syrup. Combine 1 tablespoon lemon juice and 1½ tablespoons agave syrup. Bring to a simmer; remove from heat.

BLUEBERRY MUFFINS

Start to Finish: 45 minutes
Yield: 12 muffins

¾ cup brown rice flour
¾ cup rice flour
½ cup tapioca starch
1 teaspoon baking soda
2 teaspoon baking powder
1¼ teaspoon xanthan gum
¼ teaspoon salt
½ cup sugar

3 tablespoons butter, room temperature
2 tablespoons nonfat plain yogurt
1 egg, beaten
¾ cup buttermilk
1 teaspoon vanilla extract
⅔ cup blueberries, frozen

1. Preheat oven to 350°F. Line muffin cups with paper cupcake liners.

2. Combine rice flours, tapioca starch, baking soda, baking powder, xanthan gum, salt, and sugar. Mix well.

3. Cut butter into flour mixture until it resembles corn meal.

4. Combine yogurt, egg, buttermilk, and vanilla. Gently fold into dry ingredients, forming a very thick, almost pastelike batter.

5. Fold in blueberries and scoop into muffin tins.

6. Bake for 15 minutes or until the top is slightly browned and a skewer inserted in the center comes out clean. Cool 5 minutes in muffin tins; then remove to a rack to cool.

Variations:
• Replace blueberries with frozen raspberries or with ½ cup dried cherries or cranberries.

Nutrition Facts per Serving: 150 calories, 2.8 g protein, 3 g fat (1.5 g saturated fat), 30 g carbohydrate, 1.5 g fiber, 27 mg cholesterol, 250 mg sodium, 22 glycemic load

FRUIT & NUT ENERGY BARS

Start to Finish: 1 hour
Yield: 9 servings

1	cup rolled oats	1	cup dried fruit in ½-inch pieces
1	cup unsweetened puffed cereal	¼	cup agave syrup
¼	cup pumpkin seeds, toasted	3	tablespoons brown sugar
½	cup assorted nuts, toasted	2	tablespoons plain nonfat yogurt
1	tablespoon oat bran	1	teaspoon vanilla extract
½	cup wheat germ, toasted		Nonstick cooking spray as needed
½	teaspoon ground cinnamon		
1	pinch salt		

1. To toast the oats, seeds, and nuts: Place each in a single layer on a sheet pan. Do not place on the same sheet pan since they all take varying amounts of time. Bake in a 300°F oven for 5–10 minutes or until the oats are slightly brown, the pumpkin seeds start to pop, and the nuts are slightly browned.

2. Spray a 9-inch by 9-inch pan with cooking spray.

3. Preheat oven to 275°F.

4. Combine oats, cereal, pumpkin seeds, nuts, bran, wheat germ, cinnamon, salt, and fruit in a large bowl.

5. Place agave syrup and brown sugar in a saucepan. Over medium heat, bring to a low simmer; cook 2–3 minutes or until sugar dissolves. Be careful not to overreduce. Stir in yogurt and vanilla.

6. Pour hot syrup over oat mixture. Mix well to lightly coat everything with syrup.

7. Spread in an even layer in the prepared pan. Place a lightly sprayed piece of parchment paper on top and press firmly into the pan, being sure to push the mixture into all corners.

8. Bake in oven for 30 minutes or until the edges are golden brown. Remove from oven. Place pan on a wire rack; let sit for 5 minutes. Using parchment or plastic, again press firmly into the pan. Let sit until completely cooled.

9. Once cool, cut into 9 squares. Store in an airtight container.

> **CULINARY NOTES**
>
> • Make sure the bars are allowed to cool completely in the pan. This allows the ingredients to firm up and stick together.
>
> • If you are in a humid climate, if the bars become soft, place them in a 275°F oven and bake for 15 minutes to dry them out again.

Variations:

• Use this as a basic recipe for energy bars. Instead of rolled oats, you can use barley or rye flakes. Instead of pumpkin seeds, use sunflower or sesame seeds. For the assorted nuts, use slivered almonds, walnuts, cashews, hazelnuts, or peanuts. For the dried fruits, use dried cherries, raisins, golden raisins, papaya, mango, pears, or apples.

Nutrition Facts per Serving: 270 calories, 8 g protein, 10 g fat (1.5 g saturated fat), 42 g carbohydrate, 6 g fiber, 0 mg cholesterol, 70 mg sodium, 12 glycemic load

SONOMA GRANOLA

Start to Finish: 1 hour 10 minutes
Yield: 5 servings, ½ cup each

1 cup rolled oats—not instant

¼ cup oat bran or wheat bran

1 tablespoon flax seeds, coarsely ground

½ cup nuts, slivered or whole

1 tablespoon assorted seeds (such as sunflower and pumpkin), hulled

2 tablespoons coconut, flaked

½ teaspoon ground cinnamon

¼ teaspoon ground ginger

1 pinch nutmeg

1 pinch salt

3 tablespoons agave syrup

3 tablespoons applesauce

1 tablespoon brown sugar

½ teaspoon vanilla extract

1 tablespoon extra-virgin olive oil

½ cup assorted dried fruit in ¼-inch to ½-inch pieces

1. Preheat oven to 300°F.

2. Combine oats, bran, flax seeds, nuts, seeds, coconut, spices, and salt in a bowl.

3. In another bowl, combine agave syrup, applesauce, brown sugar, vanilla, and olive oil. Add wet ingredients to the dry ingredients; mix well. Scoop onto a sheet pan and spread in a ¼-inch-thick layer. Bake for 45 minutes to 1 hour, stirring every 20 minutes, until golden brown. The granola will seem a little soft when it is finished cooking. It will dry up as it cools. Add the dried fruit once the granola is cool.

Variations:

- **Nuts:** Use almonds (slivered or coarsely chopped), cashews, peanuts, hazelnuts (peeled and coarsely chopped), walnuts, or pecans (in quarters or halves).

- **Seeds:** Use sesame seeds, hulled sunflower seeds, or hulled pumpkin seeds.

- **Dried fruits:** Use dried cranberries, raisins, golden raisins, cherries, papaya, mango, apple, figs, plums, or peaches.

CULINARY NOTES

- For a wheat-free version, replace wheat bran with oat bran.
- When selecting nuts for granola, choose ones that are cut approximately the same size.
- An easy way to chop nuts is to place a towel on top of them, and crush them with a rolling pin or the bottom of a pot. Be careful not to crush them into a fine powder.

Nutrition Facts per Serving: **60** calories, **1.5** g protein, **3** g fat (**0** g saturated fat), **8** g carbohydrate, **2** g fiber, **0** mg cholesterol, **20** mg sodium, **6.3** glycemic load

HEARTY LENTIL SOUP

Start to Finish: 60 minutes
Yield: 6 servings

1 medium onion, chopped

1 medium carrot, chopped

3 cloves garlic, minced (1½ teaspoons)

2 tablespoons extra-virgin olive oil

8 cups reduced-sodium chicken broth

1½ cups brown or French lentils, rinsed and drained

1 medium tomato, seeded and chopped

3 tablespoons fresh flat-leaf parsley, chopped

1 tablespoon lemon juice

½ teaspoon cumin seeds, toasted and ground, or ½ teaspoon ground cumin

½ teaspoon fennel seeds, toasted and ground, or ½ teaspoon fennel seeds, finely crushed

Kosher salt (optional)

Freshly ground black pepper (optional)

1. In a 6- to 8-quart Dutch oven, cook onion, carrot, and garlic in hot oil about 10 minutes or until tender.

2. Add broth and lentils. Bring to boiling; reduce heat. Cover and simmer about 30 minutes or until lentils are tender.

3. Stir in tomato, parsley, lemon juice, cumin, and fennel seeds. If desired, season to taste with kosher salt and pepper. Ladle into bowls.

CULINARY NOTES

• Add a pinch of salt to the lentils at the beginning of cooking. This will help them keep their shape. Salt will strengthen the skin on beans, which is great if you're cooking lentils, but not if you're cooking beans long and slow.

• To toast seeds, heat a small skillet over medium heat. Add seeds. Cook about 2 minutes or until toasted and aromatic, shaking skillet frequently. Place toasted seeds in a spice grinder and process until finely ground.

Nutrition Facts per Serving: 240 calories, 17 g protein, 5 g total fat (1 g saturated fat), 33 g carbohydrate, 16 g fiber, 0 mg cholesterol, 775 mg sodium, 8 glycemic load

SMOKY WHITE BEAN & TOMATO SOUP

Start to Finish: 30 minutes   Yield: 6 servings

3 slices smoked bacon
1 cup onion, diced
1 tablespoon garlic, minced
1 tablespoon mixed oregano and thyme, minced
1 pinch chile flakes
1 cup canned tomatoes, chopped

1 15.5-ounce can cannellini or Great Northern beans, with liquid
3 cups chicken stock
¼ teaspoon salt
1 pinch black pepper

1. Heat a 2-quart saucepan over medium heat; add raw bacon and cook 4 minutes until crispy. Crumble bacon.

2. Add the onion and cook 3–4 minutes until translucent.

3. Add the garlic, herbs, and chile flakes; cook for 1 minute.

4. Add the tomatoes and cook for 2 minutes.

5. Add the beans with their liquid, chicken stock, salt, and pepper, and bring to a simmer. Cook for 15 minutes.

Nutrition Facts per Serving: **150** calories, **9** g protein, **4** g fat (**1** g saturated fat), **19** g carbohydrate, **4** g fiber, **10** mg cholesterol, **640** mg sodium, **4** glycemic load

BLACK BEAN BURRITO

Start to Finish: 15 minutes
Yield: 8 servings

1   16-ounce can fat-free refried beans or pinto beans

1   tablespoon olive oil

8   eggs

8   flour tortillas

½   cup cheddar cheese, shredded

1   cup fresh tomato salsa (pico de gallo)

1   avocado, diced

½   cup scallions, sliced

1   lime, juiced

Salt and pepper to taste

1. Heat beans in a medium saucepan. Set aside.

2. Heat a nonstick large pan over medium heat. Add olive oil and eggs; using a spatula, stir until eggs are scrambled. Season with salt and pepper.

3. Spread 3 tablespoons of beans in the lower section of each tortilla; top with cheese and eggs. Place salsa, avocado, and sliced scallions on top; drizzle with fresh lime juice.

4. Fold in ½ inch on the left and right sides of the tortilla to keep the filling inside as you roll the tortilla and filling from the lower end into a burrito.

5. Warm completed burritos in the oven for 5-10 minutes at 300°F.

Nutrition Facts per Serving: 400 calories, 16 g protein, 19 g fat (5 g saturated fat), 37 g carbohydrate, 6 g fiber, 200 mg cholesterol, 700 mg sodium

LATIN-STYLE SAUTÉED CORN

*Start to Finish: 20 minutes, if using frozen corn
and purchased red peppers   Yield: 4 servings*

1 tablespoon extra-virgin olive oil	½ cup roasted red peppers, diced
2 teaspoons garlic, chopped	½ cup scallions, chopped
¼ teaspoon cumin seeds	1 teaspoon lime juice
4 cups corn kernels, cut from cob or frozen	Salt and pepper to taste

1. In a large skillet, heat the extra-virgin olive oil over medium heat. Add garlic and cumin; cook until aromatic.

2. Add corn and turn heat to high. Sauté for 3–4 minutes or until the corn is warmed through and lightly toasted.

3. Add red pepper and scallions; toss to warm. Season with lime juice, salt, and pepper.

Variations:

- Add 1 teaspoon chopped chipotle in adobo sauce to add some spice.
- Add chopped cilantro.
- Omit cumin and lime; add basil and lemon juice.

CULINARY NOTE

The corn can be a   COOK 1X · EAT 2X   ingredient if you have enough leftover corn on the cob from a previous meal.

Nutrition Facts per Serving: 200 calories, 6 g protein, 6 g fat (.7 g saturated fat), 35 g carbohydrate, 5 g fiber, 0 mg cholesterol, 110 mg sodium, 16 glycemic load

Nectarine, Arugula, & Goat Cheese Salad

Start to Finish: 15 minutes   Yield: 4 servings

3 cups arugula, washed

2 cups hearts of romaine, shredded

3 tablespoons Sherry Honey Vinaigrette (page 200)

1 nectarine, ripe, cut in ¼-inch wedges

¼ cup goat cheese, cut in 1-inch pieces

2 tablespoons sliced almonds, toasted

Salt and pepper to taste

1. Combine arugula and romaine in a bowl. Sprinkle with salt and pepper. Add vinaigrette; toss well. Gently fold in nectarine slices, then goat cheese. Be careful not to overmix or the goat cheese will break up.

2. Garnish with toasted almonds.

Variations:

- Substitute a peach for the nectarine.
- Substitute watercress, mizuna, or tatsoi for the arugula.
- Substitute feta cheese for the goat cheese. Reduce amount to 2 tablespoons.

CULINARY NOTES

- The arugula is a delicate green. Do not mix or dress the salad ahead of serving time or the arugula will wilt. It adds a peppery bite to the salad that offers a great contrast to the sweetness of the nectarines.

- The goat cheese can be added on top of the salad instead of mixing it in the salad.

Nutrition Facts per Serving: 210 calories, 4 g protein, 15 g fat (2 g saturated fat), 13 g carbohydrate, 2 g fiber, 7 mg cholesterol, 50 mg sodium, 7 glycemic load

California Chicken Salad

Start to Finish: 35 minutes
Yield: 6 servings

1 pound cooked chicken breast, cubed

2 Granny Smith apples, cored and chopped

1 cup celery, peeled and chopped (2 stalks)

½ cup scallions, chopped

2 tablespoons fresh flat-leaf parsley, chopped

¼ cup light dairy sour cream

¼ cup red wine vinegar

3 tablespoons mayonnaise or salad dressing

½ teaspoon kosher salt

¼ teaspoon freshly ground black pepper

¼ cup chopped walnuts, toasted

6 cups mixed salad greens, torn

1. In a large bowl combine chicken, apples, celery, scallions, and parsley.

2. In a small bowl, combine sour cream, red wine vinegar, mayonnaise, kosher salt, and pepper. Add to chicken mixture. Stir in walnuts.

3. Divide greens among 6 serving plates; top with chicken mixture.

> **CULINARY NOTE**
>
> Leftover cooked or smoked chicken can be a COOK 1X · EAT 2X ingredient.

Variations:

- Add 1 teaspoon curry powder and ¼ cup golden raisins to the mayonnaise mixture.
- Replace the sour cream with yogurt.
- Replace walnuts with toasted chopped almonds.
- Add 1 teaspoon cinnamon and ¼ cup raisins and replace walnuts with toasted cashews.

Nutrition Facts per Serving: **258** calories, **26** g protein, **12** g total fat (**2** g saturated fat), **11** g carbohydrate, **3** g fiber, **70** mg cholesterol, **288** mg sodium, **6** glycemic load

CHICKEN, TOMATO, BASIL, & PENNE SALAD

Start to Finish: 20 minutes, if using leftover pasta Yield: 4 servings (1½ cups each)

1   tablespoon extra-virgin olive oil

1   tablespoon garlic, sliced

3   cups whole-wheat penne pasta or Barilla Plus Pasta, cooked

3   tablespoons red wine vinegar

2   cups tomatoes, seeded, diced

1   cup chicken, cooked, shredded

1½ cups baby spinach, cut in 1-inch pieces

3   tablespoons capers, rinsed, roughly chopped

1   tablespoon basil, chopped

2   scallions, chopped

1. Place olive oil and garlic in a small pan. Cook over low heat until garlic is tender, about 5 minutes. Place cooked penne in a bowl. Toss with 1 tablespoon vinegar. Add cooked garlic and oil.

2. Add tomatoes, chicken, spinach, capers, basil, and scallions. Add the remaining vinegar and toss well. Adjust seasoning with salt and pepper.

CULINARY NOTES

- Use leftover pasta and chicken.
- If using freshly cooked pasta, after the pasta is drained, toss it with the vinegar and garlic while it is still warm.
- Other whole grain or Barilla Plus pastas can be used in place of penne. Orzo, riso, gemelli, and macaroni all work well for this salad.
- If the salad is prepared in advance, combine all ingredients but the spinach. Add the spinach just before serving. Also, adjust the season just before serving as the pasta will absorb a lot of salt and acid as it sits.
- Leftover chicken can be a COOK 1X · EAT 2X ingredient.

Nutrition Facts per Serving: **157** calories, **11** g protein, **6** g fat (**1** g saturated fat), **14** g carbohydrate, **3** g fiber, **25** mg cholesterol, **240** mg sodium, **3** glycemic load

Toasted Quinoa, Chicken, Corn, & Avocado Salad

Start to Finish: 25 minutes   Yield: 4 servings (1½ cup each)

1   cup cucumbers, peeled, seeded, diced

2   cups quinoa, cooked

1   cup chicken, cooked, shredded

1   cup red pepper, seeded, diced

¾   cup corn kernels, toasted

2   scallions, chopped

2   tablespoons cilantro, chopped

4   tablespoons Simple Lemon Vinaigrette (page 204)

½   avocado, diced

Salt and pepper to taste

1. Place cucumbers in a bowl. Lightly season with salt and pepper. Let sit for 5 minutes. Drain.

2. Add quinoa, chicken, red pepper, corn, scallions, and cilantro. Gently mix. Add the vinaigrette and adjust seasoning with salt and pepper. Fold in the avocado.

CULINARY NOTES

- To avoid mushing the avocado, it should be the last thing added to the salad. Do not mix after it is added.

- Leftover chicken and quinoa can be   COOK 1X · EAT 2X   ingredients.

Variation:

- For a spicier salad, add 1 teaspoon chopped chipotle in adobo sauce or chopped fresh jalapeño.

Nutrition Facts per Serving: 250 calories, 14 g protein, 13 g fat (2 g saturated fat), 30 g carbohydrate, 5 g fiber, 26 mg cholesterol, 89 mg sodium, 9 glycemic load

CHICKEN & BLACK BEAN WRAP

Start to Finish: 10 minutes
Yield: 1 serving

2   tablespoons Black Bean-
Smoked Chile Spread
(page 186)

1   8-inch whole-wheat
flour tortilla

3   ounces cooked skinless
chicken or turkey breast,
chopped (about ½ cup)

1   cup romaine or whole
fresh baby spinach leaves,
shredded or torn

¼   cup chopped fresh cilantro

1   tablespoon bottled salsa

Place spread on one side of the tortilla.
Top with chicken, romaine, cilantro,
and salsa. Roll up.

CULINARY NOTE

Leftover chicken can be a
COOK 1X· EAT 2X ingredient.

Nutrition Facts per Serving: 322 calories, 38 g protein, 8 g total fat (2 g saturated fat),
24 g carbohydrate, 14 g fiber, 72 mg cholesterol, 554 mg sodium

GRILLED BEEF & HUMMUS WHOLE-WHEAT PITA

Start to Finish: 15 minutes   Yield: 4 sandwiches

4 whole-wheat pitas
8 ounces chickpea hummus
2 ounces feta cheese, crumbled
8 ounces leftover grilled beef skirt steak, flank steak, or tenderloin, sliced

1 tomato, sliced
1 cup baby lettuce
Lemon juice to taste
Salt and pepper to taste

1. Lightly toast pita bread. Cut each in half. Spread 2 ounces of hummus in each pita. Sprinkle with ½ ounce feta.

2. Season the sliced beef, tomato, and lettuce with a little salt, pepper, and lemon juice. Add to pita.

> **CULINARY NOTE**
>
> Leftover beef can be a COOK 1X · EAT 2X ingredient.

Variations:

- Replace beef with chicken, pork, or grilled vegetables.
- Replace lettuce with arugula.
- Replace tomatoes with cherry tomatoes.
- Replace feta cheese with parmesan or goat cheese.

Nutrition Facts per Serving: 400 calories, 28 g protein, 15 g fat (5 g saturated fat), 47 g carbohydrate, 8 g fiber, 60 g cholesterol, 580 mg sodium, 25 glycemic load

ROASTED PORK TACOS
WITH PEACH SALSA

Start to Finish: 30 minutes   *Yield: 4 servings*

1   cup cabbage, shredded fine

¼   cup red onion, slice thin, rinsed

½   cup chicken stock

½   teaspoon Spanish paprika

¼   teaspoon ground cumin

½   teaspoon chipotle in adobo sauce, chopped fine

1   pound roast pork, cut into ¼–½-inch by 1-inch pieces (page 342)

8   corn tortillas

1   tablespoon cilantro, chopped

1   tablespoon lime juice

½   cup Peach Salsa (page 193)

½   avocado, cut into 8 slices

Salt and pepper to taste

> **CULINARY NOTE**
> Leftover pork can be a COOK 1X · EAT 2X ingredient.

1. Combine cabbage and red onion in a colander. Sprinkle with salt and pepper. Let sit for 15 minutes while you prepare remaining ingredients.

2. Place chicken stock, paprika, cumin, and chipotle in a sauté pan. Add the pork and heat until warmed through.

3. Heat the tortillas on a griddle until soft.

4. Gently press the cabbage to remove excess moisture. Move to a bowl and add the cilantro and lime juice. Adjust seasonings.

5. To assemble tacos: Lay a tortilla on a flat surface. Top with 2 ounces warm pork mixture; place cabbage mixture on top. Place 1 tablespoon salsa and a slice of avocado on top.

Variation:

- Replace the pork with chicken or fish.

Nutrition Facts per Serving: 415 calories, 35 g protein, 15 g fat (4.5 g saturated fat), 34 g carbohydrate, 5 g fiber, 90 mg cholesterol, 300 mg sodium, 13 glycemic load

SONOMA MINESTRONE
WITH PESTO

Start to Finish: 2 hours (1½ hours to simmer)   Yield: 8 cups

½ tablespoon extra-virgin olive oil

1 cup onions, diced

½ cup celery, diced

2 tablespoons garlic, chopped

1 tablespoon thyme, chopped

3 cups braising greens, 1-inch pieces

1 cup zucchini, chopped

1 cup eggplant, chopped

½ cup mushrooms, sliced

1 bay leaf

½ cup farro or spelt

6 cups water or chicken stock

1 16-ounce can cannellini, drained

2 teaspoons lemon zest

2 tablespoons Pesto (page 190)

1 tablespoon parmesan cheese, shaved

Salt and pepper to taste

1. Heat a 2-quart saucepot over medium heat. Add extra-virgin olive oil, onions, celery, garlic, and thyme. Season with salt and pepper, and sauté for 5 minutes or until translucent, but not browned.

2. Add braising greens, zucchini, eggplant, mushrooms, bay leaf, farro, and water. Bring to a simmer and cook for 1½ hours.

3. Adjust seasonings with salt and pepper. Add cannellini and zest; bring back to a simmer.

4. Serve with 1 teaspoon of pesto and shaving of parmesan cheese.

CULINARY NOTES

• This soup is a long, slow cook. It can be prepared in a crockpot. Follow step one; add the ingredients in step two. Place in the crockpot and cook for 2½–3 hours or until the farro is tender. Add the beans and cook 30 minutes.

• Use any assortment of braising greens, such as collards, beet greens, mustard greens, chard, spinach, or kale.

Nutrition Facts per Serving: 175 calories, 11 g protein, 4 g fat (1 g saturated fat), 25 g carbohydrate, 5.5 g fiber, 1.8 mg cholesterol, 250 mg sodium, 5 glycemic load

BALSAMIC ROASTED BEET SALAD
WITH MINT & FETA CHEESE

Start to Finish: 1 hour 20 minutes   Yield: 4 servings

1 pound red or yellow beets, tops completely cut off	3 tablespoons extra-virgin olive oil
½ cup water	4 cups mixed salad greens
1 tablespoon olive oil	1 tablespoon mint, chopped
3 tablespoons balsamic vinegar	¼ cup feta cheese or goat cheese, crumbled
1 teaspoon lemon juice	Salt and pepper to taste
½ teaspoon garlic, mashed to a paste	

1. Preheat oven to 375°F. Place unpeeled beets, water, and 1 tablespoon olive oil in a small baking dish. Season with salt and pepper. Cover tightly with foil and bake for 45 minutes to 1 hour or until the beets are easily pierced with a knife. If the beets are not cooked through and the water has completely evaporated, add a little more and cover tightly until done. Cool slightly; then peel, and cut into eighths.

2. For the balsamic vinaigrette: Combine the balsamic vinegar, lemon juice, and garlic in a small bowl. Whisk in extra-virgin olive oil. Season with salt and pepper. Set aside.

3. In a large bowl, combine greens, mint, beets, salt and pepper to taste. Drizzle with vinaigrette, and toss to coat. Divide evenly among four plates. Top each plate with 1 tablespoon feta cheese.

- The water in the pan with the beets helps them cook more quickly by steaming the beets during three-quarters of the cooking time. It should evaporate by the last 15 minutes so the beets can take on a roasted flavor. The amount of time it takes to cook the beets will depend on their size.
- Check the beets after 40 minutes by poking them in the thickest part. The knife should easily pierce the beet.
- Peel the beets while they are still warm. It is easiest to peel them by holding them with a paper towel and rubbing the skin off. If the beets are roasted through, the skin will come off easily. If the beets are difficult to peel, they could probably cook a little longer.
- Toss the beets with the vinaigrette while still warm. They will absorb the dressing more readily when warm.

Variations:

- One 16-ounce can whole beets, drained and sliced, may be substituted for fresh beets.
- Replace feta cheese with goat cheese or fresh mozzarella.
- Replace mint with basil and add 1 tablespoon sliced kalamata olives.

Nutrition Facts per Serving: 200 calories, 4 g protein, 15 g fat (3 g saturated fat), 15 g carbohydrate, 5 g fiber, 8 mg cholesterol, 200 mg sodium, 5 glycemic load

BROCCOLI SALAD
WITH DRIED FIGS, WALNUTS, & MINT

Start to Finish: 25 minutes   Yield: 4 servings

1   pound broccoli,
    florets and stems

1   tablespoon salt

2   ounces dried figs,
    cut in half lengthwise,
    then in ¼- inch pieces

1   ounce walnuts,
    lightly toasted

2   scallions, sliced thin
    on a bias

1   tablespoon mint, chopped

5   tablespoons champagne
    vinaigrette

Salt and pepper to taste

1. Fill a 2-quart pot with water. Bring to a boil. Add 1 tablespoon salt; bring back to a boil.

2. Add the broccoli florets and cook until crisp-tender. Place in ice water to shock. Let cool for 3–5 minutes; drain well.

3. Peel and trim the broccoli stems. Cut stems in half lengthwise; slice ⅛ inch thin on a bias.

4. Combine the broccoli florets, stems, and the remaining ingredients in a bowl. Toss well.

CULINARY NOTES

- Add the vinaigrette just before serving or the salad will discolor.
- Use fresh figs when available, if desired.

Variations:

- Replace broccoli with cauliflower.
- Replace dried figs with dried cherries or golden raisins.
- Replace walnuts with pecans or hazelnuts.
- Add 1 ounce goat cheese.

Nutrition Facts per Serving: 180 calories, 5 g protein, 11 g fat (1.5 g saturated fat), 20 g carbohydrate, 6 g fiber, 0 mg cholesterol, 30 mg sodium, 5 glycemic load

BUCKWHEAT CREPES

Start to Finish: 30 minutes plus at least 3 hours to rest
Yield: 12 crepes (6 servings, 2 crepes per serving)

¾ cup low-fat milk
1 egg
1 teaspoon sugar
1 pinch salt
1 tablespoon yogurt
¼ cup buckwheat flour

¼ cup whole-wheat, all-purpose flour
Nonstick cooking spray as needed
Salt and pepper to taste
8 ounces crepe filling (see pages 298–299)

1. Whisk the milk and egg until smooth. Add sugar, salt, yogurt, and flours; whisk until smooth. Cover and refrigerate at least three hours or overnight.
2. Remove the batter from the refrigerator about an hour before cooking. Stir it well (it will have separated slightly).
3. Cut seven pieces of 7-inch-square parchment paper to separate crepes until they are filled.
4. Heat a Teflon pan over medium-low heat. Spray with cooking spray. Pour 2 tablespoons of batter into the center of the pan, swirling the pan to distribute the batter quickly and evenly. The crepes should be thin. Cook for 1 minute, or until the surface is cooked through. Gently slide onto a dinner plate using a spatula. Place a piece of parchment paper on top. Continue with the remaining batter, stirring the batter periodically.
5. Fill crepes with desired filling. Place on a parchment-lined sheet pan and warm in the oven, or place on a plate and heat in the microwave until just warm through. Serve 2 crepes per portion.

CULINARY NOTES

- The gluten in the batter must be allowed to rest after stirring to ensure a tender crepe.

- The crepes can be made in advance and frozen.

Nutrition Facts per Serving: 65 calories, 4 g protein, 1.5 g fat (.5 g saturated fat), 10 g carbohydrate, 1.3 g fiber, 40 mg cholesterol, 30 mg sodium, 3.5 glycemic load

BUCKWHEAT CREPES FILLINGS

Start to Finish: 15 minutes
Yield: 6 portions, enough for 12 crepes

GRILLED VEGETABLES AND RICOTTA

12 ounces ricotta cheese

12 ounces grilled vegetables,
cut into ½-inch pieces

Salt and pepper to taste

3 tablespoons Pesto
Vinaigrette (page 198)

1. Spread 1 ounce of ricotta cheese on half of each crepe. Top with grilled vegetables. Season with salt and pepper. Fold other side of crepe over the vegetables.

2. Place on a parchment-lined sheet pan and warm in the oven, or place on a plate and heat in the microwave until just warm through.

3. Drizzle with Pesto Vinaigrette. Serve 2 crepes per portion.

> **CULINARY NOTE**
> Leftover grilled vegetables can be
> COOK 1X · EAT 2X
> ingredients.

Nutrition Facts per Serving (includes amounts for the crepes): 137 calories, 12 g protein, 2.5 g fat (1 g saturated fat), 17 g carbohydrate, 3 g fiber, 45 mg cholesterol, 330 mg sodium, 0 glycemic load

CHICKEN, ROASTED RED PEPPERS, & CAPERS

12 ounces chicken, cooked,
shredded

¾ cup roasted red peppers,
jarred

1½ tablespoons capers

3 tablespoons grated
parmesan cheese

3 tablespoons Pesto
Vinaigrette (page 198)

Salt and pepper to taste

1. Combine chicken, red peppers, capers and cheese. Divide among 8 crepes, putting filling on half of each crepe and folding over the other half.

2. Place on a parchment-lined sheet pan and warm in the oven, or place on a plate and heat in the microwave until just warm through.

3. Drizzle with Pesto Vinaigrette. Serve 2 crepes per portion.

Nutrition Facts per Serving (including amounts for the crepes): 180 calories, 20 g protein, 5.5 g fat (1.5 g saturated fat), 13 g carbohydrate, 2 g fiber, 80 mg cholesterol, 480 mg sodium, 0 glycemic load

SPINACH AND MUSHROOM

4½ ounces low-fat ricotta cheese

4½ ounces goat cheese

3 tablespoons grated parmesan cheese

1½ tablespoons extra-virgin olive oil

6 ounces mushrooms, sliced

1½ tablespoons garlic, chopped

6 cups spinach, chopped

salt and pepper to taste

1. Combine the ricotta, goat cheese, and parmesan cheese in a bowl.

2. Heat a sauté pan. Add the oil and mushrooms; sauté for 5 minutes or until golden brown and tender. Push mushrooms to the sides of the pan. Add the garlic to the center, and cook for 10 seconds until aromatic. Add a pinch of salt and pepper; toss with mushrooms and garlic. Add spinach and cook until the spinach is wilted. Divide in 8 portions.

3. Spread half of each crepe with the cheese mixture. Top with the spinach mixture. Fold over.

4. Place on a parchment-lined sheet pan and warm in the oven, or place on a plate and heat in the microwave until just warm through.

5. Drizzle with Pesto Vinaigrette or romesco vinaigrette. Serve 2 crepes per portion.

Nutrition Facts per Serving (including amounts for crepes): 220 calories, 15 g protein, 13.5 g fat (1.5 g saturated fat), 16 g carbohydrate, 2.5 g fiber, 60 mg cholesterol, 360 mg sodium, 0 glycemic load

Concord Grape & Arugula Salad

Start to Finish: 15 minutes   Yield: 4 servings

2 cups arugula

2 cups romaine leaves, shredded

1 cup concord grapes, cut in half, seeded if necessary

1 teaspoon lemon zest

3 tablespoons Concord Grape Balsamic Vinaigrette (page 195)

¼ cup slivered almond, toasted

2 tablespoons blue cheese, crumbled

Salt and pepper to taste

Place the arugula and romaine in a bowl. Add grapes and lemon zest. Season with salt and pepper; then dress with vinaigrette. Divide between 4 plates. Top with almonds and blue cheese.

CULINARY NOTE

Cutting the grapes in half makes them easier to eat. Seasoning the greens before dressing allows them to take on the flavor of the salt and pepper more readily than after they are coated with vinaigrette.

Variations:

- Replace arugula with watercress, endive, or red leaf lettuce.
- Replace concord grapes with red, green, or black seedless grapes.
- Replace grapes with peaches or nectarines.
- Replace Concord Grape Balsamic Vinaigrette with Balsamic Vinaigrette (page 204).

Nutrition Facts per Serving: **150** calories, **5** g protein, **10** g total fat (**2** g saturated fat), **12** g carbohydrate, **2.5** g fiber, **5** mg cholesterol, **100** mg sodium, **3** glycemic load

GRAIN MEDLEY
WITH MEDITERRANEAN SEASONINGS

Start to Finish: 55 to 85 minutes (depending on grains used)   Yield: 8 servings

2 stalks celery,
   cut into 1-inch pieces
1 large carrot,
   cut into 1-inch pieces
1 small onion,
   cut into 1-inch pieces
2 bay leaves
10 fresh thyme sprigs
10 fresh flat-leaf parsley sprigs

8 ounces (about 1¼ cups)
   mixed grains (such as
   kamut; spelt; triticale;
   brown rice; wild rice;
   brown, French, or green
   lentils; regular barley;
   and/or quinoa),
   rinsed and drained
3 cups water
¼ teaspoon kosher salt
¼ teaspoon freshly ground
   black pepper

1. Cut a 12-inch square from a double thickness of 100% cotton cheesecloth. Place celery, carrot, onion, bay leaves, thyme, and parsley in center of the cheesecloth square. Bring up corners and tie with 100% cotton string.

2. In a 2- to 3-quart saucepan, combine desired grains, water, and cheesecloth bag. Bring to boiling; reduce heat. Cover and simmer for 30 to 60 minutes or until grains are tender. Remove from heat. Let stand, covered, for 5 minutes. Discard cheesecloth bag, allowing any liquid to drain off. Drain any excess liquid from grains. Stir in kosher salt and pepper.

CULINARY NOTE

You can cook kamut, spelt, triticale, brown rice, and wild rice together; they will take 45 to 60 minutes to cook. You can cook lentils, barley, and quinoa together; they will take about 30 minutes to cook. If you want to combine shorter-cooking grains with longer-cooking grains, cook the longer-cooking grains for 20 to 30 minutes and then add the shorter-cooking grains and cook about 30 minutes more or until tender.

Nutrition Facts per Serving: **103** calories, **4** g protein, **1** g total fat (**0** g saturated fat), **20** g carbohydrate, **4** g fiber, **0** mg cholesterol, **64** mg sodium, **8** glycemic load

GRAIN MEDLEY
WITH SOUTHWESTERN SEASONINGS

Start to Finish: 30 minutes   Yield: 4 servings

½ cup fresh or frozen corn kernels

1 teaspoon extra-virgin olive oil

1 cup cooked quinoa

½ cup cooked brown or wild rice

½ cup canned black beans, rinsed and drained

½ cup red bell pepper, finely chopped

½ cup green bell pepper, finely chopped

½ cup cucumber, seeded and finely chopped

2 tablespoons scallion, thinly sliced

2 tablespoons lime juice

1 tablespoon extra-virgin olive oil

1½ teaspoons fresh jalapeño or serrano chile pepper, finely chopped

1½ teaspoons fresh cilantro, chopped

Kosher salt

Freshly ground black pepper

1. Thaw corn, if frozen. Heat a large nonstick skillet over medium-high heat. Add the corn and 1 teaspoon oil. Cook and stir about 5 minutes or until browned and toasted. Transfer to a large bowl.
2. Add the quinoa, rice, black beans, bell peppers, cucumber, scallion, lime juice, 1 tablespoon oil, jalapeño, and cilantro. Mix well; season to taste with kosher salt and black pepper.

CULINARY NOTE

Look for quinoa at a health food store or in the grains section of a large supermarket. To cook quinoa, in a small saucepan add ⅓ cup quinoa to ⅔ cup boiling water. Cover and simmer about 20 minutes or until quinoa is tender and water is absorbed.

Nutrition Facts per Serving: **174** calories, **6** g protein, **6** g total fat (**1** g saturated fat), **28** g carbohydrate, **4** g fiber, **0** mg cholesterol, **154** mg sodium, **8** glycemic load

ROAST CAULIFLOWER
WITH CAPERS & GARLIC

Start to Finish: 30–40 minutes depending on size of florets   Yield: 4 servings

1 head cauliflower	1 tablespoon capers, chopped
2 tablespoons extra-virgin olive oil	1 tablespoon lemon juice
1 tablespoon garlic, sliced thin	2 teaspoons parsley
	Salt and pepper to taste

1. Cut the cauliflower into 1-inch slabs, then into 1-inch florets. Keep them about the same size for even cooking.

2. Heat a sauté pan over medium heat. Add extra-virgin olive oil and cauliflower in a single layer. Cook until the cauliflower is golden brown; turn over and continue to brown, about 25 minutes. Or place the cauliflower in a 350°F oven and roast, turning periodically until golden brown.

3. Add the garlic; cook until aromatic. Add the capers, lemon juice, and parsley. Toss well; adjust seasoning with salt and pepper.

Variations:
- Replace cauliflower with potatoes, Brussels sprouts, or celery root in the winter.

Nutrition Facts per Serving: **100** calories, **3** g protein, **7** g fat (**1** g saturated fat), **8** g carbohydrate, **3** g fiber, **0** mg cholesterol, **108** mg sodium, **0** glycemic load

ROASTED ZUCCHINI

Start to Finish: 35 minutes
Yield: 4 servings

2 cloves garlic, minced (1 teaspoon minced)	½ teaspoon freshly ground black pepper
1 tablespoon extra-virgin olive oil	¼ teaspoon kosher salt
1 tablespoon chopped fresh rosemary or ½ teaspoon dried rosemary, crushed	1½ pounds (about 6 cups) zucchini and/or yellow summer squash, sliced ½ inch thick

1. Preheat oven to 425°F.

2. In a small saucepan, cook garlic in hot oil over medium heat for 30 seconds. Stir in rosemary, pepper, and kosher salt.

3. Place zucchini in a 13-inch by 9-inch by 2-inch baking pan; add oil mixture. Toss to coat. Roast, uncovered, for about 20 minutes or until crisp-tender, stirring once.

Variations:

- As soon as the zucchini are removed from the oven, stir in ½ cup roasted diced red peppers or 1 tablespoon pesto or ¼ cup chopped sun-dried tomatoes and 1 tablespoon grated parmesan cheese.

CULINARY NOTES

- Use zucchini and squash during the spring and summer when they are in season.
- Zucchini and summer squash can be slightly bitter. Be sure to season well with salt and pepper, which will adjust the bitterness.

Nutrition Facts per Serving: 61 calories, 2 g protein, 4 g total fat (1 g saturated fat), 6 g carbohydrate, 2 g fiber, 0 mg cholesterol, 138 mg sodium, 1 glycemic load

SONOMA STUFFED ARTICHOKES

Start to Finish: 1½ hours   Yield: 4 servings

4   tablespoons whole-wheat
    bread crumbs
1   tablespoon parsley, chopped
½   tablespoon extra-virgin
    olive oil
4   large artichokes
2   tablespoons lemon juice
2   teaspoons olive oil

1   tablespoon garlic, minced
2   cups chicken stock,
    vegetable stock, or water
4   cups artichoke filling
    (page 306)
Fresh dill, parsley, thyme,
    oregano to taste, chopped
    (optional)
Salt and pepper to taste

1. Preheat oven to 375°F.

2. Combine bread crumbs, parsley, and extra-virgin olive oil. Season with salt and pepper. Set aside.

3. Cut the top 1 inch off the top of each artichoke. Remove the outer layer of small tough leaves from the base. Trim the stem flush with the base of the artichokes so they will sit flat. Using scissors, trim the spiky tips from the leaves. Starting from the outside layers, gently push back the leaves to loosen. Pull open the leaves at the center until you see the lighter colored leaves around the heart. Gently pull out those leaves, exposing the choke.

4. Using a melon baller or spoon, scoop out and discard the choke. Season inside of artichokes with ½ tablespoon of lemon juice, salt, and pepper.

5. Spoon ½ cup of filling into the center of the artichoke. Place the remaining stuffing between the outside leaves.

6. Heat 2 teaspoons oil in a large skillet over medium high. Add the garlic; sauté 10 seconds or until aromatic. Add the chicken stock and 1½ tablespoons lemon juice. Bring to a simmer. Carefully stand the stuffed

> **CULINARY NOTE**
>
> Select large artichokes for easier handling. Each artichoke will hold about 1 cup of stuffing.

artichokes upright in the pan. Cover, place in the oven, and bake until tender, about 50 minutes. The artichokes will be ready when the heart can be easily pierced with a knife. Remove the cover, top with bread crumb mixture, and bake for 15 minutes or until golden brown. Remove artichokes from braising liquid. Add fresh chopped herbs to the braising liquid; season with salt and pepper.

7. Serve with a small bowl of the braising liquid for a dipping sauce if desired.

Filling:

TOMATO, FETA, CAPERS, AND OREGANO

1 tablespoon extra-virgin olive oil

1½ cup onions, diced

1 tablespoon garlic, chopped

8 ounces feta cheese, crumbled

3 cups tomatoes, chopped

3 tablespoons capers, rinsed, coarsely chopped

4 tablespoons coarse bulgur, rinsed

3 tablespoons oregano, chopped

1 teaspoon lemon zest

Salt and pepper to taste

1. Heat olive oil in a small sauté pan. Add the onions and cook over medium heat until translucent. Add the garlic and cook until aromatic. Set aside to cool.

2. Combine the onion mixture, feta, tomatoes, capers, bulgur, oregano, and lemon zest. Season with salt and pepper. Divide the filling into 4 portions.

CULINARY NOTE

When using the Tomato, Feta, Capers, and Oregano stuffing, bake the artichoke covered until the bulgur is tender, approximately 20 minutes. Remove the cover and sprinkle with the bread crumbs. Bake for 10 minutes or until the bread crumbs are golden brown.

Nutrition Facts per Serving: **389** calories, **13** g protein, **19** g total fat (**9** g saturated fat), **40** g carbohydrate, **11** g fiber, **33** mg cholesterol, **250** mg sodium, **4** glycemic load

SPICY BLACK BEAN & CORN CHOWDER

Start to Finish: 45 minutes   Yield: 6 appetizer servings

1 tablespoon olive oil

1 cup onion, chopped

1 teaspoon garlic, minced

½ teaspoon ground cumin

1 teaspoon chili powder

1 pinch favorite dry chile or chipotle powder, to taste

1 cup red peppers, chopped

1 cup green peppers, chopped

2 15-ounce cans black beans or reduced-sodium black beans, with liquid

1 cup sweet potato, peeled and diced

1 cup frozen corn kernels, thawed

2 cups cleaned baby spinach

1 teaspoon fresh lime juice

Salt and black pepper to taste

Optional Toppings

1 tablespoon fresh cilantro, chopped

2 tablespoons salsa fresca (purchased)

2 tablespoons low-fat yogurt

1. Place olive oil in a saucepan. Add onions and cook until caramelized.

2. Add garlic and spices; cook until aromatic. Add peppers; sauté 5 minutes.

3. Add beans with liquid. Bring to a simmer; cook 10 minutes. Add sweet potato; simmer 10 minutes or until tender.

4. Add corn and spinach. Bring to a simmer until the spinach wilts.

5. Adjust seasoning with lime juice, salt, and pepper. Add optional toppings, as desired.

Nutrition Facts per Serving: **220** calories, **16** g protein, **9** g fat (**2.5** g saturated fat), **18** g carbohydrate, **4** g fiber, **30** mg cholesterol, **500** mg sodium, **4** glycemic load

STEAMED SPAGHETTI SQUASH

Start to Finish: 1 hour
Yield: 4 servings

| 1 spaghetti squash (3 pounds) | Water |
| | Salt and pepper to taste |

1. Preheat oven to 400°F.
2. Cut squash in half; scoop out
seeds with a spoon. Season with
salt and pepper. Place 2 tablespoons
water in the cavity of each half.

CULINARY NOTES

Can be served hot as a side
vegetable or cold as a salad.

Place in a baking dish and add ½ cup of water to the bottom of the pan.
Cover tightly with foil and bake in the oven for 40–50 minutes or until
the squash is soft enough to pull the flesh from the skin in strands. The
squash may still be a bit crunchy, but should pull easily from the skin.
3. Gently pull at the flesh with a fork to separate it into spaghetti
strands. Season with salt and pepper.

Variations:

- Sprinkle with 3 tablespoons of lemon juice, 1 tablespoon extra-virgin
  olive oil, and 1 tablespoon each chopped basil and parsley.

- Add 2 tablespoons capers, 1 tablespoons chopped oregano,
  1 cup chopped tomatoes, 1 tablespoon extra-virgin olive oil, and
  3 tablespoons red wine vinegar.

- Add 1 cup chopped tomatoes, 1 tablespoons chopped cilantro,
  3 tablespoons lime juice, 1 tablespoon extra-virgin olive oil, 1 teaspoon
  toasted ground cumin, and 1 tablespoon chopped chipotle in adobo
  sauce or chipotle powder.

- Add 4 tablespoons white balsamic vinegar and 2 tablespoons toasted
  almonds; garnish with 2 ounces of gorgonzola or blue cheese.

Nutrition Facts per Serving: **100** calories, **2** g protein, **2** g fat (**0** g saturated fat),
23 g carbohydrate, **3** g fiber, **0** mg cholesterol, **55** mg sodium, **17** glycemic load

TOASTED BARLEY SALAD
WITH FRESH HERBS, TOMATO, & ZUCCHINI

Start to Finish: 30 minutes   Yield: 10 servings

Developed by Chef Andy Wild for The New Sonoma Diet

1½ cups chicken stock
1 cup barley, toasted
1 cup parsley, minced
¼ cup cilantro, minced
¼ cup pine nuts, toasted
2 tablespoons water
1 lemon, zested and juiced

3 tablespoons extra-virgin olive oil
1½ cups zucchini, seeded and diced
2 cups cherry tomatoes, cut in half
¼ cup red onion, diced
¼ cup dry jack cheese

1. Bring the chicken stock to a boil and add the barley; cover, reduce heat, and simmer 15 minutes. Remove from heat; let stand, covered, for 5 minutes.

2. Combine in a large bowl the minced herbs, pine nuts, water, lemon zest and juice, olive oil, zucchini, tomatoes, and onion. Mix well. Sprinkle with cheese.

Nutrition Facts per Serving: 380 calories, 12 g protein, 16 g fat (3 g saturated fat), 53 g carbohydrate, 14 g fiber, 4.5 mg cholesterol, 188 mg sodium, 19 glycemic load

WATERMELON, ARUGULA, & FETA SALAD

Start to Finish: 15 minutes   Yield: 4 servings, 1 cup each

2   cups watermelon, cut in
    1-inch pieces

2   cups arugula

2   tablespoons Balsamic
    Vinaigrette, page 204

¼   cup feta cheese or
    goat cheese

Salt and pepper to taste

Place watermelon and arugula in a bowl. Toss with vinaigrette, salt, and pepper. Garnish with feta cheese.

Variations:

- Use canteloupe, canary, or Crenshaw melons in place of watermelon.

- Use goat cheese in place of feta cheese.

CULINARY NOTE

Watermelons are fruits that do not ripen once harvested. It is best to use the watermelon as soon as you purchase it.

Nutrition Facts per Serving: 65 calories, 2 g protein, 3 g fat (1.5 g saturated fat), 7 g carbohydrate, .5 g fiber, 8.5 mg cholesterol, 165 mg sodium, 3.6 glycemic load

WHEAT BERRY TABBOULEH

*Start to Finish: 1 hour 25 minutes, including cooking time
for wheat berries   Yield: 6 servings*

2⅔ cups cooked wheat berries (page 246)
¾ cup tomato, chopped
¾ cup cucumber, chopped
½ cup fresh parsley, chopped
¼ cup scallions, thinly sliced
1 tablespoon fresh mint, chopped

3 tablespoons extra-virgin olive oil
3 tablespoons lemon juice
¼ teaspoon kosher salt
Sliced cucumber (optional)
Sliced lemon (optional)

1. In a large bowl combine cooked wheat berries, tomato, chopped cucumber, parsley, scallions, and mint.

2. For dressing, in a screw-top jar combine oil, lemon juice, and kosher salt. Cover and shake well. Drizzle dressing over wheat berry mixture; toss to coat.

3. To serve, if desired, arrange sliced cucumber and lemon around edge of bowl.

CULINARY NOTE

Make-ahead directions: Prepare the salad and add the dressing; cover and chill for up to 24 hours. To serve, if desired, arrange sliced cucumber and lemon around edge of bowl.

Nutrition Facts per Serving: 142 calories, 7 g total fat (1 g saturated fat), 0 mg cholesterol, 86 mg sodium, 17 g carbohydrate, 2 g fiber, 3 g protein, 6 glycemic load

WILD MUSHROOM & BARLEY RISOTTO

Start to Finish: 1 hour 35 minutes   Yield: 5 servings

1½ ounces fresh chanterelle, stemmed oyster, and/or stemmed shiitake mushrooms, sliced

1 large shallot, finely chopped (½ cup)

1 clove garlic, minced (½ teaspoon)

1 tablespoon extra-virgin olive oil

⅓ cup dry white wine

3¾ cups chicken stock or reduced-sodium chicken broth

½ cup regular barley

Fresh flat-leaf parsley, chopped

1. In a large skillet cook mushrooms, shallot, and garlic in hot oil over medium heat for 5 to 10 minutes or until mushrooms are tender and lightly browned. Add wine. Bring to boiling; reduce heat. Simmer, uncovered, about 5 minutes or until liquid is nearly evaporated.

2. Meanwhile, in a medium saucepan bring chicken stock to boiling; reduce heat. Keep hot over very low heat.

3. Add barley to mushroom mixture; stir to coat. Add 1 cup of the hot stock to the barley mixture. Cook over medium heat until liquid is absorbed, stirring occasionally. (This should take about 15 minutes. If the liquid absorbs too quickly, reduce the heat.) Repeat with 2 cups more of the hot stock, adding 1 cup at a time and cooking until all the liquid is absorbed before adding more, stirring occasionally. (This should take about 30 minutes.)

4. Stir in the remaining hot stock. Cook until the barley is slightly creamy and just tender. (This should take about 15 minutes. Increase the heat slightly if the mixture is too wet.) Sprinkle with parsley.

Nutrition Facts per Serving: **145** calories, **5** g protein, **3** g total fat (**0** g saturated fat), **23** g carbohydrate, **4** g fiber, **0** mg cholesterol, **366** mg sodium, **6** glycemic load

ASIAN SATAY SKEWERS
WITH BLACK BEAN SAUCE

Start to Finish: 1 hour 10 minutes   Yield: 6 servings

For satay:

1   pound boneless, skinless chicken breasts cut in ½-inch by 2-inch strips
1   cup low-sodium teriyaki sauce
1   tablespoon ginger, minced
1   tablespoon garlic, minced
1   teaspoon sesame oil
1   pack wooden skewers, 6-inch long
Salt and black pepper, to taste
1   12-inch sheet aluminum foil

For sauce:

½   15-ounce-can black beans, drained and rinsed
½   15.8 ounce can Great Northern beans, drained and rinsed
1   cup frozen shelled soybeans, thawed and ready to eat
½   cup scallions, chopped
2   tablespoons ginger, finely chopped
2   tablespoons cilantro, chopped
2   tablespoons sugar
3   tablespoons lime juice
¼   cup low-sodium soy sauce
1   teaspoon garlic, finely chopped
1   serrano chile, chopped * (optional)
2   teaspoons sesame oil

1. For the satay: Season chicken with salt and pepper.

2. Combine teriyaki sauce, ginger, garlic, and sesame oil in a medium bowl.

3. Toss the sauce with the chicken. Let marinate for at least 45 minutes. Weave meat onto skewers. Discard marinade.

4. Preheat the grill to medium hot. Fold a 12-inch sheet of heavy-duty foil in thirds lengthwise. Place on the grill by the edge.

5. Place satays on the grill laying meat end over fire, and the wood end on the piece of foil. This will help keep the exposed wood from burning.

6. For the sauce: Combine beans, soybeans, green onions, ginger and cilantro into a medium bowl. Mix well.

7. In a small bowl, combine sugar, lime juice, and soy sauce.

8. Mix until the sugar dissolves. Add garlic, Serrano chile, and sesame oil. Let sit for 5 minutes.

9. Add soy sauce mixture to the beans, gently toss to coat.

10. Serve the satays with bean salad. Drizzle some of the liquid from the salad on top of the satays.

Variations:

- You can substitute skirt steak, flank steak, or London broil for the chicken. Cut the meat against the grain into ¼-inch thick by 2-inch long pieces.

CULINARY NOTE

* Because hot chile peppers contain oils that can burn your skin and eyes, wear rubber or plastic gloves when working with them. If your bare hands do touch the chile peppers, wash your hands well with soap and water.

Nutrition Facts per Serving: **230** calories, **22** g protein, **22** g fat (**4** g saturated fat), **26** g carbohydrate, **7** g fiber, **0** mg cholesterol, **1000** mg sodium, **6** glycemic load

BABY GREENS
WITH APPLES, CHICKEN, & WALNUTS

Start to Finish: 25 minutes   Yield: 4 servings

Developed by Chef Andrew Wild for The New Sonoma Diet

2 tablespoons lemon juice

2 tablespoons shallots, finely chopped

1 tablespoon white wine vinegar

2 tablespoons extra-virgin olive oil

¼ teaspoon kosher salt

⅛ teaspoon freshly ground black pepper

6 cups mixed salad greens, torn

3 Granny Smith apples, cored and cut into bite-size strips

¾ cup fresh flat-leaf parsley leaves

½ cup cucumber, sliced

¼ cup walnut pieces, toasted

12 ounces cooked skinless chicken breast halves, sliced, or 8 hard-cooked eggs, peeled and halved

1. For vinaigrette, in a small bowl combine lemon juice, shallots, and vinegar. Let stand for 5 minutes. Whisk in oil, kosher salt, and pepper until well mixed.

> **CULINARY NOTE**
>
> For extra flavor, top each serving with a tablespoon of goat cheese.

2. In a large bowl combine the greens, apples, parsley leaves, cucumber, and walnuts. Add vinaigrette; toss lightly to coat. Divide among 4 serving plates. Top with chicken or eggs. Serve immediately.

Nutrition Facts per Serving: 327 calories, 29 g protein, 15 g total fat (2 g saturated fat), 20 g carbohydrate, 5 g fiber, 72 mg cholesterol, 203 mg sodium, 6 glycemic load

CALABRIAN-STYLE CHICKEN IN PARCHMENT

Start to Finish: 45 minutes   Yield: 4 servings

Developed by Chef Andrew Wild for The New Sonoma Diet

1   pound boneless skinless chicken breast

2   tablespoons olive oil

2   tablespoons fresh oregano, minced

2   tablespoons fresh thyme, minced

2   tablespoons fresh flat-leaf parsley, minced

1   lemon, zest and juice

2   tablespoons Calabrian chile peppers, sliced in rounds (about 4 chiles)

1   tablespoon capers

10 ounces broccoli rabe, chopped

2   tablespoons sun-dried tomatoes in oil, julienned

1   cup canned artichoke hearts, drained and quartered

Salt and freshly ground black pepper to taste

1. Preheat oven to 400°F.

2. Cut the chicken breast into 12 ½-inch slices.

3. In a large bowl combine the remaining ingredients and toss to coat completely with the fresh herbs and olive oil.

4. Lay out 4 half sheets of parchment paper. In the center of each sheet place 3 slices of chicken; top with an equal amount of the vegetable mixture. Fold the paper over and crimp and fold the edges to form a seal.

5. Place the packs on a sheet pan. Bake for 30 minutes. Remove from the oven and serve immediately.

Variation:

- For a fresh summer version, omit the broccoli rabe and sun-dried tomatoes and add 1 cup cherry tomatoes and 10 ounces asparagus, sliced thin.

Nutrition Facts per Serving: 450 calories, 24 g protein, 24 g fat (5 g saturated fat), 40 g carbohydrate, 10 g fiber, 49 mg cholesterol, 600 mg sodium, 0 glycemic load

CHICKEN EN PAPILLOTE
WITH VEGETABLES

Start to Finish: 55 minutes   Yield: 4 servings

1   pound skinless, boneless chicken breast halves

2   tablespoons extra-virgin olive oil

1   tablespoon fresh oregano, chopped, or 1 teaspoon dried oregano, crushed

1   tablespoon fresh thyme, chopped, or ½ teaspoon dried thyme, crushed

1   teaspoon lemon zest

2   tablespoons lemon juice

½   teaspoon kosher salt

¼   teaspoon freshly ground black pepper

10   ounces fresh asparagus, trimmed and cut into 2-inch pieces (2 cups)

6   ounces pea pods, trimmed (2 cups)

1   cup canned artichoke hearts, drained and quartered, or

1   cup frozen artichoke hearts, thawed and quartered

1   cup cherry tomatoes, halved

2   tablespoons fresh flat-leaf parsley, chopped

Parchment paper

½   cup scallions, sliced

1. Preheat oven to 400°F.

2. Cut chicken breasts crosswise into ½-inch slices. In a medium bowl combine oil, oregano, thyme, lemon zest, lemon juice, kosher salt, and pepper. Add chicken to bowl and toss to coat. Let stand while preparing vegetables.

3. In a large bowl combine asparagus, pea pods, artichoke hearts, cherry tomatoes, and parsley. Tear four 20-inch by 12-inch pieces of parchment paper; fold each in half crosswise and crease. Open up again. On half of one parchment sheet, arrange one-fourth of the vegetable mixture. Top with one-fourth of the chicken pieces. Top with one-fourth of the scallions. To make packet, fold parchment paper over chicken and vegetables. Crimp and fold edges to seal; twist corners. Repeat to make 4 packets.

4. Place 2 packets on each of 2 baking sheets. Bake on separate racks for about 20 minutes or until chicken is no longer pink. (To test, carefully open the packets and peek.) Serve packets immediately.

CULINARY NOTES

- Cooking en papillote is similar to steaming or baking in a bag. If you do not have parchment paper, use foil, but be wary of letting high-acid ingredients sit in the foil for more than 1 hour.
- When using paper, be sure to seal the edges tightly so the pouch does not open up when steaming.

Variations:

- Add 1 cup of white cannellini beans to the vegetable mixture.
- **Latin Variation:** Replace lemon peel and juice with lime peel and juice. Add 1 teaspoon chopped chipotle in adobo sauce to marinade. Add sliced zucchini in place of pea pods.

Nutrition Facts per Serving: 249 calories, 31 g protein, 8 g total fat (1 g saturated fat), 13 g carbohydrate, 6 g fiber, 66 mg cholesterol, 498 mg sodium, 2 glycemic load

ENFRIJOLADAS WITH CHICKEN, CORN, & ROASTED PEPPERS

Start to Finish: 30 minutes; 45 if using sweet potato filling Yield: 4 servings

½ tablespoon olive oil

1 cup onion, diced

1 tablespoon garlic, minced

2–3 teaspoons chipotle in adobo sauce, chopped

1 14–16-ounce can refried pinto beans

2 cups chicken stock

1 cup corn, frozen, thawed

½ pound chicken, cooked, shredded

½ cup canned green chiles, roasted, diced

½ cup red pepper, roasted, diced

2 tablespoons scallion, chopped

1 tablespoon cilantro, chopped

2 tablespoons lime juice

Salt and pepper to taste

8 corn tortillas

½ cup salsa fresco— homemade or store-bought

1. Heat the olive oil in a sauté pan; add onions and cook until slightly caramelized. Add garlic; cook until aromatic. Add chipotle, beans, and chicken stock. Bring to a simmer. Cook for 10 minutes; let cool slightly. Place in a blender or food processor and blend until smooth. Adjust seasoning. Pour bean puree into a pie pan or flat pan.

2. Heat a skillet over medium high heat. Add corn to dry pan; sauté for 1–2 minutes or until slightly browned. Add the chicken, chiles, and red pepper. Sauté 1–2 minutes until the chicken is warmed through. Add the scallion, cilantro, and lime juice. Adjust seasonings with salt and pepper. Divide into 8 portions.

3. To assemble: Heat the tortillas in a dry sauté pan until slightly browned. Dip whole tortilla in the bean puree; place on a small plate. Place one portion of filling down the center of the tortilla in a straight line. Roll the tortilla around the filling, and place seam side down on the

Nutrition Facts per Serving: 450 calories, 28 g protein, 12 g fat (3 g saturated fat), 55 g carbohydrate, 11 g fiber, 45 mg cholesterol, 800 mg sodium , 18 glycemic load

plate. Continue with the rest of the tortillas. Pour remaining bean puree over the enfrijoladas. Serve with a spoonful of salsa fresca.

Filling Variations:

- Use black beans instead of pinto beans.

- Use leftover roasted vegetables or grilled vegetables in place of the corn.

- Use leftover cooked shrimp in place of the chicken.

CULINARY NOTES

- Don't be afraid to season the filling assertively with lime and salt. The bean puree is rich and will need the acid and salt to cut through the richness.

- Leftover roasted or grilled veggies, cooked chicken, or shrimp can be COOK 1X · EAT 2X ingredients.

SMOKY SWEET POTATO, CARROT, & CHICKEN

Start to Finish: 20 minutes   Yield: 4 servings

1	tablespoon extra-virgin olive oil	1	cinnamon stick
½	cup onion, diced	1	cup chicken stock
1	tablespoon garlic, chopped	2	cups chicken, cooked, shredded
1	tablespoon chipotle in adobo sauce, chopped	1	tablespoon cilantro, chopped
1	cup carrots, chopped		Lime juice as needed
1	cup sweet potato, cut in ½-inch pieces		Salt and pepper to taste

Heat oil in a medium saucepan over medium heat. Add onions and garlic; cook until slightly caramelized. Add the chipotle, carrots, and sweet potato. Cook for 5 minutes over medium-low heat. Add cinnamon stick and chicken stock. Bring to a simmer. Cook until the vegetables are almost tender. Add chicken; cook until the vegetables are tender and chicken is warmed through. Remove cinnamon stick; stir in cilantro. Season with lime juice, salt and pepper.

Nutrition Facts per Serving: 450 calories, 28 g protein, 12 g fat (3 g saturated fat), 58 g carbohydrate, 10 g fiber, 47 mg cholesterol, 500 mg sodium, 18 glycemic load

GREEK CHICKEN SALAD
WITH WHITE BEANS

Start to Finish: 20 minutes   Yield: 1 serving

1   tablespoon sun-dried
    tomatoes, diced or cut up

Boiling water

2   cups mixed salad greens,
    torn

3   ounces cooked skinless
    chicken breast, sliced

¼   cup canned cannellini
    beans (white kidney beans),
    rinsed and drained

1   tablespoon feta cheese,
    crumbled

1   tablespoon slivered
    almonds, toasted

1   tablespoon Red Wine
    Vinaigrette (page 199)

1. Place dried tomatoes in a small bowl.
Add enough boiling water to cover; let
stand for 5 minutes. Drain well.

2. Meanwhile, arrange salad greens
on a serving plate. Top with chicken,
cannellini beans, feta cheese, and
almonds. Sprinkle with drained
tomatoes. Drizzle with Red Wine
Vinaigrette.

CULINARY NOTES

- Save the water from
  rehydrating the
  tomatoes and use in
  tomato soups or sauces.

- Leftover prepared
  chicken or pork can
  be COOK 1X·EAT 2X
  ingredients.

Variations:

- Replace chicken with marinated pork. Use Sherry Vinaigrette (page
  200) in place of Red Wine Vinaigrette.

- Toss the chicken and cannellini beans with 1 teaspoon Spanish paprika,
  salt, and pepper.

Nutrition Facts per Serving: **326** calories, **35** g protein, **15** g total fat (**3** g saturated fat),
16 g carbohydrate, **6** g fiber, **80** mg cholesterol, **442** mg sodium, **5** glycemic load

GRILLED CHICKEN
WITH TOMATO-BEAN SALAD

Start to Finish: 25 minutes plus 8 to 24 hours for marinating Yield: 4 servings

4   4-ounce skinless, boneless
    chicken breast halves
Kosher salt
Freshly ground black pepper
¾ cup Charmoula Marinade
    (see page 176)
2   medium green and/or
    red bell peppers,
    seeded and chopped

1   15- to 16-ounce can
    garbanzo beans (chickpeas),
    rinsed and drained
1   large tomato, chopped
½ cup onion, finely chopped
½ resh serrano chile pepper,
    seeded and finely chopped
    (optional)
2   tablespoons chopped fresh
    flat-leaf parsley

1. Season chicken with kosher salt and black pepper. Place chicken in a self-sealing plastic bag set in a shallow dish; add ¼ cup of Charmoula Marinade. Seal bag; turn to coat chicken. Marinate in the refrigerator for 8 to 24 hours, turning bag occasionally.

CULINARY NOTE

Leftover prepared chicken can be a COOK 1X·EAT 2X ingredient.

2. Drain chicken, discarding marinade. For a charcoal grill, place chicken on the rack of an uncovered grill directly over medium coals. Grill for 12 to 15 minutes or until chicken is no longer pink (170°F), turning once halfway through grilling. For a gas grill, preheat grill. Reduce heat to medium. Place chicken on grill rack over heat. Cover and grill as above.

3. Meanwhile, in large bowl combine bell peppers, garbanzo beans, tomato, onion, serrano pepper (if desired), and remaining ½ cup Charmoula Marinade. Season to taste with kosher salt and black pepper. Divide garbanzo bean mixture among 4 serving plates. Add a chicken breast half to each plate. Sprinkle with parsley.

Nutrition Facts per Serving: 433 calories, 33 g protein, 19 g total fat (3 g saturated fat), 34 g carbohydrate, 8 g fiber, 66 mg cholesterol, 907 mg sodium, 0 glycemic load

MEDITERRANEAN TABBOULEH SALAD
WITH CHICKEN

Start to Finish: 60 minutes   Chill: 4 to 24 hours   Yield: 6 servings

1 ½ cups water

½ cup bulgur

2 medium tomatoes, chopped

1 cup cucumber, seeded and finely chopped

1 cup flat-leaf parsley, finely chopped

⅓ cup scallions, thinly sliced

¼ cup fresh mint, chopped, or 1 tablespoon dried mint, crushed

⅓ to ½ cup lemon juice

¼ cup extra-virgin olive oil

¾ teaspoon kosher salt

½ teaspoon freshly ground black pepper

12 large romaine leaves

18 ounces grilled or broiled skinless, boneless chicken breast halves, sliced

1. In a large bowl combine the water and bulgur. Let stand for 30 minutes. Drain through a fine sieve, using a large spoon to push out excess water. Return bulgur to bowl. Stir in tomatoes, cucumber, parsley, scallions, and mint.

2. For dressing, in a screw-top jar combine lemon juice, oil, kosher salt, and pepper. Cover and shake well. Pour dressing over the bulgur mixture (tabbouleh). Toss lightly to coat. Cover and chill for 4 to 24 hours, stirring occasionally. Bring to room temperature before serving.

3. For each serving, place 2 romaine leaves on a serving plate. Top each with ⅔ cup of the tabbouleh mixture and 3 ounces of the cooked chicken.

Nutrition Facts per Serving: **298** calories, **30** g protein, **13** g total fat (**2** g saturated fat), **17** g carbohydrate, **5** g fiber, **72** mg cholesterol, **324** mg sodium, **3** glycemic load

CULINARY NOTES

- To grill chicken breast halves, lightly sprinkle chicken with kosher salt and freshly ground black pepper. For a charcoal grill, place chicken on the rack of an uncovered grill directly over medium coals. Grill for 10 to 12 minutes or until chicken is no longer pink (170°F), turning once halfway through grilling. For a gas grill, preheat grill. Reduce heat to medium. Place chicken on grill rack over heat. Cover and grill as above.

- To broil chicken breast halves, lightly sprinkle chicken with kosher salt and freshly ground black pepper. Place chicken on the unheated rack of a broiler pan. Broil chicken 4 to 5 inches from the heat for 12 to 15 minutes or until chicken is no longer pink (170°F), turning once halfway through broiling.

- Grains absorb seasoning as they sit, so reseason the salad before serving.

- Leftover prepared chicken, fish or shrimp can be COOK 1X · EAT 2X ingredients.

Variations:

 GLUTEN FREE : Replace bulgur and water with 1 cup cooked quinoa.

Roast Chicken
WITH ROASTED VEGETABLES

Start to Finish: 1½ hours   Yield: 4–6 servings

(about 4 ounces of chicken, 1 cup vegetables, and ½ cup whole grain per serving)

1 ounce olive oil	1 ounce olive oil
1 ounce white wine	2 cups turnips, peeled, cut in ¾ inch pieces*
1 tablespoon Dijon mustard	
2 tablespoons rosemary, chopped	2 cups carrots, peeled, cut in ¾-inch pieces**
1 tablespoon garlic, chopped	2 cups cauliflower, cut in 1½-inch florets
1 whole chicken, giblets and excess fat removed	Salt and pepper to taste

1. Place a shallow roasting pan with a rack in the oven. Preheat oven to 375°F.

2. Combine 1 ounce olive oil, wine, mustard, rosemary, and garlic. Season with salt and pepper.

3. Gently loosen the skin from the breast and legs of the chicken, being careful not to tear the skin. Rub ¾ of rosemary mixture underneath the skin of the chicken. Rub the remaining ¼ all over the skin. Season the chicken well with salt and pepper.

4. Place the chicken on the rack in the roasting pan in the oven. Cook for 10 minutes.

5. Toss the veggies with 1 ounce olive oil. Place around the chicken in the bottom of the pan. Every 10–15 minutes, baste the chicken with the juices and fat that have accumulated in the bottom of the pan, and turn the vegetables. Roast another 45–50 minutes until the juice runs clear or until the chicken is 165°F. at the thigh or approximately 160°F. at the breast.

6. Let rest in a warm place for 15 minutes prior to carving.

Nutrition Facts per Serving: 320 calories, 38 g protein, 12 g fat (2 g saturated fat), 15 g carbohydrate, 4 g fiber, 115 mg cholesterol, 300 mg sodium, 4.5 glycemic load

Variations:

MEDITERRANEAN VARIATION

Replace rosemary with ¾ tablespoon each of oregano, thyme, and marjoram, chopped.

Replace vegetables for roasting with

1 cup carrots, peeled, cut in ¾-inch cubes	2 cups celery root, peeled, cut in ¾-inch cubes
2 cups fennel, cut into ¾-inch cubes	

Serve chicken with 1 cup of the vegetables and ½ cup of quinoa or whole-grain rice of choice.

(Use squash, fennel, and mushrooms in Wave 1.)

Nutrition Facts per Serving: **286** calories, **38** g protein, **9** g fat (**1.7** g saturated fat), **13** g carbohydrate, **3.7** g fiber, **115** mg cholesterol, **240** mg sodium, **6.2** glycemic load

ASIAN VARIATION

Replace oil, white wine, mustard, rosemary, and garlic mixture with

2	tablespoons soy sauce	½	tablespoon sugar
2	teaspoons ginger, chopped	½	tablespoon rice vinegar
1	scallion, chopped	1	teaspoon sesame oil

Replace vegetables for roasting with

2	cups mushrooms, cut in quarters	1	cup sweet potatoes, peeled, cut in ¾-inch cubes
1	cup carrots, peeled, cut in ¾-inch cubes	2	cups daikon, peeled, cut in ¾-inch cubes

Serve chicken with 1 cup of the vegetables and ½ cup of brown rice.

Nutrition Facts per Serving: 340 calories, 38 g protein, 13 g fat (2.4 g saturated fat), 16 g carbohydrate, 3.7 g fiber, 115 mg cholesterol, 480 mg sodium, 4.6 glycemic load

LATIN VARIATION

Replace oil, white wine, mustard, rosemary, and garlic mixture with

1	tablespoon garlic, chopped	1	teaspoon Mexican oregano
½	teaspoon ground cumin	2	tablespoons lime juice
1	teaspoon chipotle in adobo sauce, chopped		

Replace vegetables for roasting with

2	cups carrots, peeled, cut in ¾-inch cubes	2	cups summer squash, cut in ¾-inch cubes
2	cups chayote, peeled, seed removed, cut in ¾-inch cubes		

Serve chicken with 1 cup of the vegetables, 1 corn tortilla, and red or green salsa.

Nutrition Facts per Serving: 275 calories, 38 g protein, 10 g fat (1.3 g saturate fat), 8 g carbohydrate, 6 g fiber, 118 mg cholesterol, 600 mg sodium, 2.1 glycemic load

ROMAINE & WATERCRESS SALAD
WITH TOASTED ALMONDS & DIJON VINAIGRETTE

Start to Finish: 30 minutes   Yield: 4 servings

¼ cup red wine vinegar

2 tablespoons finely chopped shallots

1 clove garlic, minced (½ teaspoon)

1½ teaspoons Dijon mustard

3 tablespoons extra-virgin olive oil

¼ teaspoon kosher salt

⅛ teaspoon freshly ground black pepper

1 pound romaine, cored and thinly sliced crosswise

4 ounces watercress or fresh spinach, large stems removed

2 medium carrots, halved lengthwise and thinly sliced

1 medium red bell pepper, seeded and chopped

2 scallions, thinly sliced

¼ cup sliced almonds, toasted

12 ounces cooked skinless chicken breast halves, sliced, or 8 hard-cooked eggs, peeled and sliced

1 tablespoon Asiago or parmesan cheese, finely shredded

CULINARY NOTE
Leftover prepared chicken can be a COOK 1X·EAT 2X ingredient.

1. For the vinaigrette, in a small bowl combine vinegar, shallots, and garlic. Let stand for 5 minutes. Whisk in mustard. Add oil in a thin, steady stream, whisking constantly until combined. Stir in kosher salt and black pepper.

2. In a large bowl combine romaine, watercress or spinach, carrots, bell pepper, scallions, and almonds. Add the vinaigrette; toss to coat. Divide among 4 serving plates.

3. Top servings with chicken or egg slices and sprinkle with cheese. Serve immediately.

Variation:

- **Latin Style:** Substitute Simple Spicy Lime Cilantro Vinaigrette (page 201). Replace the carrot with 1 cup chopped jicama and ½ cup cooked corn. Replace almonds with toasted pepita seeds.

Nutrition Facts per Serving: **334** calories, **32** g protein, **18** g total fat (**3** g saturated fat), **13** g carbohydrate, **5** g fiber, **73** mg cholesterol, **294** mg sodium, **3** glycemic load

SIMPLE CHICKEN TACOS
WITH ROASTED TOMATO JALAPEÑO SALSA

Start to Finish: 30 minutes   Yield: 4 portions

1 cup cabbage, shredded fine

¼ cup red onion, sliced thin, rinsed

1 pound roast chicken, bones removed, shredded into ¼-inch to ½-inch pieces

1 cup Roasted Tomato Jalapeño Salsa (page 194)

½ teaspoon chipotle in adobo sauce, chopped fine (optional)

8 corn tortillas

1 tablespoon cilantro, chopped

1 tablespoon lime juice

½ avocado, cut into 8 slices

Salt and pepper to taste

1. Combine cabbage and red onion in a colander. Sprinkle with salt and pepper. Let sit for 15 minutes while you prepare remaining ingredients.

2. In a sauté pan, combine roast chicken with ½ cup tomato salsa and optional chipotle. Heat until warmed through.

3. Heat the tortillas on a griddle until soft.

4. Gently press the cabbage to remove excess moisture. Transfer to a bowl and add the cilantro and lime juice. Adjust seasonings.

5. To assemble tacos: Lay tortillas on a flat surface. Top each with 2 ounces warm chicken mixture; place cabbage mixture on top. Place 1 tablespoon salsa and a slice of avocado on top.

CULINARY NOTES

• For an easy meal, use leftover roast chicken and store-bought salsa. But if you have the time, prepare the Roasted Tomato Jalapeño Salsa (page 194)—it's well worth the effort!

• Use leftover chicken, pork, fish, or shrimp as COOK 1X· EAT 2X ingredients.

Nutrition Facts per Serving (tacos with Roasted Tomato Jalapeño Salsa): **350** calories, 32 g protein, 11 g fat (3 g saturated fat), **30** g carbohydrate, 5 g fiber, **85** mg cholesterol, 227 mg sodium, 11 glycemic load

Sonoma Salad
WITH TOMATOES & FETA

Start to Finish: 20 minutes   Yield: 4 servings

8 cups mixed salad greens, torn

12 ounces cooked skinless chicken or turkey breast, lean beef, or pork, sliced

1 cup cherry tomatoes, halved

½ cup cucumber, halved and sliced

¼ cup small fresh basil leaves

1 recipe Red Wine Vinaigrette (page 199)

Kosher salt

Freshly ground black pepper

¼ cup feta or goat cheese, crumbled (1 ounce)

1 tablespoon pine nuts, toasted

In a very large bowl combine greens, meat, tomatoes, cucumber, and basil. Drizzle with Red Wine Vinaigrette. Toss to coat. Season to taste with kosher salt and pepper. Top with feta cheese and pine nuts. Serve immediately.

Variations:

- Replace chicken with water-packed tuna in 1-inch pieces.

- Replace mixed greens with half baby spinach and half shredded romaine lettuce.

CULINARY NOTE

Leftover prepared tuna, chicken or other lean meats can be COOK 1X · EAT 2X ingredients.

- Replace cucumber with ¼-inch slices of hearts of palm and ½ cup thinly sliced red peppers.

- Replace cucumber with ½ cup artichoke hearts, cooked, and ½ cup sliced red and yellow peppers. Replace pine nuts with chopped toasted almonds.

Nutrition Facts per Serving: **267** calories, **30** g protein, **13** g total fat (**3** g saturated fat), **6** g carbohydrate, **2** g fiber, **80** mg cholesterol, **318** mg sodium, **1** glycemic load

WHEAT BERRY CHICKEN PAELLA
WITH CHICKPEAS & ZUCCHINI

Start to Finish: 1 hour 10 minutes   Yield: 4 servings

¾ pound boneless chicken legs, skin and excess fat removed, cut into 2-inch pieces

2 teaspoons Spanish paprika

1 tablespoon extra-virgin olive oil

½ cup onion, diced

3 cups chicken stock

1 tablespoon garlic, minced

2 ounces Spanish chorizo, cut in quarters lengthwise, then in ⅛-inch pieces

1 pinch saffron (optional)

1 15-ounce can tomatoes, diced, drained

½ cup arborio or Spanish rice

1 cup cooked wheat berries (page 246)

1 teaspoon lemon zest

½ cup canned chickpeas plus liquid

1 cup zucchini, sliced in quarters lengthwise, then in ¼-inch-wide pieces

1 tablespoon parsley, chopped

Salt and pepper to taste

1. Season chicken with salt, pepper, and 1 teaspoon Spanish paprika.

2. Heat a large sauté pan or paella pan over medium heat. Add the extra-virgin olive oil and the chicken. Cook over medium high to brown the chicken on all sides. The chicken should be golden brown all over, but still raw when finished. Remove the chicken from the pan. Set aside on a plate, reserving all juice that comes out.

3. Add the onions and cook over medium heat for 3 minutes. Add ¼ cup chicken stock to deglaze pan, reducing until stock is almost dry. Add garlic, chorizo, remaining paprika, and saffron; cook for 30 seconds. Add tomatoes; heat for 4 minutes.

4. Stir in rice and wheat berries. Add remaining chicken stock, lemon zest, and chickpeas; bring to a simmer. Adjust seasoning with salt and pepper. Return the chicken and any juices to the pan, gently burying it in the grains. Loosely cover and cook for 30 minutes over medium-low heat, stirring periodically to prevent sticking to the bottom of the pan.

(Alternatively, the paella can be baked covered in a 350°F oven.) When most of the liquid has been absorbed and the rice is almost cooked through, mix in the zucchini, and cook until the rice is tender. (If the liquid has been absorbed and the rice is still hard, add more stock until the rice is cooked through.)

5. The paella is done once the rice is tender and the liquid has been absorbed. Let rest for 5 minutes. Sprinkle parsley on top.

Variations:

- Substitute cooked spelt, kamut, farro, or barley (not pearled barley) for the wheat berries.
- Substitute pork tenderloin or loin for the chicken. Add during the last 15 minutes of cooking.
- Substitute shrimp for the chicken. Do not brown the shrimp. Place seasoned raw shrimp on top of the paella during the last 15 minutes of cooking. Cook covered, and check shrimp periodically. You can also sauté or grill the shrimp separately and lay it on top.
- Substitute white beans or cannellini beans for the chickpeas.
- Substitute green beans, romano beans, or assorted squash for the zucchini.
- Add 1 tablespoon fresh chopped thyme, or oregano before adding the stock.

CULINARY NOTES

- The wheat berries should be cooked in advance but can still be a little firm when added to the paella.
- The paella should be cooked in a shallow pan, no deeper than 1 1/2-inches.
- When preparing for a large group of people, the paella can also be cooked on the grill or over an open fire. This gives it a great smoky flavor.

Nutrition Facts per Serving: 450 calories, 33 g protein, 15 g fat (3.7 g saturated fat), 50 g carbohydrate, 7.5 g fiber, 80 mg cholesterol, 590 mg sodium, 18 glycemic load

CUBAN-STYLE FLANK STEAK

Start to Finish: 1 hour, plus 3 hours in a crock pot
Yield: 6 servings

1½ pounds flank steak, excess fat removed
1 tablespoon paprika
2 teaspoons coriander
1 tablespoon chile powder
1 tablespoon extra-virgin olive oil
1 cup onion, sliced
2 tablespoons garlic, chopped
½ teaspoon cumin seeds
1 teaspoon oregano, dried
2 cups red pepper and yellow pepper, sliced
1 4-ounce can green chiles, chopped (New Mexico Hatch chiles)
1 28-ounce can tomatoes, diced
1 cup chicken stock
salt and pepper to taste

1. Season the meat with salt and pepper.
2. Combine the paprika, coriander, and chile powder. Sprinkle on seasoned meat. Let sit for 15 minutes.
3. Heat a sauté pan over medium heat. Add extra-virgin olive oil and meat. Sear on both sides. Remove meat from pan. Add onion and garlic to pan. Sauté until onion is slightly caramelized. Add cumin seeds and oregano; cook 30 seconds. Add peppers, green chiles, tomatoes, and stock. Bring to a simmer. Pour into crock pot, bury flank steak in liquid. Cook on low for 3 hours or until the meat is tender and able to shred.
4. Tear meat into strips with a fork. Mix with the peppers and broth. Serve with corn tortillas or rice.

CULINARY NOTE

- By seasoning the meat with salt and pepper first and letting it sit, you are allowing the salt to penetrate the flesh of the meat, allowing for a fuller flavor. It is important to season the meat before applying the spices. This prevents the spices from seeming gritty when the meat is eaten. The meat can be seasoned overnight if desired.

- COOK 1X·EAT 2X in salads, frittatas, omelets, wraps, or sandwiches.

Nutrition Facts per Serving: 250 calories, 28 g protein, 8 g fat (3 g saturated fat), 18 g carbohydrate, 5 g fiber, 34 mg cholesterol, 250 mg sodium, 0 glycemic load

MUSHROOM & CHARD–STUFFED FLANK STEAK

Start to Finish: 1 hour, plus 4–5 hours for cooking   Yield: 4 servings

1½ pounds flank steak, excess fat removed, at least 8 inches wide by 7 inches long

1 tablespoon extra-virgin olive oil

1 cup mushrooms, sliced

½ cup onion, diced

1 tablespoon garlic, chopped

4 cups chard, chopped 1-inch pieces

¼ cup coarse bulgur

¼ cup chicken stock

1 tablespoon extra-virgin olive oil

1 cup onion, diced

1 tablespoon garlic, chopped

1 cup canned tomatoes, diced

1 bay leaf

½ cup chicken stock

1 yard twine

Salt and pepper to taste

1. Season meat with salt and pepper; set aside.

2. Heat a large sauté pan over medium-high heat. Add 1 tablespoon extra-virgin olive oil and mushrooms; sauté for 4 minutes. Add ½ cup of onions and 1 tablespoon garlic; sauté for 2 minutes. Add chard. Cook for 4 minutes or until just wilted. Add bulgur and ¼ cup of chicken stock. Season well. Remove from heat, spread in the pan, and cool in the refrigerator.

3. Once the filling is cooled, lay the flank steak on a cutting board. Notice how the grain of the meat runs lengthwise down the meat. Place the filling down the center of the meat, running with the grain. Roll the meat around the filling. Wrap the twine around the meat and tie about 1 inch from the end of the roll. Continue tying at 1½-inch intervals. Don't worry about any filling that falls out; just push it back in.

4. Heat the sauté pan over medium heat. Add 1 tablespoon extra-virgin olive oil. Add the beef. Sear each side of the meat. Remove from pan.

Nutrition Facts per Serving: 440 calories, 41 g protein, 21 g fat (7 g saturated fat), 21 g carbohydrate, 5 g fiber, 69 mg cholesterol, 330 mg sodium, 2.5 glycemic load

5. Add 1 cup onion and 1 tablespoon garlic to sauté pan; cook 2 minutes. Add tomatoes, bay leaf, and ½ cup chicken stock. Bring to a simmer. Place tomato mixture in a crock pot. Place meat on top. Cover and cook for 4–5 hours or until the meat is tender.

6. Remove meat from pan. Let rest for 10 minutes. Slice against the grain.

7. Remove excess grease from the sauce by using a large spoon to skim the top layer of the sauce. Pour sauce into 4 soup plates. Top each with 2 slices of meat.

> **CULINARY NOTE**
>
> Flank steak is a long, fibrous muscle. It is important to place the filling along the grain of the meat and wrap the meat around the filling so that when you slice the cooked meat, you are slicing across the grain.

Variation:

SPINACH, RED PEPPER, & ALMOND STUFFING

1 tablespoon extra-virgin olive oil	½ cup toasted almonds, chopped
½ cup onion, diced	¼ cup coarse bulgur
1 tablespoon garlic, chopped	¼ cup chicken stock
1 cup roasted red peppers, diced	Salt and pepper to taste
3 cups baby spinach, chopped 1-inch pieces	

Heat a large sauté pan over medium-high heat. Add 1 tablespoon extra-virgin olive oil, onion, and garlic; sauté for 2 minutes. Add red peppers. Heat 1 minute to warm. Add spinach and cook to wilt, 2 minutes. Add almonds, bulgur, and chicken stock. Season well with salt and pepper. Remove from heat, spread in pan, and cool in the refrigerator.

Nutrition Facts per Serving: 270 calories, 8 g protein, 17 g fat (1.8 g saturated fat), 24 g carbohydrate, 8 g fiber, 0 g cholesterol, 250 mg sodium, 2.5 glycemic load

GRILLED MOROCCAN PORK TENDERLOIN KABOBS

Start to Finish: 45 minutes plus 1 to 2 hours for marinating Yield: 4 servings

2 tablespoons fresh flat-leaf parsley, chopped

2 tablespoons lemon juice

1 tablespoon extra-virgin olive oil

8 cloves garlic, minced (4 teaspoons)

1 tablespoon fresh oregano, chopped, or 1 teaspoon dried oregano, crushed

1½ teaspoons coriander seeds, ground, or 1 teaspoon ground coriander

1 teaspoon paprika

1 teaspoon fresh ginger, grated

½ teaspoon freshly ground black pepper

¼ teaspoon kosher salt

¼ teaspoon cayenne pepper or crushed red pepper

¼ teaspoon ground turmeric

1 pound pork tenderloin, cut into 1-inch cubes

2 cups seedless green grapes

skewers

1. For marinade, in a large bowl stir together parsley, lemon juice, oil, garlic, oregano, coriander seeds, paprika, ginger, black pepper, kosher salt, cayenne pepper, and turmeric until combined. Add pork cubes and grapes. Stir gently until pork and grapes are coated. Cover and marinate in the refrigerator for 1 to 2 hours.

2. On eight 12-inch skewers, alternately thread pork and grapes, leaving a ¼-inch space between pieces. For a charcoal grill, place kabobs on the rack of an uncovered grill directly over medium coals. Grill for 10 to 12 minutes or until pork is just slightly pink in center, turning occasionally to brown evenly. For a gas grill, preheat grill. Reduce heat to medium. Place kabobs on grill rack over heat. Cover and grill as above.

CULINARY NOTE

- If using wooden skewers, soak in enough water to cover for at least 1 hour before using.

- COOK 1X·EAT 2X in salads, frittatas, omelets, wraps, or sandwiches.

Nutrition Facts per Serving: **211** calories, **25** g protein, **7** g total fat (**2** g saturated fat), **12** g carbohydrate, **1** g fiber, **73** mg cholesterol, **170** mg sodium, **1** glycemic load

HERBED PORK TENDERLOIN

Start to Finish: 1 hour, plus 2 to 4 hours for marinating
Yield: 8 servings

2 12-ounce pork tenderloins	1 tablespoon extra-virgin olive oil
Kosher salt (optional)	1 tablespoon soy sauce
Freshly ground black pepper (optional)	2 3-inch sprigs fresh rosemary
2 tablespoons balsamic vinegar	2 3-inch sprigs fresh marjoram
2 tablespoons dry sherry	2 3-inch sprigs fresh thyme
1 tablespoon cracked black pepper	2 cloves garlic, minced (1 teaspoon)
	2 tablespoons extra-virgin olive oil

1. If desired, season meat with kosher salt and ground black pepper. Place meat in a large self-sealing plastic bag set in a shallow dish. Set aside.

2. For marinade, in a small bowl stir together vinegar, sherry, cracked black pepper, 1 tablespoon oil, soy sauce, rosemary, marjoram, thyme, and garlic. Pour over meat. Seal bag; turn to coat meat. Marinate in the refrigerator for 2 to 4 hours, turning bag occasionally.

3.   Preheat oven to 425°F.

4. Drain meat, reserving marinade. In a large skillet heat the 2 tablespoons oil. Brown meat quickly on all sides in hot oil (about 5 minutes).

5. Place meat in a shallow roasting pan. Pour marinade over meat. Insert an oven-safe meat thermometer into the thickest portion of one of the tenderloins. Roast, uncovered for 15 minutes. Spoon pan juices over meat. Roast for 10 to 15 minutes more or until thermometer registers 155°F. Cover roast with foil and let stand for 15 minutes.

6. The temperature of the meat after standing should be 160°F. Transfer meat to a serving platter, reserving pan juices. Strain juices and pour over meat.

Nutrition Facts per Serving: 159 calories, 18 g protein, 8 g total fat (2 g saturated fat), 2 g carbohydrate, 0 g fiber, 55 mg cholesterol, 155 mg sodium, 0 glycemic load

LATIN ROAST PORK TENDERLOIN
WITH PINTO BEANS & ZUCCHINI

Start to Finish: 1 hour   Yield: 4 servings

1 tablespoon extra-virgin olive oil

1 pound pork tenderloin in Latin Marinade (see recipe on page 339)

1 cup onions, chopped

1 tablespoon garlic, chopped

1½ teaspoon chile powder

1 14-ounce can tomatoes, chopped

1 14-ounce can pinto beans, drained, liquid reserved

1 cup chicken stock

2 cups zucchini, cut in quarters lengthwise, cut ¼-inch-wide pieces

4 cups baby spinach or braising greens

Salt and pepper to taste

1. Preheat oven to 400°F.

2. Heat a sauté pan over medium heat. Add one tablespoon extra-virgin olive oil and pork tenderloin. Cook until lightly browned. Turn tenderloin over and move to the side of the pan. Add onions to the side of the pan where the pork had browned. Add 1 tablespoon of the bean liquid. Add garlic and chile powder; stir. Let pork continue to brown. Once brown, remove pork from pan. Add tomatoes and pinto beans; stir to coat. Place pork on top of beans and place in hot oven. Roast for 15–20 minutes or until the pork is 143°F (turn at 8 minutes).

3. Remove pork from pan and let rest in a warm spot. Add zucchini and chicken stock. Bring to a boil. Stir in the spinach. Adjust seasoning with salt and pepper. Slice pork ¼ inch thick on bias.

4. To serve: Place 1½ cup of beans mixture on a plate. Top with 4 ounces of sliced pork on top.

Nutrition Facts per Serving: 320 calories, 31 g protein, 10 g total fat (2 g saturated fat), 31 g carbohydrate, 8.5 g fiber, 65 mg cholesterol, 650 mg sodium, 4 glycemic load

Latin Marinade
FOR ROAST PORK TENDERLOIN

Start to Finish: 20 minutes   Yield: 4 servings

1   pound pork tenderloin, fat trimmed

1½ teaspoon garlic, mashed to a paste

1   tablespoon extra-virgin olive oil

1½ teaspoon chile powder

½   teaspoon ground cumin

1   teaspoon paprika

1   pinch cinnamon

1   teaspoon oregano, chopped

1   teaspoon red wine vinegar

Salt and pepper to taste

1. Season pork with salt and pepper.

2. Mash garlic to a paste with a pinch of salt. Add remaining ingredients and stir to mix. Spread all over pork tenderloin. Let sit for 15 minutes to overnight.

CULINARY NOTE

This is a good option for several COOK 1X · EAT 2X recipes.

OVEN-FRIED PORK CUTLETS

Start to Finish: 1 hour
Yield: 4 servings

4   pork loins, fat and sinew
     removed, cut ½ inch thick,
     4 ounce pieces
1   egg white
¼   cup buttermilk
1   tablespoon Dijon mustard
1   teaspoon Spanish paprika

½–1 teaspoon hot sauce
1   cup whole-wheat
     bread crumbs
⅓   cup parmesan cheese
1   teaspoon chili powder
¼   teaspoon garlic powder
Salt and pepper to taste
Nonstick cooking spray

1. Preheat oven to 450°F.

2. Season the pork with salt and pepper. Let sit while you prepare the egg white.

3. Whisk the egg white and a pinch of salt until foamy; stir in buttermilk, mustard, paprika, and hot sauce. Add seasoned pork and let marinate for at least 15 minutes.

4. Combine the bread crumbs, parmesan cheese, chili powder, garlic powder, and salt and pepper in a shallow pan. Dip the pork into the bread crumb mixture one piece at a time, being sure to coat the entire piece.

5. Place the pork on an elevated rack on a sheet pan. Spray generously on both sides with cooking spray. Place on the top shelf of the oven and bake for 5 minutes. Turn the pork and continue to cook for 5 minutes on the other side.

6. Turn the oven to broil and cook for 1 minute on each side until browned and the juices run clear. The internal temperature of the pork should be 143°F.

7. Serve immediately.

Nutrition Facts per Serving: 250 calories, 30 g protein, 6 g fat (2.3 g saturated fat), 18 g carbohydrate, 2 g fiber, 60 mg cholesterol, 600 mg sodium, 8 glycemic load

Pan Pork Chops
WITH DRIED CHERRY & BALSAMIC VINEGAR SAUCE

Start to Finish: 45 minutes   Yield: 4 servings

From Chef Dave Bush at St. Francis Winery & Vineyards
Suggested Wine Pairing: 2007 Zinfandel, Wild Oak, Sonoma County

4 pork chops
2 tablespoons extra-virgin
   olive oil
½ cup chicken broth
½ cup tart dried cherries

¾ cup balsamic vinegar
1 tablespoon honey
2 tablespoons unsalted butter
Salt and black pepper to taste

1. Preheat oven to 375°F.

2. Season both sides of the pork chops with salt and black pepper. Preheat a heavy-bottomed sauté pan over medium-high heat. Add olive oil to the preheated sauté pan. Place the pork chops in the hot olive oil and sear both sides until dark and caramelized. Place the pan with the chops in the preheated oven. Cook the chops for 10–12 minutes for medium or until desired doneness. Remove the pan from the oven and place the chops on a serving platter to rest.

3. Return the sauté pan to the stove over medium-high heat. Add the chicken broth and dried cherries to the pan and reduce by half. Add the balsamic vinegar and the honey to the reduced chicken broth and reduce by half again. Finish the sauce by adding the butter while the sauce is boiling, whisking until the butter is fully incorporated.

4. Spoon the sauce and cherries over the chops and serve immediately.

St. Francis Winery & Vineyards, located in the heart of Sonoma Valley, produces big, bold, full-bodied wines that deliver on flavor. Each wine is produced from 100% hand-picked Sonoma County fruit and is a direct expression of the winemaking philosophy of "maximum extraction, minimal intervention."

Nutrition Facts per Serving: 330 calories, 16 g protein, 19 g fat (7 g saturated fat), 22 g carbohydrate, 1 g fiber, 68 mg cholesterol, 100 mg sodium

ROAST PORK TENDERLOIN
WITH GRILLED PEACH SALSA

Start to Finish: 40 minutes   Yield: 4 servings

1   teaspoon Spanish paprika, smoked or plain
½   teaspoon ground coriander
1   teaspoon lemon zest
1½ tablespoons sherry vinegar
½   teaspoon garlic, chopped
1   tablespoon olive oil
1   pound pork tenderloin, fat removed
2   peaches, cut in half, pits removed

1   pinch sugar
2   scallions, chopped
¼   teaspoon fresh ginger, grated or chopped
1   cup cherry tomatoes cut in half, or chopped tomatoes
1   teaspoon fresh mint
1   tablespoon extra-virgin olive oil
Salt and pepper to taste

1. Combine paprika, coriander, lemon zest, ½ tablespoon sherry vinegar, garlic, and 1 tablespoon olive oil. Mix well. Season pork with salt and pepper. Coat with spice mixture.

2. Season peaches with salt, pepper, and 1 pinch of sugar. Place peaches on a hot grill. Cook until charred, but not cooked through. Remove skin, and chop into ¼-inch pieces. Gently combine with scallions, ginger, cherry tomatoes, mint, 1 tablespoon sherry vinegar, and 1 tablespoon extra-virgin olive oil.

3. Grill or roast pork until internal temperature reaches 140°F, about 20 minutes. Let rest for 10 minutes. Slice on a bias, ¼ inch thick.

4. Serve grilled pork with the peach salsa.

CULINARY NOTE

COOK 1X· EAT 2X

in salads, frittatas, omelets, wraps, or sandwiches.

Nutrition Facts per Serving: 239 calories, 23 g protein, 12 g fat (3 g saturated fat), 8 g carbohydrate, 2 g fiber, 71 mg cholesterol, 60 mg sodium

ALMOND-CRUSTED SALMON

Start to Finish: 20 minutes
Yield: 4 servings

1 pound salmon fillet, skinned, cut in 4-ounce portions

2 tablespoons whole-wheat bread crumbs

2 teaspoons extra-virgin olive oil

2 tablespoons almonds, lightly toasted, coarsely chopped

2 teaspoons parsley, chopped

1 teaspoon thyme, chopped

Salt and pepper to taste

1 tablespoon olive oil or canola oil

1. Season salmon with salt and pepper. Set aside.

2. Combine the bread crumbs and extra-virgin olive oil. Mix just to coat. Add chopped almonds and herbs. Season with salt and pepper. Spread on a plate.

3. Gently press each portion of seasoned salmon into almond mixture to coat one side. Place crumb side up on a plate.

4. Heat a Teflon pan over medium heat. Add oil; then place the fish, crumb side down, in the pan. Cook about 2 minutes or until the crumbs are golden brown. Carefully turn the fish and cook 2–4 more minutes until the fish is just cooked through. Remove from the pan.

CULINARY NOTE

- If the bread crumbs are browning too quickly on the salmon, turn down the heat and cook for a longer time on the second side. You can also brown the fish on both sides, then finish it on a pan in a 350°F oven.

- COOK 1X· EAT 2X in salads, frittatas, omelets, wraps, or sandwiches.

Variation:

- Replace salmon with halibut, snapper, or black bass.

Nutrition Facts per Serving: 289 calories, 24 g protein, 20 g fat (4.5 g saturated fat), 3 g carbohydrate, 1 g fiber, 55 mg cholesterol, 81 mg sodium, 2.5 mg omega-3, 1.5 glycemic load

HALIBUT & SUMMER VEGETABLES EN PAPILLOTE

Start to Finish: 45 minutes   Yield: 4 servings

4 4- to 5-ounce fresh or frozen halibut steaks

2 tablespoons extra-virgin olive oil

2 cloves garlic, thinly sliced

Parchment paper

2 medium tomatoes, sliced ¼ inch thick

1 medium fennel bulb, cored and sliced

Kosher salt

Freshly ground black pepper

12 ounces zucchini, bias-sliced ¼ inch thick

12 ounces yellow summer squash, bias-sliced ¼ inch thick

¼ cup pitted kalamata olives, quartered

2 teaspoons finely shredded lemon peel

3 tablespoons lemon juice

2 tablespoons thinly sliced fresh basil or 2 teaspoons dried basil, crushed

1. Preheat oven to 400°F.

2. Thaw halibut, if frozen. Rinse halibut; pat dry with paper towels. In a small saucepan, heat oil over low heat. Add garlic; cook for 5 minutes, watching carefully so garlic does not brown. Set aside.

3. Tear four 20-inch by 12-inch pieces of parchment paper; fold each in half crosswise and crease. Open up again. On half of one parchment sheet, arrange one-fourth each of the tomato and fennel slices; sprinkle lightly with kosher salt and pepper. Drizzle with some of the oil and garlic mixture. Top with one-fourth of the zucchini and yellow squash; sprinkle again with kosher salt and pepper. Top with one-fourth of the olives and one piece of halibut. Sprinkle again with kosher salt and pepper; sprinkle with some of the lemon peel, lemon juice, and basil. To make packet, fold paper over fish and vegetables. Crimp and fold edges to seal; twist corners. Repeat to make 4 packets.

4. Place packets in a shallow baking pan. Bake about 15 minutes or until fish flakes easily when tested with a fork. (To test, carefully open the packets and peek.) Serve immediately.

En Papillote Variations:

Substitute shrimp or chicken for fish.

CHARMOULA-MARINATED FISH

Omit the lemon juice, lemon peel, and basil. Marinate the fish in
Charmoula Marinade (see page 176) for 15 minutes. Sprinkle each layer
of vegetables with 1 teaspoon excess marinade. Place fish on top. Top
with 1 teaspoon capers. Crimp and fold packets.

MEDITERRANEAN-MARINATED FISH

Omit the lemon juice, lemon peel, and basil. Marinate the fish in
Mediterranean Herb Marinade (see page 178). Place on top of vegetables.
Pour 1 tablespoon excess marinade on top of vegetables. Crimp and
fold packets.

TILAPIA WITH SALSA

Omit the lemon juice, lemon peel, fennel, olives, and basil. Marinate fish
in Simple Spicy Lime Cilantro Vinaigrette (see page 201). Combine
1 cup corn kernels, ¼ cup diced roasted red peppers, and 1 tablespoon
chopped scallions. Season with salt and pepper. Set aside. Sprinkle
the tomatoes with vinaigrette, salt, and pepper. Sprinkle zucchini and
summer squash with vinaigrette, salt, and pepper. Place fish on top of
squashes and top with corn and pepper mixture. Sprinkle with
1 teaspoon vinaigrette. Crimp and fold packets.

Nutrition Facts per Serving: **249** calories, **27** g protein, **11** g total fat (**1** g saturated fat),
13 g carbohydrate, **4** g fiber, **36** mg cholesterol, **648** mg sodium, **2** glycemic load

MEDITERRANEAN TUNA & CAPER SALAD

Start to Finish: 25 minutes   Yield: 4 servings

2   Roma tomatoes, chopped

2   tablespoons capers, drained

2   tablespoons extra-virgin olive oil

2   tablespoons balsamic vinegar

⅛   teaspoon dried oregano, crushed, or ½ teaspoon fresh oregano, chopped

⅛   teaspoon kosher salt

Dash freshly ground black pepper

6   cups packaged European-style torn mixed salad greens

2   6-ounce cans chunk white tuna (in water), drained and broken into chunks

1   cup canned garbanzo beans (chickpeas), rinsed and drained

1   cup fresh green beans, blanched

¼   cup pitted kalamata olives, quartered

4   teaspoons extra-virgin olive oil

4   teaspoons balsamic vinegar

1. In a small bowl combine tomatoes, capers, 2 tablespoons oil, 2 tablespoons balsamic vinegar, oregano, kosher salt, and pepper; set aside.

> **CULINARY NOTES**
>
> • Do not mix too early or the green beans will discolor.
>
> • Use leftover cooked Sicilian Tuna Steak (page 348) as a COOK 1X · EAT 2X ingredient.

2. On four serving plates, arrange torn salad greens, tuna chunks, garbanzo beans, green beans, olives, and tomato mixture. Drizzle 4 teaspoons oil and 4 teaspoons balsamic vinegar evenly over salads.

Variations:

• Use red wine vinegar in place of balsamic vinegar.

• Add 1 cup artichoke cut in quarters

Nutrition Facts per Serving: 324 calories, 25 g protein, 16 g total fat (2 g saturated fat), 21 g carbohydrate, 5 g fiber, 36 mg cholesterol, 775 mg sodium, 5 glycemic load

MEDITERRANEAN WHITE WINE POACHED FISH

Start to Finish: 30 minutes   Yield: 4 servings

For Mediterranean poaching broth:
1 pinch saffron
1 cup white wine
1 teaspoon extra-virgin olive oil
1 cup onions, sliced thin
1 tablespoon garlic, chopped
1 cup fennel, sliced thin

1 teaspoon fennel seeds
1 pinch chile flakes
1 15-ounce can tomatoes, chopped
1 bay leaf
1 tablespoon orange zest
2 cups fish or chicken stock
Salt and pepper to taste
1 pound fish

1. Combine saffron and white wine.

2. Heat oil in a sauce pot over medium heat. Add onions, garlic, fennel, fennel seeds, and chile flakes. Sweat until translucent. Add white wine; reduce by half. Add tomatoes, bay leaf, and orange zest; cook 2 minutes. Add stock; bring to a simmer. Cook for 15 minutes or until the flavors meld. Use to poach fish or chicken.

CULINARY NOTES

- Make this broth ahead without the herbs. It will freeze well.
- COOK 1X· EAT 2X in salads, frittatas, omelets, wraps, or sandwiches.

3. Add fish in a single layer. Cover and simmer for 5 to 6 minutes or until fish flakes easily when tested with a fork. Using a slotted spatula, carefully transfer fish to a platter. Serve with sauce and vegetables.

Variation:

- Add 1 can white cannellini beans, drained, and 2 cups spinach to the poaching liquid.

Nutrition Facts per Serving: 150 calories, 7 g protein, 3 g fat (.5 g saturated fat), 25 g carbohydrate, 5 g fiber, 0 mg cholesterol, 300 mg sodium, 8 glycemic load

SICILIAN TUNA STEAK

Start to Finish: 45 minutes
Yield: 4 servings

1 pound fresh or frozen tuna steaks, 1 inch thick

1 small onion, chopped

2 cloves garlic, minced (1 teaspoon)

1 tablespoon extra-virgin olive oil

2 pounds Roma tomatoes, seeded and chopped, or one 28-ounce can diced tomatoes, drained

½ cup dry white wine

¼ to ½ teaspoon crushed red pepper

¼ cup pitted ripe olives

2 tablespoons capers, rinsed and drained

2 tablespoons fresh basil, chopped, or 2 teaspoons dried basil, crushed

1 tablespoon fresh mint, chopped, or 1 teaspoon dried mint, crushed

¼ teaspoon kosher salt

⅛ teaspoon freshly ground black pepper

1 tablespoon lemon juice

> **CULINARY NOTE**
>
> Make leftover tuna steak a COOK 1X · EAT 2X ingredient for Mediterranean Tuna and Caper Salad (page 346).

1. Thaw tuna, if frozen. Cut tuna into four portions, if necessary. Rinse tuna; pat dry with paper towels. Set aside.

2. In a large skillet cook onion and garlic in hot oil over medium heat until onion is tender. Add tomatoes, wine, and crushed red pepper. Bring to boiling; reduce heat. Simmer, uncovered, for 7 minutes. Add olives and capers. If using dried basil and mint, add them here.

3. Sprinkle tuna with kosher salt and black pepper. Add tuna to skillet on top of tomato mixture. Cover and cook over medium heat for 5 minutes. Uncover and cook for 10 to 15 minutes more or until tuna flakes easily when tested with a fork and is slightly pink in the center.

4. Transfer tuna pieces to four serving plates. Spoon tomato mixture over tuna. If using fresh basil and mint, sprinkle them on top. Drizzle with lemon juice.

Nutrition Facts per Serving: 233 calories, 29 g protein, 6 g total fat (1 g saturated fat), 12 g carbohydrate, 3 g fiber, 51 mg cholesterol, 377 mg sodium, 6 glycemic load

VERACRUZ-STYLE FISH

Start to Finish: 35 minutes
Yield: 4 servings

1 pound boneless, skinless salmon, halibut, or snapper

1 tablespoon extra-virgin olive oil

1 cup onion, thinly sliced

1 tablespoon garlic, minced

1 4-ounce can roasted green chile strips, drained

1 28-ounce can tomatoes, chopped, drained

1 tablespoon oregano, chopped

3 tablespoons capers, rinsed

¼ cup golden raisins

3 tablespoons green olives, pitted, sliced

¾ cup vegetable or fish stock

Salt and pepper to taste

1. Season fish with salt and pepper. Set aside.

2. Heat a large sauté pan over high heat. Add olive oil and swirl to coat pan; then immediately add the fish. Sear until golden brown; flip to sear on the other side. Remove fish from pan and place on a rack over a plate to catch juices. The fish should be raw to rare.

3. Return the pan to the heat. Add onions; cook over high heat for 2 to 3 minutes, stirring periodically. Add garlic, chiles, and tomatoes; sauté for 2 minutes. Add oregano, capers, raisins, olives, and stock. Bring to a simmer. Simmer for 4 minutes or until the flavors meld and the raisins plump.

4. Return the fish and any accumulated juices to the pan, and bury in the sauce. Cover and cook over low heat for 3–4 minutes or until the fish is cooked through. Taste broth and adjust seasoning.

5. Spoon a portion of the sauce into a soup plate or pasta bowl. Top with a piece of fish and a little more sauce.

> **CULINARY NOTE**
>
> COOK 1X·EAT 2X in salads, frittatas, omelets, wraps, or sandwiches.

Nutrition Facts per Serving: 350 calories, 33 g protein, 14 g fat (2 g saturated fat), 23 g carbohydrate, 4 g fiber, 80 mg cholesterol, 800 mg sodium, 8 glycemic load

ALMOND CHERRY BISCOTTI

Start to Finish: 1 hour 15 minutes
Yield: 3 dozen cookies (2 cookies per serving)

¾ cup unbleached
   all-purpose flour

½ cup whole-wheat
   pastry flour

½ cup sugar

1 teaspoon baking powder

¼ teaspoon salt

½ cup almonds, slivered,
   toasted

½ cup dried cherries

1 egg

1 egg white

½ teaspoon lemon zest or
   orange zest

½ teaspoon vanilla

1 tablespoon yogurt

1. Preheat oven to 325°F. Line sheet pan with parchment paper.

2. Combine the flours, sugar, baking powder, and salt in a bowl. Add the nuts and dried fruit.

3. In a separate bowl, whisk together the egg, egg white, zest, vanilla, and yogurt. Slowly add the egg mixture to the flour mixture; mix until well blended into a sticky, moist dough, 1–2 minutes.

4. To shape: Slightly wet your hands, and place the dough onto the prepared baking sheet. Shape the dough into two 2¼-inch by 10-inch rectangles, wetting your hands as needed. Press and shape the dough as evenly as possible.

5. Bake for 25 minutes or until the dough is golden brown on top and slightly dark around the edges. Cool for 15 minutes.

> **CULINARY NOTE**
>
> Do not mix the eggs and yogurt until just adding to the dry ingredients or the eggs will curdle from the acid in the yogurt.

6. Transfer the biscotti to a cutting board, removing it from the parchment with a large metal spatula if necessary. Using a serrated knife, cut the biscotti crosswise into 1/3-inch-thick slices. Return the slices to the baking sheet, arranging them cut side down.

7. Bake until the biscotti are light golden brown and feel dry, 12–14 minutes. Transfer to a rack to cool.

8. They will crisp up as they dry. Store in an airtight container.

Variations:

- Replace almonds with other nuts such as pine nuts, walnuts, or pistachios.
- Replace cherries with other dried fruits such as cranberries, apricots, pears, or apples.

Nutrition Facts per Serving: **80** calories, **2** g protein, **7.5** g fat (**.1** g saturated fat), **14** g carbohydrate, **1** g fiber, **8** mg cholesterol, **58** mg sodium, **4** glycemic load

SPICED GINGER COOKIES

Start to Finish: 30 minutes, plus 3 hours to chill
Yield: 4 dozen cookies (2 cookies per serving)

¾ cup whole-wheat
   pastry flour
1 cup unbleached
   all-purpose flour
1 tablespoon bran
1½ teaspoons ground ginger
1 teaspoon ground cinnamon
¼ teaspoon ground nutmeg
½ teaspoon baking soda
¼ teaspoon salt

¼ teaspoon freshly ground
   black pepper
¼ cup unsalted butter,
   completely softened at
   room temperature
⅓ cup packed
   dark brown sugar
1¼ cup nonfat yogurt
1 large egg yolk
3 tablespoons molasses

1. Combine the flours, bran, ginger, cinnamon, nutmeg, baking soda, salt, and pepper in a medium bowl.

2. In a stand mixer bowl or using a hand mixer, beat the butter and brown sugar on medium speed until light and fluffy, about 3 minutes. Add the yogurt, egg yolk, and molasses and mix until well blended, about 1 minute.

3. Add the flour mixture to the butter mixture and mix on medium-low speed until the dough is well blended.

CULINARY NOTES

- This dough needs to chill for a few hours so it will slice thinly and bake evenly. If not given time to chill, the dough may be too sticky to handle and will spread when baking.

- The ginger flavor intensifies over time. These cookies will hold well in an airtight container. The dough also freezes well.

4. Place the dough onto an unfloured work surface; gently knead until it comes together. Shape into two 9-inch-long logs about 1 inch in diameter. Wrap in plastic. Refrigerate until firm, about 3 hours.

5. Preheat the oven to 350°F. Line two large sheet pans with parchment or nonstick baking liners.

6. Unwrap the dough and use a thin, sharp knife to cut the logs into ¼-inch slices. Arrange the slices about 1 inch apart on the prepared sheet pans. Bake one sheet at a time until the cookies are slightly brown on the bottoms and around the edges, 8 to 10 minutes. Place sheet pan on a rack to cool for 10 minutes. Transfer the cookies to a rack and let cool completely. When cool, store in airtight containers.

Nutrition Facts per Serving: **80** calories, **1.5** g protein, **2.5** g fat (**1.2** g saturated fat), **12** g carbohydrate, **6** g fiber, **14** mg cholesterol, **60** mg sodium, **4** glycemic load

CHERRY ALMOND CLAFOUTIS

Start to Finish: 1 hour 20 minutes
Yield: 12 servings

Nonstick cooking spray as needed

1 tablespoon flour

3 cups small fresh cherries (about 1 pound), pitted

½ cup sliced almonds, toasted

3 large eggs

½ cup sugar

3 tablespoons whole-wheat all-purpose flour

¾ cup low-fat milk

½ teaspoon vanilla

1 pinch salt

1. Preheat oven to 375°F.

2. Spray a 9-inch cast-iron skillet or gratin dish. Sprinkle with ½–1 tablespoon flour just to coat. Turn pan upside down and pat out excess flour.

3. Sprinkle cherries and half the almonds over the bottom of the pan.

4. Combine remaining ingredients in a mixing bowl, and using a hand mixer or stand mixer, whisk for 5 minutes, or until slightly aerated. Pour over cherries and almonds.

5. Bake for 20 minutes; sprinkle with remaining almonds. Bake 20–25 minutes more until puffed and golden-brown and a toothpick inserted in the center comes out clean.

6. Transfer to a rack and let cool for 30 minutes. Serve warm or at room temperature, spooned onto individual serving plates.

Variations:

- Replace cherries with blueberries, peaches, or other fruits, but do not use high-acid fruits such as citrus or pineapple.
- Replace almonds with hazelnuts, pistachios, or walnuts.

Nutrition Facts per Serving: 112 calories, 3.5 g protein, 3 g fat (.5 g saturated fat), 18 g carbohydrate, 1 g fiber, 50 mg cholesterol, 60 mg sodium, 8 glycemic load

FLOURLESS CHOCOLATE CAKE

Start to Finish: 1 hour
Yield: 12 servings

4 ounces good-quality bittersweet chocolate (72% cacao), in small pieces	¼ teaspoon salt
¼ cup butter	½ teaspoon vanilla
¼ cup nonfat yogurt	1¼ cups finely chopped almonds
3 eggs	1 tablespoon powdered sugar
⅓ cup white sugar	3 cups fresh raspberries, blueberries, or strawberries

1. Preheat oven to 325°F. Spray a 9-inch round cake pan with nonstick cooking spray. Line the bottom of the pan with parchment paper and spray again on top of the parchment paper. Place chocolate and butter in a bowl. Place over a pot of barely simmering water. Gently heat until the chocolate is melted. Whisk in yogurt and set aside.

2. In a large mixing bowl, beat eggs and sugar with an electric mixer until thick and fluffy, about 4 minutes on high speed. Stir in salt and vanilla. Add nuts; then gently fold in chocolate. Do not overmix. Pour into prepared pan. Bake 30–35 minutes or until a toothpick inserted in the center of the cake comes out clean. Dust with powdered sugar and serve with ¼ cup of fresh seasonal fruit.

CULINARY NOTES

- Do not melt the chocolate over boiling water or the chocolate may scorch. Gentle heat is best, and stir periodically.

- Whip the eggs and sugar until light in color and full of air. This leavens the cake and gives it a light texture.

Variations:

- Replace almonds with ground pistachios.
- Replace almonds with ground hazelnuts.

Nutrition Facts per Serving: **207** calories, **5** g protein, **14** g fat (**5** g saturated fat), **17** g carbohydrate, **4** g fiber, **63** mg cholesterol, **97** mg sodium, **5.8** glycemic load

CREAMY LIME RICOTTA TART

Start to Finish: 45 minutes, 2–3 hours to chill
Yield: 1 9-inch tart (12 servings)

15 ounce container low-fat ricotta cheese (about 1½ cups)

3 ounces low-fat cream cheese, at room temperature

⅓ cup sugar

2 tablespoons whole-wheat all-purpose flour

¼ teaspoon salt

3 large egg yolks

1 tablespoon finely grated lime zest

1 tablespoon lime juice

1 9-inch Graham Cracker Tart Crust (page 360)

¾ cup fresh raspberries

Strips of lime zest, for garnish (optional)

1. Preheat oven to 350°F.

2. Place ricotta and cream cheese in a large bowl. Using an electric mixer, beat on medium speed until well blended and no lumps remain, about 2 minutes. Add the sugar, flour, and salt and continue beating until well blended, about 1 minute. Stir in the egg yolks, lime zest, and lime juice. Use a rubber spatula to scrape the filling into the crust and spread evenly.

3. Bake the tart until the filling just barely jiggles when the pan is nudged, 25 to 30 minutes. Let cool completely on a rack. Refrigerate the tart in the pan until chilled and firm, 2 to 3 hours. Place fresh raspberries around the edge of the tart. Garnish with strips of lime zest.

Variation:

• Replace lime zest and lime juice with lemon.

CULINARY NOTE

Make sure the cream cheese is soft and at room temperature. It will be easier to mix. Cold cream cheese is more likely to create lumps, causing you to overwhip the cheese mixture.

Nutrition Facts per Serving: **190** calories, **6** g protein, **9** g fat (**3** g saturated fat,) **23** g carbohydrate, **1** g fiber, **67** mg cholesterol, **280** mg sodium, **12.5** glycemic load

Nectarine Blueberry Galette

*Start to Finish: 1½ hours, assuming pie dough
is chilled and ready to roll   Yield: 12 servings*

3 cups nectarines, washed, seed removed, cut into ¼-inch wedges

1 cup blueberries

4 tablespoons applesauce

2 tablespoons brown sugar

1 teaspoon lemon zest

½ teaspoon vanilla (optional)

1 tablespoon cornstarch

1 pinch salt

dough for 11-inch Whole-Wheat Pie Crust (page 361)

1 tablespoon graham cracker crumbs

1 tablespoon sliced almonds, lightly toasted

1 tablespoon agave syrup

Parchment paper

Nonstick cooking spray

1. Preheat oven to 425°F.

2. Combine nectarines, blueberries, applesauce, sugar, lemon zest, vanilla, cornstarch, and salt in a bowl.

3. Lightly spray 2 ½-sheets of parchment paper (12–14-inch) with cooking spray. Place pie dough between the 2 sheets of parchment and roll pie crust ⅛ inch thick. To prevent sticking, periodically peel the parchment papers from the dough and then replace dough between them. Once the dough is the desired thickness, remove top sheet, keeping the pie crust on the bottom sheet of parchment paper. Place on a sheet pan.

4. Sprinkle graham cracker crumbs in a 10-inch circle on the pie crust. Scoop the fruit mixture into the center of the pie crust, leaving a 1-inch rim around the outside. Be sure to capture all the juice. Using the parchment paper, gently fold the 1-inch rim over the edge of the fruit all around the galette. Sprinkle the sliced almonds on top.

Nutrition Facts per Serving: **185** calories, **2.5** g protein, **8** g fat (**2** g saturated fat), **26** g carbohydrate, **2.5** g fiber, **5** mg cholesterol, **120** mg sodium

5. Bake galette on the bottom rack of the oven for 50 minutes, turning halfway through the cooking time. The fruit juices should bubble and thicken; the crust should start to brown lightly.

6. Remove from oven, brush edge of tart with agave syrup, and let cool for 20 minutes.

CULINARY NOTE

The pie crust is a delicate dough. Rolling the piecrust between the two pieces of parchment paper makes it easier to transfer to the baking sheet and also prevents the dough from sticking to the rolling pin.

Variations:

- Replace fruit with any seasonal fruits: strawberries and rhubarb, raspberries, apricots, plums, or peaches. Apples and pears may be used in the winter but will need to be peeled and sliced ⅛ inch thick.

- The galette can also be made with gluten-free Pie Dough (page 359).

Nutrition Facts per Serving (made with gluten-free Pie Dough): 250 calories, 3 g protein, 9 g fat (3 g saturated fat), 44 g carbohydrate, 4 g fiber, 60 mg cholesterol, 160 mg sodium, 10.5 glycemic load

PIE DOUGH

Start to Finish: 10 minutes, plus 60 minutes to chill
Yield: 1 15-inch piecrust circle, 8 servings

½ cup brown rice flour
½ cup white rice flour (Asian, nonglutinous)
½ cup tapioca starch
¼ cup potato starch
1 pinch salt
1 teaspoon sugar
2 teaspoons xanthan gum

2 tablespoons cold butter, cut in ¼-inch pieces
2 tablespoons canola or safflower oil, cold
1 egg
1 teaspoon white vinegar
3 tablespoons cold water
Parchment paper
Nonstick cooking spray

1. Combine the rice flours, starches, salt, sugar, and xanthan gum. Cut in the cold butter with a pastry cutter or fork until it is the size of chocolate chips, not too small.

2. Combine oil, egg, vinegar, and water; add to flour mixture. Mix enough to bring the dough together. Knead 1 minute. Gather dough into a ball and form a flat disk. Wrap in plastic wrap and chill in refrigerator for 30 minutes or overnight.

CULINARY NOTE

Do not overwork the dough or the crust will be tough. Add only enough water so the dough comes together. It should barely hold together and not be wet.

3. To roll: Lightly spray 2 half-sheets of parchment paper (12 inches by 14 inches) with cooking spray. Place pie dough between the 2 sheets of parchment and roll pie crust ⅛ inch thick. To prevent sticking, periodically peel the parchment papers from the dough and then replace dough between them. Once the dough is the desired thickness, remove top sheet, keeping the pie crust on the bottom sheet of parchment paper. Place on a sheet pan for a galette, or flip dough over into a pie pan and peel off the parchment. Gently press into the pie pan. Chill for 30 minutes prior to baking.

Nutrition Facts per Serving: 180 calories, 2 g protein, 6 g fat (1.5 g saturated fat), 28 g carbohydrate, 1.5 g fiber, 35 mg cholesterol, 100 mg sodium, 15 glycemic load

GRAHAM CRACKER TART CRUST

Start to Finish: 20 minutes
Yield: 1 9-inch tart shell (12 servings)

¾ cup graham cracker crumbs
¼ cup almonds, finely ground
1 tablespoon oat bran
2 teaspoons sugar

1 tablespoon butter, soft or melted
1 tablespoon nonfat yogurt
1 pinch salt
Nonstick cooking spray

1. Preheat oven to 350°F.

2. Combine all ingredients in a bowl. Mix well.

3. Spray a 9-inch tart shell with a removable bottom with cooking spray. Pour crust mixture into the tart shell. Place a piece of plastic wrap on top and firmly press the crust into a thin, even layer on the bottom and sides of the tart shell.

4. Bake for 10 minutes or until just slightly toasted.

CULINARY NOTES

- Using the plastic wrap, press crust evenly into the tart shell, making sure to press into the corners. If the shell is not firmly pressed into the pan, it is likely to crumble once removed from the pan.

- To remove the tart from the pan, gently push the bottom of the tart shell from the mold. Use 1 or 2 large offset spatulas to slide the tart onto a flat plate.

Nutrition Facts per Serving: 45 calories, 2 g protein, 2.5 g fat (.75 g saturated fat), 5.5 g carbohydrate, .5 g fiber, 2.5 mg cholesterol, 39.5 mg sodium, 2 glycemic load

WHOLE-WHEAT PIE DOUGH OR GALETTE CRUST

Start to Finish: 10 minutes, plus 30 minutes to chill   Yield: 1 pie crust*

½ cup whole-wheat pastry flour	2 tablespoons cold butter, cut in ¼-inch pieces
½ cup unbleached all-purpose flour	2 tablespoons canola or safflower oil, cold
1 teaspoon sugar	½ teaspoon white vinegar
¼ teaspoon baking powder	2–4 tablespoons cold water
2 tablespoons oat bran or wheat bran	Parchment paper
1 pinch salt	Nonstick cooking spray

1. Mix the flours, sugar, baking powder, oat bran, and salt in a large bowl. Cut in the cold butter with a pastry cutter or fork until it is the size of mini chocolate chips.

2. Stir in oil and vinegar. Add just enough cold water to bring the dough together. It should still be a little dry.

3. Gather dough into a ball and form a flat disk. Wrap in plastic wrap and chill in refrigerator for 30 minutes or overnight.

4. To roll: Lightly spray 2 half-sheets of parchment paper (12–14 inches) with cooking spray. Place pie dough between the 2 sheets of parchment and roll ⅛ inch thick. To prevent sticking, periodically peel the parchment papers from the dough and then replace dough between them. Once the dough is the desired thickness, remove top sheet of parchment paper, keeping the pie crust on the bottom sheet. Place on a sheet pan for a galette, or flip the dough over into a pie pan and peel off the parchment; gently press into the pie pan. Chill for 30 minutes before baking.

CULINARY NOTES

- Do not overwork the dough or the crust will be tough. After you add the water, the dough should barely hold together and not be wet.

* (serves 12)

Nutrition Facts per Serving: **60** calories, **1** g protein, **4.5** g fat (**1.2** g saturated fat), **8** g carbohydrate, **1** g fiber, **5** mg cholesterol, **60** mg sodium, **1** glycemic load

CONCORD GRAPE & LIME SORBET

Start to Finish: 4 hours to overnight   Yield: 4 servings

4   cups concord grapes
1   pinch salt
¼   cup water

⅔   cup agave syrup
1½ tablespoons lime juice
1   teaspoon lime zest

1. Set up a large ice bath.

2. Place grapes, salt, and water in a saucepan over medium heat. Cook 4–5 minutes until the grapes start to burst and release their juice. Reduce heat to low and simmer for 4 minutes or until the grapes break apart and the juice is dark purple; gently stir and mash the grapes as they cook. Pass the mixture through a food mill, then through a mesh strainer, using the back of a ladle to push the juice through. Place over an ice bath to cool.

3. Once the mixture is cool, stir in agave syrup, lime juice, and zest.

4. Place in refrigerator and chill. Process in an ice cream machine according to manufacturer's directions.

Variations:

- Add 1 tablespoon fresh herbs such as mint, lemon verbena, or thyme.

CULINARY NOTES

- An ice bath is a bowl of ice with just enough water to come to the top of the ice. The bowl should be large enough so if you place something in the ice water, the water will not spill over the sides.

- If you do not have an ice cream machine, freeze sorbet mixture in ice cube trays until solid. Unmold cubes and place in a food processor with a chopping blade. Process in batches until fairly smooth, but still icy. Scrape down sides periodically while processing and store batches in freezer.

- Chill the serving bowls or dishes that you use.

Nutrition Facts per Serving: 200 calories, 6 g protein, 3 g fat (0 g saturated fat), 55 g carbohydrate, 9 g fiber, 0 mg cholesterol, 85 mg sodium, 3 glycemic load

GRAPEFRUIT MINT SORBET

Start to Finish: 1 hour
Yield: 4 servings

3 cups fresh grapefruit juice,
    no seeds

⅓ cup agave syrup

⅓ cup sugar

1 pinch salt

½ cup mint leaves

1 tablespoon lime
    or lemon juice

1. Place grapefruit juice, agave syrup, sugar, and salt in a blender. Blend until smooth and sugar has dissolved.

2. Bruise mint leaves and add to grapefruit mixture. Add the lemon or lime juice. Let blender container sit for 30 minutes in refrigerator.

3. Process in ice cream machine according to manufacturer's directions.

CULINARY NOTES

- If you do not have an ice cream machine, freeze sorbet mixture in ice cube trays until solid. Unmold cubes and place in a food processor with a chopping blade. Process in batches until fairly smooth, but still icy. Scrape down sides periodically while processing and store batches in freezer.

- For a refreshing beverage of "agua fresca," add 4 cups water to ¼ cup of the grapefruit mix.

Variations:

- Substitute tangerine or orange juice for the grapefruit juice.

Nutrition Facts per Serving: 150 calories, 1 g protein, 0 g fat (0 g saturated fat), 40 g carbohydrate, 1 g fiber, 0 mg cholesterol, 5 mg sodium, 22 glycemic load

MANGO APPLE GRANITA
WITH BASIL

Start to Finish: 4 hours to overnight   Yield: 4 servings

2   cups mango,
    frozen or fresh, peeled,
    cut in 1-inch chunks
½   cup apple juice
½   cup water

1   tablespoon lemon juice
1   pinch salt
⅓   cup agave syrup
4   large basil leaves

1. Combine all ingredients in a blender. Blend until smooth and the basil is in small pieces.

2. Pour into a 9-inch by 13-inch glass or metal pan. Place pan on a level surface in the freezer. Freeze, stirring and scraping with a large fork every 30 minutes, moving the frozen edges to the center and breaking up any lumps. Continue to do this until the granita is firm, but not frozen solid, approximately 3 hours depending on how deep the granita mixture is in the pan and how cold your freezer is.

3. Cover the pan with plastic and freeze overnight. When ready to serve, place a fork at the top of the dish and pull it toward you in rows. Move from one end of the pan to the other; rotate the pan and repeat.

4. Serve immediately in chilled bowls.

Variations:

- Substitute mint, Thai basil, lemon verbena, or rosemary for the basil. Add just enough to flavor the granita, as rosemary can be over-powering.
- Substitute fresh or frozen peaches or nectarines for the mangos.

Nutrition Facts per Serving: 75 calories, .5 g protein, 0 g fat (0 g saturated fat), 15 g carbohydrate, 1.5 g fiber, o mg cholesterol, 4 g sodium, 11 glycemic load

TROPICAL FRUIT POPS

Start to Finish: 15 minutes, plus freezing for 6 hours
Yield: 8 large or 12 small pops

½ cup boiling water
1 4-serving-size package
  sugar-free gelatin
  (lemon, mixed fruit, or
  strawberry flavor)

1 15¼-ounce can
  crushed pineapple
2 medium bananas,
  cut into chunks

1. In a 1- or 2-cup glass measure, stir together the boiling water and the gelatin until gelatin dissolves. Pour into a blender. Add undrained pineapple and banana chunks. Cover and blend until smooth.

2. Pour a scant ½ cup of the fruit mixture into each of eight 5- to 6-ounce paper or plastic drink cups. (Or pour a scant ⅓ cup into each of twelve 3-ounce cups.) Cover each cup with foil. Using the tip of a knife, make a small hole in the foil over each cup. Insert a wooden stick into the cup through the hole. Freeze about 6 hours or until firm.

3. To serve, remove foil and quickly dip the cups in warm water to soften the fruit mixture and loosen the sides of the pops from the drink cups.

Nutrition Facts per large pop: 65 calories, 1 g protein, 0 g total fat (0 g saturated fat), 15 g carbohydrate, 1 g fiber, 0 mg cholesterol, 29 mg sodium, 12 glycemic load

REFERENCES

Citations for PARADOX LOST, page 10

Trichopoulou, A., C. Barnia, and D. Trichopoulos. Anatomy of health effects of Mediterranean diet: Greek EPIC prospective cohort study. *British Medical Journal* 338:B2337, 2009. DOI:10:1136 / bmj.b2337.

Sanchez-Villegas., A, M. Delgado-Rodriguez, A. Alonso, et al. Association of the Mediterranean dietary pattern with the incidence of depression. *Archives of General Psychiatry* 66:1090–1098, 2009.

Martinez-Gonzalez, M.A., C. de la Fuente-Arrillaga, J.M. Nunez-Cordoba, et al. Adherence to Mediterranean diet and risk of developing diabetes: Prospective cohort study. *British Medical Journal* 336: 1348–1351, 2008. [PMID: 18511765]

Romaguera, D., et al. Adherence to Mediterranean diet is associated with lower abdominal obesity in European men and women. *Journal of Nutrition* 139:1728–1737, 2009.

Schaffer, S., J. Podstawa, F. Visioli, et al. Hydroxytyrosol: Rich olive mill wastewater extract protects brain cells in vitro and ex vivo. *Journal of Agricultural and Food Chemistry* 55(13):5043–5049, 2007.

Gu, Y., J.W. Nieves, Y. Stern, et al. Food combination and Alzheimer disease risk: A protective diet. *Archives of Neurology* 67(6):699–706, 2010.

Esposito, K., M.I. Maiorino, M. Ciotola, et al. Effects of a Mediterranean-style diet on the need for antihyperglycemic drug therapy in patients with newly diagnosed type 2 diabetes: A randomized trial. *Annals of Internal Medicine* 151: 306–314, 2009.

Citation for THE SONOMA SPIRIT, page 11

Kokkinos, A., C.W. le Roux, K. Alexiadou, et al. 2009. Eating slowly increases the postprandial response of the anorexigenic gut hormones, peptide YY and glucagon-like peptide-1. *Journal of Clinical Endocrinology and Metabolism* 95(1):333–337, 2010.

Citation for A GLASS A DAY, page 15

Wang, L., I.-M. Lee, J.E. Manson, et al. Alcohol consumption, weight gain, and risk of becoming overweight in middle-aged and older women. *Archives of Internal Medicine* 170(5):453–461, 2010.

Citations for TO LOSE WEIGHT, page 12

Fulkerson, J.A., M. Kubik, M. Story, et al. Are there nutritional and other benefits associated with family meals among at-risk youth? *Journal of Adolescent Health* 45(4):389–395, 2009. Epub May 28, 2009.

Burgess-Champoux, T.L., N. Larson, D. Neumark-Sztainer, et al. Are family meal patterns associated with overall diet quality during the transition from early to middle adolescence? *Journal of Nutrition Education and Behavior* 41(2):79–86, 2009.

Larson, N.I., M.C. Nelson, D. Neumark-Sztainer, et al. Making time for meals: Meal structure and associations with dietary intake in young adults. *Journal of the American Dietetic Association* 109(1):72–79, 2009.

Eisenberg, M.E., D. Neumark-Sztainer, and S. Feldman. Does TV viewing during family meals make a difference in adolescent substance use? *Preventive Medicine* 48(6):585–587, 2009. Epub April 14, 2009.

Citations for LEAN AND MEAN PROTEIN, page 16

Layman, D.K., E.M. Evans, D. Erickson, et al. A moderate-protein diet produces sustained weight loss and long-term changes in body composition and blood lipids in obese adults. *Journal of Nutrition* 139:514–521, 2009.

Heaney, R.P., and D.K. Layman. Protein quality assessment: Impact of expanding understanding of protein and amino acid needs for optimal health. *American Journal of Clinical Nutrition* 87(suppl):1576S–1581S, 2008.

Citations for WHEN TO STOP, page 23

Willcox, B.J., D.C. Willcox, and M. Suzuki. *The Okinawa Program.* New York: Clarkson Potter, 2001.

Wansink, B., and M.M. Cheney. Super bowls: Serving bowl size and food consumption. *JAMA* 293, 14:1727–1728, 2005.

Citations for ALMONDS AND DARK CHOCOLATE, page 29

Douglas, L., and M.E. Sanders. Probiotics and prebiotics in dietetics practice. *Journal of the American Dietetic Association* 108:510, 2008.

Gibson, G. Prebiotics as gut microflora management tools. *Journal of Clinical Gastroenterology* 42(suppl):S75, 2008.

Citations for BLUEBERRIES, page 36

Wolfe, K.L., and Liu, R.H. Structure-activity relationships of flavonoids in the cellular antioxidant activity assay. *Journal of Agricultural and Food Chemistry* 56(18):8418–8426, 2008.

Prior, R.L., L. Gu, X. Wu, et al. Plasma antioxidant capacity changes following a meal as a measure of the ability of a food to alter *in vivo* antioxidant status. *Journal of the American College of Nutrition* 26, 2: 170–181, 2007.

Shukitt-Hale, B., F.C. Lau, A.N. Carey, et al. Blueberry polyphenols attenuate kainic acid-induced decrements in cognition and alter inflammatory gene expression in rat hippocampus. *Nutritional Neuroscience* 11(4):172–182, 2008.

Kalea, A.Z., K. Clark, D.A. Schuschke, et al. Dietary enrichment with wild blueberries (*Vaccinium angustifolium*) affects the vascular reactivity in the aorta of young spontaneously hypertensive rats. *Journal* of *Nutritional Biochemistry* 21(1):14–22, 2010.

Grace, M.H., D.M. Ribnicky, P. Kuhn, et al. Hypoglycemic activity of a novel anthocyanin-rich formulation from lowbush blueberry, *Vaccinium angustifolium Aiton*. *Phytomedicine* 16(5):406–415, 2009.

Citations for GRAPES, page 40

Anselm, E., M. Chataigneau, M. Ndiaye, et al. Grape juice causes endothelium-dependent relaxation via a redox-sensitive Src- and Akt-dependent activation of eNOS. *Cardiovascular Research* 73(2):404–413, 2007.

Nantz, M.P., C.A. Rowe, C. Nieves, et al. Bioactive compounds from Concord grapes prime T cells and reduce DNA strand breaks. Paper presented at Experimental Biology meeting, San Diego, CA, April 5–9, 2008.

Dohadwala, M.M., M. Holbrook, B.H. Kim, et al. Effect of grape juice on blood pressure and blood glucose in patients with prehypertension and stage 1 hypertension. Paper presented at American Heart Association's joint conference on Cardiovascular Disease Epidemiology and Prevention / Nutrition, Physical Activity and Metabolism, March 2–5, 2010.

Citations for OLIVE OIL, page 42

Pitt, J., W. Roth, P. Lacor, et al. Alzheimer's associated AB Oligomers. *Toxicology and Applied Pharmacology* 240(2):189–197, 2009.

Estuch, R., M. Gonzalez, D. Corella, et al. Effects of a Mediterranean-style diet on cardiovascular risk factors (PRED-IMED). *Annals of Internal Medicine* 145:1–11, 2006.

Gonzales, M., C. Arigalla, J. Cordoba, et al. Adherence to Mediterranean diet and risk of developing diabetes: Prospective cohort study. *British Medical Journal* 336(7657):1348–1351, 2008.

Citations for OMEGA-3 BENEFITS, page 72

Micallef, M., I. Munro, M. Phang, et al. Plasma n-3 polyunsaturated fatty acids are negatively associated with obesity. *British Journal of Nutrition* 102:1370–1374, 2009.

Albanese, E., A. Dangour, R. Uauy, et al. Dietary fish and meat intake and dementia in Latin America, China, and India. *American Journal of Clinical Nutrition* 90:392–400, 2009.

Citation for NUTS TO YOU, page 75

Sebate, J., K. Roda, E. Ross, et al. Nut consumption and blood lipid levels: A pooled analysis of 25 intervention trials. *Archives of Internal Medicine* 10(9):821–827, 2010.

Citation for FRIENDLY BACTERIA, page 80

Kadooka, Y., M. Sato, K. Imaizumi, et al. Regulation of abdominal adiposity by probiotics in adults. *European Journal of Clinical Nutrition* 64 (6):636–643, 2010.

DIET INDEX

Water, 97, 104.
See also Agua frescas
Wave 1, 82–104
  about: overview of, 24, 25, 82–83
  alcohol restriction, 96
  beverages, 104
  changing eating habits/ attitude toward food, 82–83
  dairy food items, 103
  destructive habits eliminated by, 82–83
  duration of, 82
  eating without stress, 90–91
  exercise, 91–92
  fats, 99–100, 104
  flavor boosters, 104
  foods list, 102–104
  fruit (Tier 1), 102–103
  grains, 104
  how to fill your plate, 98–99
  kitchen cleanup, 84
  losing cravings for bread and sugar, 95–96, 157, 158.
  See also Refined foods
  meal plans (guides), 25, 101, 205–211
  nuts, 104
  plate/bowl sizes and food proportions, 92–94
  preparing for, 84–94
  protein food items, 103
  purpose of, 82–83, 95
  recipes. *See Recipe Index*
  restrictions, 95–97
  salt savvy, 89–90
  snacks, 100
  vegetables (Tier 1), 102
  way of, 95–97
  weight loss overview and, 23–25
Wave 2
  about: overview of, 24–25, 105–106
  beverages, 122
  eating guide, 106–108
  fats, 106
  fiber and, 108–110
  flavor boosters, 123
  food combinations, 113
  foods list, 120–123

fruit, 120, 121
glycemic index and, 110–113
grains, 106, 122
meal plans (guides), 25, 265–273
nuts, 122
plate/bowl sizes and food proportions, 106–108
recipes. *See Recipe Index*
snacks, 117, 126–127
sweets and, 108–109, 115
variety in, 105–106
vegetables, 120, 121
weight loss overview and, 23–25
wine and, 106, 116–119
Wave 3 (New Sonoma Diet lifestyle), 136–148
  background and overview, 2–7
  bedtime, 130, 140
  diet success, 136–137
  exercise, 142–143
  guidelines for life, 143–144
  healthy adjustments, 141–142
  if weight creeps up, 144–145
  mindful living, 145–147.
  See also Mindfulness
  nontypical foods, 141–142
  organic foods and, 147–148
  perfect weight for life ("maintenance"), 138–139
  reaping rewards, 137–138
  recipes. *See Recipe Index*
  satisfying results, 139–140
  testimonials. *See* Testimonials
Weight loss. *See also* Wave 1; Wave 2; Wave 3 (New Sonoma Diet lifestyle)
  about: overview of, 52–53, 124–125
  bedtime and, 130, 140
  challenges summarized, 124–125
  changing eating habits/ attitude toward food

and, 82–83, 125–131
crave busters, 128–129, 158
eating more slowly for, 12, 13, 24, 31, 90–91, 126, 140
exercise and, 91–92, 127, 132–135
FAQs, 156–165
fast-tracking, 124–135
guidelines for, 12–13, 21
health benefits and, 52–53
journal, 126–128
loving to eat and, 52–54
packaged food and, 127
perfect weight for life ("maintenance"), 138–139. *See also* Wave 3 (New Sonoma Diet lifestyle)
plateaus, working through, 131–135, 157
plate filling and, 126.
  See also Portion control
quick tips, 126–127
snacking and, 126–127
stress and, 129–130
target weight, 126–127
in waves, 23–25
whole grains and, 54–56
Whole foods, 14
Whole grains, 14, 48–51
breads, 57, 58–59
breakfast cereals and, 57
cereals, 57, 58
finding and buying, 55
focus on, 22
gluten and, 50–51, 59
glycemic index and, 110–113
health benefits, 56–57
list of things to stock, 86
oat flour, 59
oats, 51, 58
pasta, 50, 60, 85, 113
percent by meal, 93, 107, 108
refined grains, body fat and, 55–56
rice varieties, 59–60
sprouted, 60–62
substitutions, 61
types and characteristics, 58–60

Wave 1 percentages, 93,
99
Wave 2 percentages,
107, 108
Waves 1 and 2 list, 104,
106, 122
weight loss and, 54–56
Wine
benefits of, 14, 15,
116–119

encouragement to drink,
116
FAQs, 164–165
health benefits of,
118–119
other alcoholic drinks
instead of, 165
preserving, 106
red, 119
Sonoma way, 119

Wave 1 and, 96, 116
Wave 2 and, 106,
116–119
white, 119
Workplace cafeterias, 155

RECIPE INDEX

Chicken. *See* Poultry
Chickpeas. *See* Beans and
legumes
Chipotle Lime Marinade,
177
Chocolate
about: almonds with, 29;
benefits of, 73; dark, 29,
73; nutritional value, 73
Flourless Chocolate Cake,
(W2, W3) 355
Cioppino Seafood en
Papillote, (W1) 261–262
Citrus
about: lemon and green
tea, 40; nutritional
value, 39–40; power
combos, 40; Power
Food qualities, 39–40;
selecting, 39
Chipotle Lime Marinade,
177
Creamy Lime Ricotta
Tart, (W2, W3) 356
Lemon Poppy Seed
Pancakes, (W2, W3)
276
Lemon Vinaigrette, (W1)
229–230
Simple Spicy Lime
Cilantro Vinaigrette,
201
Coffee Rub, 182
Concord grapes. *See* Grapes
Cook Once/Eat Twice meals
about: ideas for, 242
Buckwheat Crepes
Fillings, (W2, W3)
298–299
California Chicken Salad,
(W2, W3)
287
Chicken & Black Bean
Wrap, (W2, W3) 290
Chicken & White Bean
Chile Verde with
Sonoma Pesto, (W1)
249–250
Chicken, Tomato, Basil,
& Penne Salad,
(W2, W3) 288
Greek Chicken Salad with
White Beans,
(W2, W3) 321
Grilled Beef & Hummus

Whole-Wheat Pita,
(W2, W3) 291
Grilled Chicken with
Tomato-Bean Salad,
(W2, W3) 322
Latin Marinade for Roast
Pork Tenderloin,
(W2, W3) 339
Latin-Style Sautéed Corn,
(W2, W3) 285
Mediterranean Tabbouleh
Salad with Chicken,
(W2, W3) 323–324
Mediterranean Tuna &
Caper Salad, (W2, W3)
346
Roast Chicken, Garbanzo
Bean, Red Pepper, &
Caper Salad, (W1) 251
Roast Chicken with
Roasted Vegetables
(with Mediterranean,
Asian, Latin variations),
(W2, W3) 325–327
Roasted Pork Tacos with
Peach Salsa, (W2, W3)
292
Romaine & Watercress
Salad with Toasted
Almonds & Dijon
Vinaigrette, (W2, W3)
328
Sautéed Broccoli Rabe,
(W1) 241
Simple Chicken Tacos
with Roasted Tomato
Jalapeño Salsa,
(W2, W3) 329
Sonoma Salad with
Tomatoes & Feta,
(W2, W3) 330
Toasted Quinoa, Chicken,
Corn, & Avocado Salad,
(W2, W3) 289
Toasted Quinoa Pilaf,
(W1) 244–245
Wheat Berries, (W1)
246
Corn
Grain Medley with
Southwestern
Seasonings, (W2, W3)
302
Latin-Style Sautéed Corn,
(W2, W3) 285

Spicy Black Bean
& Corn Chowder,
(W2, W3) 307
Toasted Quinoa, Chicken,
Corn, & Avocado Salad,
(W2, W3) 289
Creamy Lime Ricotta Tart,
(W2, W3) 356
Crepes and fillings,
(W2, W3) 297–299
Crusts and pie dough,
359–361
Cuban-Style Flank Steak,
(W2, W3) 333
Cucumbers
Toasted Quinoa, Chicken,
Cucumber, & Dill Salad,
(W1) 226

Dairy products
about: brands list, 172;
butter, 160; protein and,
80–81, 122; snack ideas,
100
in salads. *See* Salads
Desserts (sweets)
about: reducing cravings
for, 82, 95–96, 108–
109, 157, 158; Wave 1
and, 87, 95–96; Wave 2
and, 108–109, 112, 115
Almond Cherry Biscotti,
(W2, W3) 350–351
Cherry Almond Clafoutis,
(W2, W3) 354
Concord Grape & Lime
Sorbet, (W2, W3) 362
Creamy Lime Ricotta
Tart, (W2, W3) 356
Flourless Chocolate Cake,
(W2, W3) 355
Graham Cracker Tart
Crust, (W2, W3) 360
Grapefruit Mint Sorbet,
(W2, W3) 363
Mango Apple Granita,
(W2, W3) 364
Nectarine Blueberry
Galette, (W2, W3)
357–358
Pie Dough, (W2, W3) 359
Spiced Ginger Cookies,
(W2, W3) 352–353
Tropical Fruit Pops, (W2,
W3) 365

Graham Cracker Tart Crust,
(W2, W3) 360
Grains. *See* Breads; Quinoa;
Whole grains
Granola, Sonoma,
(W2, W3) 280–281
Grapefruit Mint Sorbet,
(W2, W3) 363
Grapes
about: antioxidant power,
41–42; juice power, 41;
nutritional value, 41–42;
Power Food qualities,
40–42; red/purple vs.
white/green, 41
Concord Grape &
Arugula Salad,
(W2, W3) 300
Concord Grape & Lime
Sorbet, (W2, W3) 362
Concord Grape Balsamic
Vinaigrette, 195
Greek Chicken Salad with
White Beans, (W2, W3)
321
Greek Salad with Grilled
Shrimp, (W1) 227–228
Greek Vinaigrette, 197
Greens. *See also* Spinach
Baby Greens with Apples,
Chicken, Walnuts,
(W2, W3) 315
Mushroom & Chard-
Stuffed Flank Steak,
(W2, W3) 334–335
in salads. *See* Salads
Grilled Asparagus Salad,
(W1) 238
Grilled Beef & Hummus
Whole-Wheat Pita,
(W2, W3) 291
Grilled Chicken with
Tomato-Bean Salad,
(W2, W3) 322
Grilled Moroccan Pork
Tenderloin Kabobs,
(W2, W3) 336
Grilled Tuna with Rosemary,
(W1) 263
Grilled Vegetable Frittata,
(W1) 219
Grilled Vegetable Rolls
Stuffed with Feta Cheese,
Pine Nuts, & Mint, (W1)
239–240

Halibut & Summer
Vegetables en Papillote,
(W2, W3) 344–345
Harissa Sauce, 188
Harissa (Tunisian Hot Chile
Paste), 187
Hearty Lentil Soup,
(W2, W3) 282
Herbed Pork Tenderloin,
(W2, W3) 337
Herb-Marinated Flank Steak,
(W1) 254
Herb seasonings.
See Seasonings
Hummus, 189

Indian-Spiced Pork Loin
with Yogurt Marinade,
(W1) 256

Jamaican Jerk Rub, 183

Latin Marinade for Roast
Pork Tenderloin,
(W2, W3) 339
Latin Roast Pork
Tenderloin with Pinto
Beans & Zucchini, (W2,
W3) 338
Latin-Style Sautéed Corn,
(W2, W3) 285
Lemon and limes. *See* Citrus
Lentils. *See* Beans and
legumes

Mango Apple Granita,
(W2, W3) 364
Marinades. *See* Seasonings
Meal plans (guides)
about, 25, 88, 101
Wave 1, 101, 205–211
Wave 2, 25, 265–273
Meat. *See also* Beef; Pork
about: lean, 77, 78;
protein and, 77–78;
Wave 2, 121–122
Salsa Verde for, 191
Mediterranean Herb
Marinade, 178
Mediterranean-Marinated
Fish, (W2, W3) 345
Mediterranean Tabbouleh
Salad with Chicken,
(W2, W3) 323–324

Mediterranean Tuna &
Caper Salad, (W2, W3)
346
Mediterranean White Wine
Poached Fish, (W2, W3)
347
Minestrone Soup, (W1)
223. *See also* Sonoma
Minestrone with Pesto
Mushrooms
Mushroom & Chard-
Stuffed Flank Steak,
(W2, W3) 334–335
Mushroom Omelet,
(W1) 220
Portobello and Blue
Cheese Wrap,
(W1) 232
Wild Mushroom &
Barley Risotto,
(W2, W3) 312
Mustard seasonings.
See Seasonings

Nectarines
Nectarine, Arugula, &
Goat Cheese Salad,
(W2, W3) 286
Nectarine Blueberry
Galette, (W2, W3)
357–358
Nuts
about: benefits of, 75–76;
butters, 160; list of
things to stock, 87;
nutritional value, 75–76;
protein and, 103; snack
ideas, 100; walnuts, 76
Fruit & Nut Energy Bars,
(W2, W3) 278–279

Olive oil
about: antioxidant power,
43; as healthy fat, 42–
43; power combo, 43;
Power Food qualities,
42–43; spinach and, 43
Omelets. *See* Eggs
Orange Roughy with
Cilantro Pesto, (W1) 264
Oven-Fried Pork Cutlets,
(W2, W3) 340

Pancakes, 212–214,
275–276

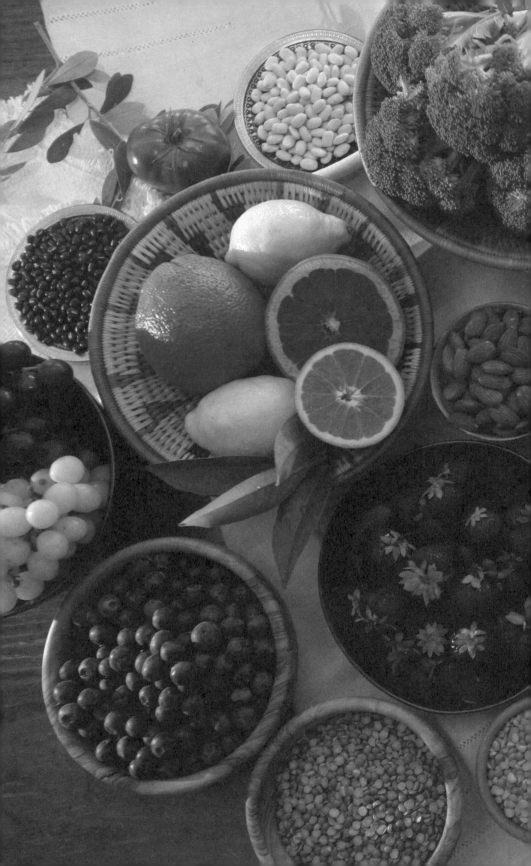